*praise for*

# THE HITE REPORT
## A Nationwide Study of Female Sexuality

"Women who read it will feel enormously reassured about their own sexuality. . . . If enough men read it, the quality of sex . . . is bound to improve. Read *The Hite Report* if you want to know how sex really is right now."
—Erica Jong, *The New York Times Book Review*

"A remarkable book . . . opens new vistas and new insights into where females 'are at' in the 1970's . . . I highly recommend it."
—Dr. Wardell Pomeroy, co-author with Dr. Alfred Kinsey, *The Kinsey Reports*

"One of the greatest causes of my success in sex."
—Peter Ustinov, *Daily Telegraph*

"Shere Hite has changed the way we think about sex."
—Barbara Walters

"Every woman should read this book."
—Gloria Steinem

"Hite's books have caused a sensation—and keep arousing passionate controversy."
—Tom Brokaw

"The only honest book about sex."
—Marlon Brando

"This groundbreaking study of female sexuality opens new vistas."
—American Association of Sex Educators, Counselors and Therapists (AASECT)

"Hite has devised a brilliant new methodology letting women speak for themselves."
—Laura Tanner, Women in Psychology

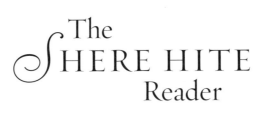

# The SHERE HITE Reader

*New and Selected Writings on
Sex, Globalization, and Private Life*

## SHERE HITE

SEVEN STORIES PRESS
New York / Toronto / London / Melbourne

Seven Stories Press
140 Watts Street
New York, NY 10013
http://www.sevenstories.com

In Canada:
Publishers Group Canada, 250A Carlton Street, Toronto, ON M5A-2L1

In the U.K.:
Turnaround Publisher Services Ltd., Unit 3, Olympia Trading Estate, Coburg Road, Wood Green, London N22 6TZ

In Australia:
Palgrave Macmillan, 627 Chapel Street, South Yarra, VIC 3141

Library of Congress Cataloging-in-Publication Data
Hite, Shere.
  The Shere Hite reader : new and selected writings on sex, globalization, and private life / Shere Hite.—1st ed.
    p. cm.
  Includes bibliographical references and index.
  ISBN-13: 978-1-58322-568-4 (pbk. : alk. paper)
  ISBN-10: 1-58322-568-4 (pbk. : alk. paper)
  1. Sex. 2. Sex customs. 3. Women—Sexual behavior. 4. Men—Sexual behavior. 5. Homosexuality. 6. Love. I. Title.

HQ21.H52 2005
306.77—dc22
                                2005011468

9 8 7 6 5 4 3 2 1

College professors may order examination copies of Seven Stories Press titles for a free six-month trial period. To order, visit www.sevenstories.com/textbook/, or fax on school letterhead to (212) 226-1411.

Book design by Jon Gilbert
Cover design by M. Astella Saw

Printed in Canada.

# Contents

## PART 2: MALE SEXUALITY AND LOVE DESCRIBED BY MEN (1981) ...111

# Acknowledgments

There are many people who have helped in these research projects over the years, so that it would hardly be possible to name them all. Yet I wish to name those who were or are most central.

Most importantly of all, I am grateful to those who participated in my research, giving so much of themselves to me, to others, and to the world. As they were asked not to sign their questionnaire replies, written in the form of essay answers to approximately 150 questions, their anonymity is protected completely; not even I know their names.

I would like to pay special tribute to members of my family and friends and those who have helped me finance and complete these projects over the years, including Cecile and Paul Rice, Rick Kwiecinski, Howard and Christine Wilson, Steve and Marina Kaufman, Martin Sage, Virgilio del Toro, Iris Brosch, Joyce Gold, Regina Ryan, Sydelle Beiner, Joyce Snyder, P. Trainotti, and many others.

I would also like to pay tribute to those who have gone out of their way to support my research in terms of professional help. Foremost among these is Barbara Seaman, of whom I wrote in 1996 (in the preface to the United States Edition of *The Hite Report on the Family*), "Some things, like the Statue of Liberty, we take for granted. Barbara Seaman, one of the most influential women in the twentieth-century women's movement, is something like that. It was Barbara who made sure that this book—already published in ten other countries—was also published in the United States, as it was Barbara who had earlier introduced me to the editor of the first Hite Report, Regina Ryan. A woman of great personal charm and energy as well as a seminal author, Seaman has written such books as *Free and Female* and *The Doctor's Case Against the Pill*; she is the cofounder of The Women's Health Network, and her work has led to congressional hearings and procedural changes on the part of the world's physicians and pharmaceutical companies. As Jane O'Reilly of *Time* magazine remarked on meeting her, "Do you know who that is? That woman has saved thousands of lives!"

Also invaluable to me, I would like to thank for their help in getting *The Hite Report on the Family* published in the United States several important writers and intellectuals who put their own reputations on the line to defend mine when it was under attack.[1] Since the previous Hite Report had sustained harsh personal attacks in 1987–1988 (often falsely drawn on "methodological grounds"—as the methodology was new, later winning awards, few at the time understood it, although today it has proven accurate, standing the test of time), some United States publishers seemed intimidated and appeared to fear publishing my new works. For example, the research on the family was published in the United States only two years after it appeared in forty-nine other countries and eleven languages, with the first publisher, Dutton, cancelling its contract after, in effect, blocking publication for two years; this situation was resolved when a petition published by *Ms. Magazine* alongside an article by Jennifer Gonnerman, as well as an in-depth fifteen-minute NBC interview by Tom Brokaw and Katie Curic, done in London, broke the silence and challenged nonpublication. The Dutton contract with the originating United Kingdom publisher, Bloomsbury (Liz Calder), was nullified, and Grove-Atlantic published the book in 1996. For their courage and support at that time I would like to express my profound gratitude to Phyllis Chesler, Naomi Weisstein, Jesse Lemisch, Barbara Ehrenreich, Kate Millett, Ruby Rohrlich, Andrea Dworkin, Gloria Steinem, Susan Faludi, Stephen Jay Gould, Barbara Seaman, Karla Jay, and Kate Colleran, who wrote and put forth a statement in my defense.[2] I would also like to thank Marcia Gillespie, Janet Wolfe, Jessica Velmans, Morgan Entrekin, Allison Draper who edited the book, Gillian Taylor, Lin Crouch, Victoria McKee, Friedrich Hoericke, my husband, and many others for their support at that time.

I would also like to thank the group of famous writers who spontaneously defended me against the painful and startling personal and "methodological" attacks of 1987–88 (leading up to the 1994–95 situation), which included an attack on the cover of *Time* magazine; they wrote a statement which they read out at the American Studies Association annual convention of 1988, including the words, "Terribly important issues that concern women's lives and health . . . are being obscured and trivialized by the media's assault on Shere Hite's new book, *Women and Love. . . .* These attacks are not so much directed against a single woman as they are directed against the rights of women everywhere."[3] Those writing this statement, signing it, and appearing included: Barbara Seaman, Phyllis Chesler, Naomi Weisstein, Barbara Ehrenreich, Kate Millett, Ruby Rohrlich, Karla Jay, Ti-Grace Atkinson and others. Atkinson and Seaman both spoke out at at that meeting at great personal cost to themselves: Atkinson's father had just died, and Seaman had been pushed down a flight of stairs earlier that week, breaking her leg, so she appeared in a cast with a crutch; Rohrlich was outspoken in her responses to reporters about "methodology," as was Laura Cottingham; further reports of the dynamics of that event are reported in *The Chronicle of Higher Education*, whose reporter covered the event, as did Louise Armstrong for the *Women's Review of Books*, in a hilarious send up of the entire media depiction of events.[4]

Financing this research over the years has taken a heavy toll, since the research was always independent and never funded by either government or industry (such as a pharmaceutical company). I personally have made many private investments, friends and family have loaned money (always paid back); however, for the most part I have relied on publishing advances (money paid up front against future earnings of royalties); in every case the publisher of a report recouped this money soon after publication. In this regard, I would like to thank Robert Gottlieb, the editor-in-chief of Alfred A. Knopf, who for ten years was my editor before he left that august publishing house.

There are many others I would like to thank who have enabled me to work and carry on my research since the 1970s, many continuing today, but alas, they are too numerous to mention. I beg friends and colleagues who have helped me during the past thirty years to understand and forgive any lapses in what must necessarily, in publishing terms, be a relatively brief synopsis of my life's relationships. I am certain that in a span of the thirty years covered by this book, I will inevitably neglect to mention someone who has been important in my work. I beg their forgiveness and understanding.

Professional colleagues in the field have always been helpful and supportive, including Dr. Mary Calderone, founder of SIECUS, one of the most important sex research groups during her active life; Dr. Leah Schaefer, former president of the Society of the Scientific Study of Sex (SSSS); Dr. Wardell Pomeroy, coresearcher with Alfred Kinsey and later president of SSSS; Dr. William Granzig, president of the American Academy of Clinical Sexology; Dr. Shirley Zussman, former president of the American Association of Sex Educators, Counselors and Therapists (AASECT) and member of the American Civil Liberties Union (ACLU); Dr. Helen Singer Kaplan; Dr. Virginia Johnson, partner with Dr. William Masters; Professor Toshiyasu Ishiwatari; Victoria McKee; Dorothy Crouch; Hermann Meller; and many others.

There have been a few notable and outstanding pieces of analysis in media around the world for each of my nine books. I cannot mention each name here, but I want to point out how important—invaluable—these informal critiques have been to me; and to those who took the time to read the works and acquaint themselves with the ideas they contained, I do say thank you.

Editors at publishing houses and newspapers have played a crucial part in helping me communicate with readers; I have learned an enormous amount from them and from my agents over the years, hopefully growing in my thinking via this process. They include Regina Ryan, Lindy Hess, Robert Gottlieb, Corona Machemer, Candida Lacey, Dale Spender, Liz Calder, Gary Pulsifer, Marilyn Abraham, Katarina Czernecki, Michael Meller, Irving "Swifty" Lazar, Calla Fricke, Lionel von dem Knesebeck, Nigel Newton, Sally Richardson, Hermann Plaza, Pedro J. Ramirez, Francesco Cevasco, Friedrich Hoericke, Nicholas Latimer, Iris Brosch, Howard Wilson, Steve Kaufmann, Nigel Billen, Clive James, Tom Mori, Keuchi Takeuchi, Yukiyasu Sezai, T. Akiyama, Sheri Safran, Tom McCarthy, Chris Peterson, Phoebe Hwang, Dan Simon, and other extremely important figures. I owe a special debt of gratitude to family, friends and my dog Rusty, who was there for me (as Reese Witherspoon says in *Legally Blonde II*) when I needed him.

Finally I would like to stress again that my thanks go especially to those who have answered my questionnaires and so improved the quality of my life during these years—during which I have grown and changed, both in my thinking and personally, as I hope will be apparent in this volume exposing my ideas as they developed from 1975 to 2005, a span of thirty years. By answering, participants demonstrated their caring for others, sharing their innermost thoughts and secrets, thus enabling me to pass on their ideas and feelings, as well as learning from them. This legacy of information is important now and will remain so in the future, even for people we cannot begin now to know or imagine.

As this research continues, I ask readers to please send me their responses to either one of my two questionnaires for women or to my questionnaire for men, or to answer the questions on growing up/family matters, all available in the Appendix. Please send them to me either by email to hite2000@hotmail.com (do not sign your reply), or by post to me c/o Seven Stories Press, 140 Watts Street, New York, NY 10013, U.S.A.

With my warmest personal greetings, and please write! I would like to hear from you.

NOTES

1   See Appendix.
2   See the text of their statement in the appendices.
3   See the full text of the statement in the appendices. See also *The Chronicle of Higher Education*'s synopsis, as well as Liz Smith's resumé in the *New York Post*, 1987.
4   See Appendix for this reference citation.

# Preface

## Toward a New Vision of Sexuality

### LETTER TO THE READER

Dear Reader,

Come with me on a journey to rethink your personal life—and maybe even your politics.

How are you feeling about your private life? Here is a new way of looking at sex and private life that could open many doors for you.

Female sexuality is a complex topic, not yet fully developed despite many changes (sometimes in false directions) in recent years. For example, as a woman, ask yourself, are you ever caught in a situation pressuring you to fake orgasm (or not say you didn't have one with a partner)? Is this your fault, or is there another reason? Can the reason be changed? A woman has not failed personally when this happens, but the situation needs to be changed. Another question: have you found the love you are looking for, or is your greatest love yet to come? Anything you want to review about your life you will find discussed here, inside a new overall framework.

Male sexuality is more subtle and diverse than we usually believe. After documenting 7,000 men of all ages in my research, I find that male sexuality is a delicate, sensitive phenomenon, not the simplistic "mechanism that drives men to thrust and implant their seed," the mechanical "lust-model" so often portrayed. Both men and women can understand male sexuality and love better with the information provided here. In fact, reading what men say here can change your life.

This book contains the essence of several research studies, the five Hite Reports (published as books between 1976 and 1994), plus current essays and theories (written between 1996 and 2005). (Details are telescoped here but are presented at length in the published reports.) This research is completely independent and was never financed by any institution or group (research is often funded by pharmaceutical companies or governments, etc.), thus there were no strings attached in any way. What you find here are the pure voices of those participating, plus my reflections, conclusions, and overview. These works have won many awards, including the AASECT (American Association of Sex Educators, Counselors and Therapists) award for distinguished service, been widely accepted around the world, as well as praised and defended by outstanding scholars and writers.[1]

The structure of what we believe about sex today can be changed by us. It was formed first in our childhoods, a combination of our bodies' changes and how the society around us told us to interpret these changes. We find ourselves "grown up" with a fixed idea of what "sex" is and what our sexuality is; we are sure we are right and that sex is "instinctive." (Don't our fantasies prove it? Didn't biology make our hormones that created our behavior?) However, these fixed ideas are part of a mental landscape that can change, if we want it to. And there are good reasons, as we shall see, for changing these fixed ideas. To prepare for change, it is helpful to look at how we grew up sexually and emotionally; thus this book contains documentation of how thousands of girls and boys grew up and first experienced their bodies; material originally published as *The Hite Report on the Family*, the fourth Hite Report.

Another area of fixed ideas relating to sex is that women change in a specific way as they age. Our religious mores based on the icons of Mary and her son Jesus, as well as Adam and Eve in the Garden, decree that women as they age should change to being less sexual (asexual) mothers who are primarily concerned with helping others/their children. An "older woman" who is "sexual" is usually depicted as "vulgar," "immodest" or lacking in taste, even grotesque or ridiculous. While there is nothing wrong with women caring for children, this one-sided view of "the female" has done much harm to women, men, and relationships and has decreased understanding between the two sexes. You can change the world by rejecting both the older view of women (the "religious tradition" decreeing that "the good-woman-at-home" is motherly, not sexual—a view reanimated today by some who view "uncovered women" as "representing the decline of civilization")—*and* the "modern pornographic woman" version of "everything is okay" (the opposite extreme of the same spectrum), in favor of forging your own personal way of life.

You can change the world by creating your own personal sexual and political view. Think and act for yourself. Please accept this book's information as my gift to you.

Change your own personal life today.

Shere Hite
December 1, 2005
hite2000@hotmail.com

# A New Sexual Culture

## SEX AND HUMAN RIGHTS

When you were a child, what were your first sexual thoughts? How did you feel about your sexuality the first time you had an orgasm? Try to remember . . .

Could we today rediscover our original feelings and deprogram our brains so that we could construct a new sexuality based on those forgotten feelings?

How can an individual know her original sexuality? I propose that we go back in time to discover the earliest meaning of our sexual feelings and desires as children. . . . Physical relationships, what we do with our bodies, are important, but we tend to forget what we originally felt and come to identify with the structure placed on us. While eroticism is undeniably important, we have inherited a very rigid version of "sex" revolving basically around "the act"—and this focus is creating some heavy performance pressures on all of us to "do it." We should remember the childhood joy we felt in discovering our bodies, our original openness to the physical world, and our desire to explore the bodies of others.

Reinventing sexuality means going back to basics: What do women want? What do men want? Is it the cliché of "male desire" we see in pornographic magazines? Is it orgasm? What about clitoral massage for female orgasm, shouldn't that be a part of it? Yes, there should be a possibility of "equal orgasms," but there should also be a new type of fluidity and spontaneity; caresses that do not always see coitus (and performance of "the act") as "the goal," a foregone conclusion. Other activities should reclaim importance: who would want "sex" without the overall head-to-toe physical contact it involves? Why is there no word for this full-body contact? Here is one example of the many undervalued lack-of-even-having-a-name erotic contacts we already enjoy, which can form part of the building blocks of a new body vocabulary.

## FEMALE SEXUALITY: IF SLEEPING BEAUTY SHOULD BEGIN TO AWAKEN ON HER OWN

Though some think that "if only men would understand female orgasm, sex would be fine," there is much more to redesigning sex—worthy as that first goal may be!

Many women now are taking sexual exchanges in a profoundly new direction, not by becoming "dominatrixes" (a media version of "the new woman"), but by focusing on discovering what pleases them as individuals, and involving their partners in these activities, rather than giving over autonomy. Rather than "playing the part" expected, or being enslaved by the ideology with its old dance steps—its choices being either "passivity" or "dominance"—many women now are showing real courage and initiative in their personal lives. Along with this change, there is a new mindset developing, a new psychology and view of the world.

However, despite this change, my research reveals that many women still feel that they have not yet fully "tried their wings" and used all they know and feel about their bodies, that there is still some distance between their sexual "abilities" and the context they are being asked to fit them into. It is almost as if women today have been taking a breather, resting after having achieved so much, before continuing on to further develop their identities, taking themselves in new directions—and the culture with them.

Women have begun an exciting reassessment and re-creation, questioning, of what it means to be human, sexual, and female. Yet the implications of women's knowledge have not yet borne fruit: while most women know how to orgasm when they stimulate themselves, most also find that they are blocked when even a beloved male partner is not ready to accept this information or rethink the "sexual dance"; they then feel unable to progress and often blame themselves for their continuing "passivity" and acceptance of the sexual status quo.

## THE "NEW WOMAN" OR "WOMEN ON TOP" CLICHÉ OF EQUALITY

Others say that the "new sexuality" (usually referring to media images of "women on top") demonstrates the collapse of established moral order, a decline in values, while still others disagree, claiming that "sexual freedom" is good, necessary for political freedom. Which is right?

Clearly sexual equality and self-determination for women, among the most important issues of our time, are having a major positive influence on society. Yet this is too often interpreted in a simplistic way—for example, proposing that equality means that since in the past men were "always on top" and "dominating," now "the new woman can be on top too!" In fact, women's increasing equality and self-confidence is having a major influence on sex but is taking sex in a different direction. What, in fact, does "equal rights" mean for sex?

Sexual equality is changing from the inside how "sex" and human relations are defined. Women see things differently today: what we are going through are merely the first stages, what we see in most media and pornography is the frenzied attempt of an "old culture" to portray women as "perverse" if they behave sexually or in a new way in bed, painting any hint of women's "rebellion" as "morally decadent," a sign of the decadence of the times! Yet according to my research, [2] women are quietly persevering with dignity to rethink the meaning of their sexual lives and desires, and they are trying to adapt their behavior in multifaceted ways to reflect their new thinking, not copying old clichés .

Once sex was thought of as a trivial topic; today we know that sex is a core issue. Sexuality is central to our value system; if women change their place in sex, declare their right to their bodies and their right to think for themselves, this declaration has far-ranging social repercussions. Whereas traditional sex was symbolic of women's position and role in society as "helpmate," with each "sexual act" a ritual performed by man and woman calculated to teach women "who they are" and their "purpose on this earth" (reproduction in the male-dominated family), while also reminding them that "man is the master" who has a right to orgasm, while the woman's needs are quite secondary, now we see women beginning to make a new version of sex and love.

What issues are being thought about now in addition to Viagra? What are the performance pressures most people worry about today?

### ORGASM PERFORMANCE PRESSURES ON WOMEN: WHAT THE FIRST HITE REPORT SAID

The biggest performance pressure on women is to have orgasm during "the act":

> *I'm afraid to admit it—but although I've had many orgasms through masturbation, I'm not sure what orgasm from vaginal intercourse is like. I've had very high feelings, but I guess since it wasn't like a masturbatory orgasm I didn't think it was an orgasm. To say this makes me feel totally inexperienced.*

> *I really don't know if I've had an orgasm with a man, unless it's just that I don't really know what to be aware of—because if it's supposed to be like when I'm masturbating, then I think not. I would like to know if that makes me abnormal. I feel deeply ashamed and inferior because I never have them during intercourse.*

> *I think that a lot of my desire to have orgasms during intercourse comes from shame and feelings of inadequacy (maybe I'm not sexy. . .). Hell, I don't know—I've been in therapy for two years and it has helped me personally, but I'm still no closer to having an orgasm during intercourse.*

Although most women can orgasm easily during masturbation, only a small minority reach orgasm regularly during coitus, according to my research and to "common wisdom." This is not a tragedy! It is an opportunity to change "sex," rethink it and renegotiate it, after centuries of a culture in which men owned women (and "sex was the way they proved it"). A woman is not "less good" if she does not have orgasm during "the act." Men will gain, too, from the richness of female sexuality.

The female body is marvelous and should be celebrated. Female orgasm happens easily for over 90 percent of women via clitoral massage or masturbation, according to my research; for most women this means a rhythmic soft massage of the clitoral or pubic area at the front of the body. Only two percent of women penetrate their vagina when stimulating themselves to orgasm—this means something! It is easy for women to orgasm with proper stimulation and sometimes to have several orgasms. Therefore how can it be true that women have "a problem" with orgasm? It is the definition of sex that has a problem and should change, not women's thoughts and bodies.

In other words, the type of stimulation women give themselves for orgasm is different from the stimulation women are supposed to want during sex with a man . . . Given women's historic status of being legally owned by men (able to have their own bank accounts only in the twentieth century, for example), "sex" reflected the old status of women. Now that is changing—yet the definition of sex lags behind.

In terms of performance, no woman should feel pressured to reach orgasm during coitus if this is not what she feels; she should be offered (or create for herself) the stimulation right for her to reach orgasm. Since most women can orgasm easily during clitoral massage—that is, external pubic/mons caressing in a rhythmic manner—this type of stimulation needs a name. Women and men need a term with which to refer to "this act"!!! Otherwise, women will continue to be pressured during "the act"/coitus, chided, "Look for your g-spot, haven't you found it yet?"

If women have orgasms easily via clitoral stimulation by hand, then it is illogical to speak of "female sexual dysfunction." Sex as we currently know it is grossly sexist and unequal—the standard scenario provides for male orgasm but not for female orgasm; thus it is oppressive to both women and men, it distorts their views of each other, but it can change!

Why have we focused on "the act" and thought women should orgasm from intercourse? The glorification of intercourse goes back a long way, perhaps two millenia, reflecting a social structure focused on reproductive sexuality. Sex has been "justified" in our prudish history as an activity that exists essentially because of a biological "sex drive" to reproduce; thus, sex (it was thought) "ought to" consist only of those acts that potentially lead to reproduction—even though today most of us use birth control.

The corollary of this glorified focus on intercourse is the villainization of other forms of sexuality and pleasurable contact—the historic horror of our culture for masturbation, for example, or even kissing and "prolonged caressing" between friends, not to mention homosexuality and lesbianism, derives from this set of assumptions.

In recent years, the g-spot has come to stand for the old concept of "vaginal orgasm"—that is, the idea that "every woman ought to be able to have orgasm via penetration—if she is a real woman!"

Publication of the *Hite Report on Female Sexuality* and discussions of female sexuality in the 1970s concluded that the definition of sex should change, that it should become more egalitarian, no longer focused on coitus as the sole "high point" or "climax of sex." Nevertheless, images of sex in pornography and popular media did not change.

Also, three years later (after publication of that research, *The Hite Report*, showing that women did not have a problem with orgasm but that the culture had a problem with its definition of "sex"), the hypothesis of an imagined (but almost never found) "g-spot" sent the message that it is not necessary to change the definition of sex in any way, that women should be able to have orgasm via coitus with the trendy new term "g-spot"—since "vaginal orgasm," the old term, had been completely ridiculed.* Society was not able so quickly to overturn centuries of belief, and so it clung in desperation to the new term.

This means, not that the vagina is not a sensitive and pleasurable organ for women, but that for most women, this pleasure does not lead to orgasm.

How should sex change? Since women can easily orgasm whenever they want via their own clitoral stimulation, this (stimulation by hand of a partner, in most cases) should become an equal "high point" to the stimulation the man receives for orgasm (whether through coitus or by oral sex or in another way). Sex should change even further than this, but how it should change is another subject, which will be treated at greater length in the future by this author. What we think of as "sex" can change even further, beyond this.

### SEXUAL EQUALITY—WHAT DOES IT MEAN?

If coitus brings men to orgasm, but not generally women, what does this imply for sex in this era of equality and human rights? To redesign sex to be more "equal," including the stimulation women need for orgasm as well as the stimulation men need, surely clitoral massage should become a focal point of sex—but what else would change? While coitus and clitoral massage to orgasm should be equally important, would orgasm still be seen as the high point of having sex? Or would feeling desire be more important?

There is an old myth that insists that masturbation causes "clitoral fixation" and "frigidity," although it is an almost guaranteed route to orgasm:

---

* The existence of a "g-spot" has now been conclusively proven to be false; see T. Himes, "The G-Spot: A Medical Myth," *American Journal of Obstetrics and Gynecology*, 185, 2001, pp. 359–62. Research coming to the same conclusion has also been done by the Royal Australian Medical Hospital and others; since this news was in the headlines just before the fateful attack on the World Trade Center in 2001, it was forgotten soon thereafter.

*I don't masturbate, because if you masturbate, you can get a fixation on your clitoris and are thus unable to come during intercourse.*

*I believe that the fact that I've been masturbating since I was ten has made it more difficult for me to orgasm vaginally.*

*Having been used to masturbating for years as a teenager and repressing my desire for actual intercourse with boys, I feel I developed a conditioned reflex that did not allow me to have a vaginal orgasm with my husband even though I enjoyed the act itself.*

The reverse is true: women who do not masturbate to orgasm are those most likely not to have orgasm during sex with a partner either. Masturbating to orgasm is an essential, excellent learning experience. Masturbation increases one's ability to orgasm in general, also during intercourse. Knowing how to masturbate to orgasm is essential to being able to have orgasm with a partner and to make sex more equal in that sense.

It is good news that almost all women can easily have orgasms, that this is not a problem; masturbation is a form of pure feedback about how women's orgasms occur, since no one teaches girls how to masturbate, they simply follow their bodies' desires. This is important information as we attempt to change the institution of sex for the better.

"Sex" as we have known it is out of date; it can now evolve into becoming something new. Women say that what is necessary is to change the way we define sex, so that both women's and men's needs are included—and this means changing the focus of sex, ending the rigid attachment to "the act" as "real sex" (everything else being merely "window-dressing" or "foreplay").

## FEELING DISHONEST: FAKING PLEASURE AND DESIRE

Can faking still be going on today? The performance pressures women feel are intense, as seen above.

According to my research, most women feel pressured to fake orgasm with men, since men in general expect certain responses from them during "the act"; most men, it seems, still assume that "if the man is sensitive and doesn't come too soon," the woman should have orgasm during coitus. However, since most women do not find that they can have orgasm during coitus (although they know perfectly well how to have orgasm via clitoral stimulation but don't feel free to say so), this causes a breakdown in communication, so that both men and women may begin to feel slightly uneasy and insecure, not knowing why. A type of dishonesty and deceit creep into sexual relationships due to the inequalities present in the antiquated definition of sex we have. This creates alienation, distrust, and suspicion between women and men—needlessly.

In fact, a woman finds herself in an awkward position if she is with a man who does not expect her to use separate clitoral stimulation to orgasm, because there is no name or accepted word for what she wants. (Yet it is a little like the elephant in the living room that no one wants to mention; that is, clitoral stimulation is important for female orgasm, as everybody knows but ignores.) If the woman decides to speak up, she has to say something like, "Uh, would you please caress my vulva and clitoral area with your hand or mouth until I reach orgasm?" This sounds, as one woman puts it, "weird, and like I'm the only one on earth who is requesting this—I must be a nut!" Many men say that they would feel "defeated" if a woman, by asking for "extra stimulation," implied that "my penis didn't do it for her."

This pressure on both the woman and the man could be avoided by making clitoral stimulation to orgasm a "normal" part of sex—with a name. Names do matter, after all. I propose adding the term "c-spot" to the sexual lexicon. Sex should include "c-spot stimulation" to orgasm (stroking and caressing the pubic or clitoral area) as a regular part of "sex." Men would do well to place their hand on top of the hand of their partner at first, in order to learn what pleases her.

Many women say that, although they want to try to reinvent sex with their partners, the person they love does not understand their body nor want to change. What should a woman do in this situation? First, she can try to understand where the man is coming from; this misunderstanding is not biological and inevitable. Here I would like to share part of what I have learned from my research on men. My analysis of male sexuality, based on seven years' research with over 7,000 individuals, led me to look at men in a new way.

## MALE SEXUALITY: OEDIPUS REVISITED[3]

What about men? Men's sexuality is little understood and is not well represented by the images of "hard penises" we have all seen and know. It is much more diverse, sensitive, and interesting than such clichés, according to my research—although many men try to put up a front and perform according to the "a real man is a hard penis" idea.

In my research for *The Hite Report on Men and Male Sexuality*, most men said, surprisingly, that they do not marry the women they most passionately love and that they are proud of this fact. They believe they did the right thing by "choosing rationally," remaining "in control of their feelings," even when they lamented their tragic "lost love." This seems to indicate that many men feel that "true love" is doomed from the start, it cannot last. Where did they learn their point of view?

Earlier research tells us that boys reach puberty—that is, experience a sexual "awakening"—between the ages of ten to twelve, when the changes in their bodies make orgasm with ejaculation possible for the first time, and most boys begin a very active masturbatory sex life. What has not been previously noted in psychological theory is that, while sexual feelings are becoming strong for boys, they also go through a moral crisis—a dark night of the soul—regarding their emotional identity, and, according to my findings, especially their relationship with their mothers.

Most boys' early sex lives are subliminally yet potently associated with feelings for their mothers. They love their mothers; their mother is the woman with whom they are most intimate. They have been kissed by her, have seen her body, felt her arms around them, know her personal habits in the bath, watched her combing her hair—and they know that sex is part of her life, or part of the hidden things they cannot know about her life.

Many boys feel especially close to their mothers, often preferring to spend more time with them than with their fathers. But then, around puberty, they learn that they must reject their mothers. They are pressured by the prevailing culture (especially at school) to change their behavior, with taunts like, "Don't hang on to your mothers' apron strings," "Don't be a wimp," "Get out of the kitchen and hang out with the boys," and so on. They are expected to demonstrate their new identity, showing that "She can't tell me what to do," distancing themselves from their mothers, and even ridiculing them sometimes publicly in front of male friends, fathers, and brothers.

This confusion carries over into sexual feelings. Dissociating themselves from their mothers while simultaneously experiencing the beginnings of strong sexual feelings causes a peculiar love-hate response to develop in many boys in relation to women: a sexuality connected to guilt and anxiety. Many learn to associate eroticism with hurting women. And when mothers, even as they are being rejected and ridiculed, keep coming back and offering more "love" and "understanding," the more hostile and difficult the boy becomes, so the pattern is reinforced. The mother's continuing nurturing is seen as a form of self-humiliation that affects how the boy will learn to define the "love" that comes from a woman.

It is not inevitably "male nature" to be ambivalent or even hostile during relationships with women. Obviously not all men are. These attitudes are part of an ideology that society endlessly reiterates to boys, especially at puberty. Pressure on boys to express disdain and contempt for their mothers, at the same time that there is pressure to begin to be "sexual" toward women—these messages together cause a traffic jam in boys' minds and short-circuit their brains (trauma), fusing the two together forever.

Clearly men do fall in love with women; the question is, what do they do in reaction to the confused mixture of feelings this can arouse? It is not necessary for the culture to break men's spirit and enjoyment of love and passion when they are boys; it doesn't have to brutalize boys by taunting them with being "momma's boys" if they refuse to segregate "male" and "female" emphatically or take a dominant posture and refuse to ostentatiously join "the male group." After all, this socially created "male" way of thinking leads to the I-must-conquer-things (such as the environment, love, work, and politics) mindset; changing this attitude would have a positive effect on society.

## "BAD GIRLS" AND "TRADITIONAL VALUES"

On the other hand, a woman who wants to change her sexual relationship can redesign her own sexual actions and assumptions, rather than expecting a man to change too. Although some may say that women have already changed sexually, the question is: are women today sleeping beauties or sexual copycats? Yes, they have changed, but how—and is this real change as women would like it?

In fact the images we see of "the new free sexual woman" in magazines and on billboards are not "the new woman" but out-of-date caricatures of old views of "sexy women." But what are the private thoughts and changes real women are making? Some women do use their bodies and initiative to go in new directions, whether in "one-night stands" or with men in long-term relationships—including men who may have thought they knew quite well "what a woman wants." This does not mean that women now are being "aggressive" or lack style, but that each woman is finding her own vocabulary and her own means of expressing her body in her own way. Sometimes this process is quiet and demure, other times it is noisy and showy.

A great distance remains between how women say they feel sexually in private and media images of women supposedly expressing erotic or sexual feelings. Hollywood films, sex videos, and internet pornography, in an effort to seem "up to date" and "modern," tend to show women being "active." They show women imitating men sexually (acting like male fantasies of women) 1960's style, wearing "provocative clothing," attempting to have orgasm from the same stimulation men do (intercourse), exhibiting lust for stereotypically male-pleasing activities (such as fellatio), and of course, being ever-young (in their twenties or at most thirties) and "beautiful." Doing everything they can to prove they are not "boring and out of date"—even if it is not the way they really feel. Women today are encouraged to be sexual in male copycat ways, not in their own ways.

These images of the supposed "new aggressive sexy woman" are causing an enormous revulsion "against sex" on the part of many women—some even turn to traditionalist religions, such as Islam, in a search for a different context or view of women; however, in fact women do not have to make a choice between "being like that" (a "pornographic woman") or being "asexual" (a "motherly woman"). Indeed, many women are quietly in private changing their sexual relationships in new ways that really matter. Still, the lurid images of women visible on so many advertising posters and in television commercials are mistakenly used at times by "fundamentalists" East and West to supposedly prove "the decadence of the secular West" and women's "sinful selfishness" or "foolish, silly consumerism." These images represent, not "who women are sexually," but rather the use and selling of women's bodies.

In reality, being active in sex has an entirely different meaning for women, a meaning that is only beginning to unfold. One of the keys to female sexuality during the next twenty years, I am sure, will be that more and more women will begin initiating a truly new type of sexuality, one that will cause a revolution in relationships. This movement has as yet barely begun—despite the courageous changes women have made in their sexual behavior and private lives so far.

In fact, women have hardly begun to show who they are sexually. Though the choices are theirs, really theirs, it can still take some time to wake up and see that one is free, in charge of one's life, that all decisions are possible.

Like Sleeping Beauty awakening, after 2,000 years of misinformation, women need a little time to think, take action, and invent a new sexual culture.

## SEX AND POLITICS, PEACE AND LOVE

Sex and the use of our bodies is a profound matter, for each of us personally, for the others we come into contact with, and for society as a whole. Legally women's bodies have historically been owned by men; today women rightly believe that they should own their own bodies and decide for themselves how to reproduce and have sex. This "private issue" is political; it is changing the world.

It is often said that "sex is political," but what does this mean precisely?

No one should think that claiming that "Sex is connected to world peace" means simplistically that "If people have more and better sex, they will be more satisfied, and therefore they will be less interested in war." While undoubtedly true, while the slogan "Sex, Peace, and Love" is good, the idea proposed here is something new: that through the physical movements of the sex act, individuals learn lessons in gender behavior and "proper psychology" that shape thinking and belief systems— that gender taught to children is largely inculcated through sexual values and moral codes as we know them; thus if we critique "what sex is," as we are doing here, we can begin to see ourselves (and "human life") as separate from this ideology, and therefore initiate a more positive future.

A new sexuality is part of an emerging new politics of planetary health, the environment, issues of globalization, and world peace. A re-created vision of sex is connected to a new international value system that is trying to emerge—a still hazy revised view of who we are as a species on the planet, what we are doing or should be doing with our lives. The central question of this new value system remains one of war and peace: Why are there so many wars? Is war an inevitable consequence of human nature? Could we be less warlike?

In its deepest sense sexuality is connected to world peace, not because of a superficial notion that "sex" is "deep," but because sexuality is key in women's growing "equality" and activity in the world, central to the definition of "who a woman is." And because sex is key to "who a man is," if a man rethinks his primary assumptions about sex, he will also revamp his ideas about himself and who he is as a man, and society will be greatly affected.

With this book I would like to turn the direction of society away from both what we think of as "the sexual revolution" and "fundamentalist religious values" to find a new direction that includes female equality and autonomy as well as greater sensuality for men, more choice, but avoids the clichés of pornographic sexuality labeled "freedom."

The sexual revolution has vulgarized sex, reflecting an older view that sex is "sinful" and "dirty" ("People who do it are animals and behave in a vulgar manner"). This is not the way forward that most of the women (and men) in my research are looking for. Indeed, this misunderstanding of "sexual freedom" and "women's liberation" is dangerous, because it seems to reinforce the idea that "sexy women are dirty and vulgar," that there are "two kinds of women, the sexy ones and the others." This is not good for women or men, and dehumanizes women (delegitimizes female sexuality and the female body) in the eyes of society. This misunderstanding is also dangerous in today's political climate, causing fundamentalists both East and West to point a finger of accusation at "the decadence of the secular West"—supposedly epitomized by images in pornography or ads showing "women in miniskirts marketing themselves to men."

Positing the choice as being between "family values" and "porno culture" is not really offering people a choice; the culture is going off track, women's revolution and achievement of their rights has been hijacked* by the sexually-free-media-speak nonsense used to sell magazines (and concurrently emphasize women's "insecurity"); the greatest performance pressure on women is to have orgasm during "the act," or pretend to. Women may still be Sleeping Beauties, still not the fully powerful beings they can be, still not fully sexually authentic, even today. Sexually men are not awake either. We need a real gender revolution, we have not really had one yet.

Female orgasm is a metaphor for political change, for very real reasons. If women determine their sexuality for themselves—to reproduce or not, to orgasm or not, to participate in sex or not—which they still have not fully done, despite the changes: this goes hand in hand with women taking political and economic power in the world. Conversely, no change means continuing to uphold the status quo: unless women underpin the family institution full-time (serving men and caring for children, offering husbands sexual pleasure without insisting on their own orgasm, perhaps making their own orgasms when alone via masturbation), the status quo will not be transformed in a basic way. Is this what we want?

In my analysis of male sexuality, "Oedipus Revisited," I have researched boys and men to show how the construction of boys' psychosexual identity at puberty and earlier carries over into men's identity as adults: if boys are brought up to think that being "a man" means being sexually "big," dominant over women, and financially powerful, or if the idea is pushed that "a real man" must be "cool and

---

* I am trying to change mentality—the male and female psyche—and thus change the society, not enhance female orgasm or "make women sexually free." The idea that my work may have beeen used to sell magazines with shrill headlines about "orgasm" fills me with horror and disgust; I am trying to give women (and men) power and a new way to live their lives and construct relationships.

tough"—though "sensitive"—then he may conclude that anyone who does not "show him proper respect" should be "taught a lesson," that the correct reaction for an adult man is an aggressive posture, not dialogue. Thus early gender training is linked to warlike thinking later.

The current belief in "sex drive" as "an inevitable hormonal mechanism" inside men now props up this system, asserting that men are "by nature" aggressive and need to be dominant, that "dominance" and "command" are inherent in men's "psychology" and "biology." However, in my thesis, the social commands to boys (their programming) is causing an exaggeratedly militaristic society; such rules are unjustified and can be changed, once they are identified (as here), thus ending a major cause of today's wars, small and large. Beginning to deconstruct "male sexuality" is thus doing two things: creating more pleasure and space for individual men, and helping society develop a more peaceful global strategy.

Most people today are concerned about how they should feel about "sex" in their private lives; they are also concerned by heated debates about sex in the news—that is, public discussions of abortion, domestic or sexual violence, equality, sexual harassment, "the veil"/ "the chador" (as "necessary for a woman to wear to express 'modesty' and 'humility,' the opposite of the 'secular minijupe'"), child pornography, sexual trafficking in women, and rape in war (as in Bosnia, Chechnya, and Rwanda), among other matters, such as President Clinton's sex life. Most people fear they have fantasies that are not "politically correct," and often cannot square their personal sexual desires with what they believe to be ethical. This dichotomy is of our own making, and can change.

No one should fear the changes: "sex" can be much "sexier" than it is, and revising sex does not mean making it "politically correct." If female orgasm happens for most women with some form of clitoral stimulation, this understanding is not boring! On the contrary, it opens up exciting new possibilities and brings into question many of our most sacred beliefs about "the act," "who men are by their nature," and "who women are"—it does not mean that people will be unerotic and "perfect."

In the end, sex and social reality are connected. The definitions of both female and male sexuality are central to our culture's social structure.

## DOUBTS ABOUT THE SEXUAL REVOLUTION

This work is not part of the sexual-revolution school of thought of the last decades, the "we must lose our inhibitions and be more natural" point of view—that is, "civilization is a veneer put on top of our natural instincts," which make us procreate sexually (a crude Darwinism) implying that how we behave in sex tells us who we are biologically and psychologically—that these "instincts" are deeper than the way we learn to behave in society and so forth.

This work affirms that sexual behavior is plastic, that it can be formed to take many shapes, that it has little shape of its own, that it is formed by a society's values and beliefs about the "proper way" of doing things. Although it is commonly believed that our "basic instincts" include an "animal desire to reproduce and have coitus"— and while in some situations this may be truly how we feel—most of the time when we have sex, this is not the goal of our actions. We have other goals in mind.

The ideology we currently impose on sex dates from earlier centuries and defines "male" and "female" in rigid Adam-and-Eve categories that then influence what we call our psychology. We can shape a much better type of identity and sexuality for both women and men by consciously rethinking our views of "sex"—creating, for example, a new sexual scenario that values both male and female orgasm/pleasure equally or one that does not focus on either male or female orgasm but offers an open road.

These ideas have a political link; human rights include the issue of sexuality. The current definition of sex is from an older value system that forces women, if they want to have a sexually intimate experience, to forget themselves and their own needs and serve another's, to ensure male orgasm by their behavior, but not female orgasm. It forces men to "perform" and obsess about the size of their penis or erections. This sexual scenario can be exchanged for one in which both partners can express more of themselves and their true emotions and identities, relate in new individual and unique ways.

This work is not "antimale" but seeks to open up a new view of "who men are" for both women and men to use in rethinking existing ideas of "male sexuality" and expanding the boundaries of what is now considered "the correct sexual expression of a real man." Although this work asserts that current definitions of sex are overly focused on male orgasm—almost in a rigid, semimilitaristic way, as in "It's part of men's training to hit the target every time"—in fact, male sexuality is a delicate and complex mixture of feelings, desires, and needs, not the simplistic mechanism for orgasm as current clichés insist.

Men and women together are beginning to re-create their sexuality to produce a new cultural base, a new landscape of the mind and body. Or they are doing this separately.

### CUPID AND PSYCHE: THE TRANSFORMATION OF SEX, TRANSFORMATION OF THE PSYCHE

Sex is a kind of cultural skywriting, large signals that something basic is happening in the culture.

At present there is something going on in our basic value system, something that makes extremists exclaim, "Civilization is collapsing" or, "Women's changes in the family are going too far," "Divorce statistics are skyrocketing out of control," and "There is too much of the wrong kind of immoral sex, sex, sex everywhere." Some of these beliefs may be partially true, but the conclusion to be drawn is not that we should return to the values of the past as fast as possible.

This book makes the case that we are in transition, not decline; that, amazingly, a new psychosexual identity seems to be emerging, a spectrum of emotions with a new perspective on "what is natural for human beings"—that is, portending a new sexual "human nature." What is emerging is not the obvious idea of "the new morality"—sex, drugs, and rock'n'roll or "decadent girls in miniskirts"; the subtle changes documented here are unseen (private, not public) and taking place in sexual relations between people of all ages and views.

Some say that the changes of the "new sexuality" demonstrate the collapse of the old moral order, a decline in values. Others insist that the new ideas are better, that "sexual freedom" is necessary in order to have political freedom. Clearly sexual equality and self-determination for women, one of the most important issues of our time, is having a major influence on, and playing an important part in, these changes. Sexual equality is a concept that is changing from the inside how "sex" and human relations are defined. Here we are examining implications of the movement for sexual equality on the meaning of "sex"; examining how the psyche and emotional terrain are changing in reaction and are likely to change further in the future.

Once thought of as a "trivial topic," sex is now understood to be a core issue. Sexuality is central to our value system; if women change their place in sex, their right to their own bodies, this change has far-ranging social repercussions. Traditional sex was symbolic of women's position and role in society as "helpmate," each "sexual act" a ritual performed by man and woman teaching them "who they are" and their "purpose on this earth" (reproduction), also reminding them that "man is the master" who has a right to orgasm, while woman's needs are secondary.

Reassessing such a fundamental institution as "sex" involves a great transformation of thinking, morality, and culture within each individual and in social institutions such as marriage and family. The questions: What is the meaning of the body and its desires? Why has sex been declared profane and "non-spiritual"? This shift has gone so far that Aretha Franklin recorded a popular song in 2000 addressing the situation of a young black girl in the United States who has been made love to (had sex) and then "dumped" by a man: "She's Still a Rose." The video shows this plot with great emotion.

It could be argued that, if, in the sixth century BC, Psyche killed Eros (that is, the mind learned to dominate the body), it could also be said that today people are trying to recombine the two, to find a philosophy of life that gracefully blends body and mind rather than setting them in conflict. Why say that "sex" is not "spiritual," not linked to the soul? (This is not to say that sex must be seen only within the context of the family, as a "serious matter.") This calls for a complete rethinking of the institution of "sex"; we can no longer say that it is "obviously" a "drive to reproduce" but want to discover what it means as individuals.

If the definition of "sex" should be changed—and the current definition of sex focused on coitus ("the act"—that is, reproductive activity) discriminates against

women just as much as policies in housing, hiring, equal pay, and so on have discriminated—this implies that changes are needed in the core value system. After
all, how can a core value system such as we have had for so long create a just society when it supports and continues (even seeks to glorify) injustice—that is, per-
petuates the second-class status of half the population? Traditional sexual values
have not done any favors to men either, despite superficial appearances.

Currently the core value system is being improved. It is impossible to "return to
the past"—and who would want to, since past values were based on inequality—nor
do we want to rush headlong into a "pornography sex culture." What we want is to
create a future that uses the best of everything we have seen so far.

Society still has a long way to go and will see many more developments throughout the new century, as a new fundamental value system evolves, and all of us play our
part in that evolution. At the moment, an accurate analysis of the change to date is
needed—"the good and the bad"—as offered here. The current global conflict
between "fundamentalist back-to-basics" views and a new international human rights
democratic-based value system will have enormous consequences for all of us.

NOTES

1  See essays in the Appendix.
2  See Appendix for the questionnaires I used.
3  See also Part 2.

# Part 1

# Female Sexuality Defined by Women
### (1976)

*This section contains excerpts of work done during the 1970s and published as* The Hite Report: A Nationwide Study of Female Sexuality.[1] *It presents extensive research based on over 3,000 women's own anonymous voices testifying about their feelings and experiences during sex and orgasm.[2] It shows that most women need some form of exterior clitoral stimulation in order to orgasm, that coitus itself does not create orgasm easily or regularly for most women, and that when it does, that orgasm feels muffled or, at the least, different from orgasm during self-stimulation or clitoral stimulation (some women need to hold their legs together in order to reach orgasm and may engage in coitus as a form of pleasure rather than having the goal of orgasm, for example). These testimonies imply that the definition of sex for women might be other than that so commonly assumed to be the "real" definition. What, Hite asks, would the direction of that new definition be?*

# The Female Orgasm as Metaphor

It was said for centuries that women have "difficulty" having orgasms; that female orgasms (if they exist!) are much weaker and not as "real" as men's; that men have orgasms more easily; that men's orgasms are stronger, their sexual organs larger and more important; and so on. That women are only "blocked" from having orgasm during intercourse (as men do) by either their own psychological fears and neuroses or men's haste in having orgasm themselves—that is, women could have orgasm during coitus if men would be "more sensitive" and "not orgasm too soon" themselves. Though these ideas are full of nonsense and error, for centuries they were considered unquestionable.

The twentieth century saw a breakthrough as women determined to gain equal rights and power in society. From fighting for the right to vote early in the century to equal-pay issues (still being fought), women made impressive advances, going on to include more hidden issues, such as sexuality and family-reproductive matters (the right to autonomy over their own bodies, birth control, and reproduction). In fact, today sexuality is still one of the principal keys to women's freedom and equal status, as the United Nations Declaration on the Rights of Women, signed by 140 countries in Beijing in 1995, makes clear. Women have come a long way in half a century from a time when the existence of women's orgasms was doubted, when women were legally (and economically) owned as property in marriage, to the present. Women beginning the new millenium are reinventing themselves, their work and love, reclaiming space to breathe, space to experiment and to discover what sexuality and love mean on their own terms, how they want to express themselves (which does not mean the style of the commercial images in current media of "the new free sexual woman, she's aggressive just like a man!"). After centuries of being force-fed a passive, reproductive role in sex, after endless public distortion of female sexuality in advertising and pornography, and after mixed experiences with personal relationships, both positive and negative, women now are claiming their own time and space, and their own right to sexual autonomy over their own bodies. This change is not easy!

A great distance remains between how women say they feel sexually, how they orgasm, and public visual images of how women experience sexuality and orgasm. Hollywood films, as well as sex videos and internet pornography, continue to show women imitating men sexually (acting like male fantasies of women): attempting to have orgasm from the same stimulation men do (from coitus—that is, intercourse), being "the new sexually active woman" by exhibiting lust for stereotypically male-pleasing activities, wearing clichéd sex-tart "provocative clothing," and of course, being ever young.

The assumption has been, and continues to be in Hollywood films and sex videos (and our minds?), that intercourse is the only "real" way to have "sex" and that "a normal woman" should orgasm during "penetration," just like a man. However, my research shows that most women, however much they may like coitus, need specific stimulation of their exterior vulva or clitoris in order to orgasm fully. This research began from the starting point of asking women themselves to describe exactly how they feel during various sexual activities and when they most often orgasm. Society has long known that it is easier for women to orgasm during self-stimulation (masturbation) than coitus and that masturbation is clitoral and exterior, not vaginal. Yet the society condemned women, as if their feelings were wrong, incorrect. For example, in the twentieth century, though both Freud and Kinsey knew that women could orgasm much more easily with clitoral stimulation (exterior stimulation) than with "vaginal penetration," both failed to draw the logical conclusion. Instead of seeing that society was oppressing women, they expected women to change; Freud believed that women should grow up to "adjust" and become mature, while Kinsey thought that when a woman had been married longer, had more experience sexually, she would achieve this result. However, today the logical conclusion is clear.

On the basis of the testimony of over 3,000 women in my first report, the facts are clear: most women can orgasm easily during clitoral or pubic-area stimulation (either by themselves or with another person, by hand or by mouth). Only one-third of women orgasm easily during the actual "act"—that is, "penetration" or intercourse (with "no hands"). (By the way, why is the beginning of intercourse almost always described as "vaginal penetration"—couldn't one as easily say "penile covering"?) For most women, the stimulation during masturbation and coitus is different. There is rarely penetration of the vagina during masturbation.

The conclusion: it is "normal" for women to orgasm from clitoral stimulation, not "immature" or "dysfunctional." The way women orgasm is something to celebrate, not to decry! It is not women who have a "problem" sexually, but society, which has had a problem accepting and understanding women's sexuality.

This does not mean that the vagina is not highly erotic and sensitive or that it cannot bring intense satisfaction to a woman. There is, for example, something very symbolic about being "penetrated" by the right partner, as men too can experience.

That most mysterious of organs—the female vulva, labia, vagina, uterus, and especially the clitoris—the intricate, elegant clitoral system, that large network that extends deep inside the female genitals and fills with blood to allow intensely vivid sensations and pleasures . . . names and information about these organs and how female sexuality functions was suppressed for long periods of history.

The understanding of female orgasm and women's own feelings and desires has improved greatly since publication of the original testimonies of women in *The Hite Report on Female Sexuality*: women today no longer believe that there is "something terribly wrong with them" if they do not reach orgasm during "the act," though they often wish they could.

The sexual system, however, is slow to change; according to many women, men often indicate by their actions that they assume a woman will orgasm from intercourse "unless she tells me something different"—putting a woman in the awkward position of asking for something with no name that must be "special," since it is not "ordinary" in the man's experience, not automatically offered (as women during "sex" expect to offer coitus). Thus there is an ongoing gap between men's idea of women and women's reality, and this undercurrent in "sex" makes emotions even more fragile than they would normally be in love and relationships. Publicity for drugs like Viagra implies that "the erect penis" is the main part of sex, and thus it does not help change these old ideas.

Although we may think of ourselves as "modern" ("we already know all that"), have you ever seen a Hollywood film or a sex video that shows clitoral stimulation by hand to orgasm? No, even in the twenty-first century movies, television programs, and pornography still imply that a "real woman" should "love" to have "a big piece of meat inside her," that this and only this should bring on roaring multiple orgasms. Such outdated media (and publicity for the drug Viagra) keep the myth alive that only coitus is "real sex." But in truth, for most women, orgasm occurs separately, during clitoral stimulation.

However, the old "vaginal orgasm" idea was about to make a return under a trendy new name. . . .

### G-SPOT OR C-SPOT? (TOWARD A NEW CONCEPTION OF SEX)

To discuss sex has become banal. People feel, "I know all that already," or, "Oh no, not sex and female orgasm again . . . !"

Why? In a world in which pornography has become part of daily life, in which it is everywhere, this attitude is understandable. There has been a media surfeit of the topic, usually done superficially.

The first *Hite Report on Female Sexuality* broke through this mumbo jumbo to show that "clitoral stimulation" is the real way that women reach orgasm, not via "vaginal orgasm," as it was called. (This meant vaginal stimulation via "the act," no hands or other "cheating" by stimulating the clitoral area.) Today the mythology of a supposed "g-spot" has taken over the territory of the outdated "vaginal orgasm," now making some people believe that one can carry on with the same old definition of sex in which women are supposed to reach orgasm via the same stimulation men do—that is, vaginal stimulation of the penis—never mind if, statistically, most women do not regularly reach orgasm in this way, although they can easily reach orgasm during masturbation, which means, in 99 percent of cases, clitoral-area massage. So what has changed except the terminology?

My research, demonstrating in thousands of women's own voices that most women can orgasm easily with clitoral-area stimulation in one form or another, thus concluding that it is the definition of sex that should change (not women's bodies!), was published first in 1976. Three years later, however, on slim research, three authors published a book that launched the idea of a hidden, mysterious "g-spot" inside the vagina that made "clitoral stimulation" unnecessary in any specific way.

The mass media proclaimed the "new truth" of a "g-spot," and women were thus told once again that they should find their "vaginal destiny"—never mind if they had difficulty having orgasm in that way. Freud was given new status, since he had pro-claimed that in order to be "well-adjusted," every woman should change her need for stimulation from the clitoris to the vagina at puberty; if she did not, she remained "juvenile," and had a "dysfunction" or "neurosis" and should be "treated" by his psychological therapy (bluntly, to find out why she hated her father . . .). Freud's old idea that women should not need or want clitoral stimulation but should be content with vaginal stimulation (he had published it in the 1920s) was dredged up again and given "scientific" status (denied to Freud while he was alive) by many doctors wanting to prop up the idea proposing that women yet again make themselves fit into the system (or be declared "abnormal").

The right of women themselves to determine their sexual identity, opened up by *The Hite Report* and other works, was shunted aside.

Despite the propaganda for the "g-spot" ("g" was chosen by the three authors for a doctor, then deceased, whose name was Graffenburg), the same percentage of women continued to not have orgasm during sex with their partners, although most could easily reach orgasm by themselves. According to *The Hite Report* and other sources, women have a very high statistical rate of success at achieving orgasm when they stimulate themselves; this almost always involves exterior rhythmic massage of the clitoral area, not self-penetration of the vagina. Yet the idea of a mythical "g-spot" continued its hold on the popular imagination, somewhat akin to a holy grail, despite women's individual experiences. The reason: it was codified, accepted as "true," by the general society; it gave permission to men to think that they were "modern" and believed in "clitoral stimulation" and "a woman's right to enjoy her-self"—although "most women should get the stimulation they need if a man has a big enough penis or if he is sensitive and caring" or "if he does it long enough."

The logical connection made by *The Hite Report* was lost when the language was cleansed of the terms "vaginal orgasm" and "clitoral orgasm" and when no new terminology was added to popularize the new information given by women themselves.

Women were not in charge of most agencies of public health, nor were most women psychiatrists or gynecologists, among other professions, so that women themselves were not in charge of disseminating this information. It was left to individual word of mouth (about a topic it had traditionally been difficult for women to speak about). Here, a new term is proposed: "c-spot" to mean clitoral-area stimulation or massage.

Today pornography does not show c-spot stimulation to orgasm, rather, it depicts "the act" of "penetration" as central to female (and male) sexuality. People, especially young women and men, try very hard to find their full satisfaction in the repetition of this act, denying themselves the diversity and pleasure of their own authentic sexual expression. (The diversion typically offered to men is to have several partners, thus making the repetition of "the act" less tedious, it would be supposed.) Young people today believe that pornography is "modern" and "shows it like it is." In fact, the act is not necessarily the centerpiece of female sexuality for various reasons, among them that it does not generally lead to orgasm, though it may often lead to emotional climax or "emotional orgasm," as named in *The Hite Report* (a feeling of a high moment of intensity, both emotional and physical).

I believe there is another, better direction for "sex," a path that was begun in 1977 but abandoned by the general culture with the slight pretext of a hypothesized "g-spot." This is the path of reorienting our complete idea of what "sex" or erotic movements and sharing of the body is. It is the path of equality between women and men during these relations, as well as the emotional context that has in the past divided men and women into the categories of "fucker" and "fuckee." (The man should be "the one who fucks," the women "the one who is fucked.")

The new ideas are the road of the future. Trying to cling to the old psychosexual views has created a quite reactionary (and even militaristic) psychology and society, not appropriate to today's atmosphere and needs. Sex can be much "sexier" in this new context and with this new content, if we leave behind an outdated fixation on a rigid scenario culminating and ending with the act of potential reproduction. We have to invent a new conception of sexual interchanges.

### IF SLEEPING BEAUTY BEGINS TO AWAKEN ON HER OWN . . .

Are women now redefining sexuality? Women are making many changes in how they see and practice intimate physical relations—how they express and share their bodies. Though the choices are theirs, really theirs, it can still take some time to wake up and see that one is free, in charge of one's life, that all decisions are possible; like sleeping beauty awaking after 2,000 years of misinformation, women need a little time to think clearly.

Women during recent years have been encouraged to be "sexually active" in "male copycat ways," not in their own ways—for example, performing actions that demonstrate intercourse is making them more and more excited (which may or may not be true), "initiating" sexual activities long defined to be "sexual" by men, or actively "acting hot" (counter to the ladies-don't-like-"sex," or the Mary-is-pure-and-good stereotype of women), wearing "sexy shocking outfits," and the like. In reality, being active in sex has an entirely different meaning for women, a mean-ing that is only beginning to unfold. For example, if women know how to reach orgasm on their own (during masturbation), why don't they touch themselves in the same way during sex with a partner, and make themselves orgasm? (Many women say that the men they know do not expect this and so do not aid in this process, perhaps by touching them or whispering words of encouragement—though they hope that this will change any day now.)

The semipornographic images of women visible on so many advertising posters and in television commercials—images sometimes used by fundamentalists to point to "the decadence of the secular West" or "the shameful lack of values in today's society"—do not represent "who women are sexually" but rather the use and selling of women's bodies by a double-standard commercialism.

It is no wonder, with female sexuality equated with what is shown in many ads, that some women today recoil, deciding that "the old ways were best," imagining that women were more respected then, whether or not this belief is historically accurate, and consequently they embrace a traditionalist version of religion and family values.

During the next hundred years, I am sure, one of the keys to female sexuality will be that women will begin initiating a new type of sexuality—something that will cause a real revolution, one that as of right now has barely begun, despite all the courageous changes people have made in their sexual behavior and private lives.

Women may have hardly begun to show who they are sexually.

## SEXUALITY AS A SOCIAL CONSTRUCTION: TOWARD A NEW THEORY OF FEMALE SEXUALITY

### DO MOST WOMEN ORGASM FROM INTERCOURSE?

*This is one of the last questions I've answered—I'm afraid to admit it—but I'm not really sure yes or no—although I've had many orgasms through masturbation, I'm not sure what orgasm from vaginal inter-course is like—I've had very high feelings, but I guess since it wasn't like a masturbatory orgasm I didn't think it was an orgasm. At first, this questionnaire made me feel totally inexperienced—but it's just that I guess I don't always think about these things during sex. Like I remem-ber when I had my first coitus I just kept thinking, "My god, I've got to remember all the details about this—the big important time of my life, when I chose to give up my virginity" and you know something—I don't really remember that much about that specific time.*

*I really don't know if I've had an orgasm with a man, unless it's just that I don't really know what to be aware of because if it's supposed to be like when I'm masturbating then I think not. I would like to know if that makes me abnormal.*

*I don't think I've ever really experienced an orgasm. In any event, not the way I've read about them. My husband's clitoral stimulation usually leads to a climax for me but never during vaginal stimulation. I keep hoping and working at it. Sometimes I tend to think maybe I'm not supposed to experience a vaginal climax. Sometimes it bothers my husband more than it does me. He really feels badly that I don't experience the same type of pleasure he does. Sometimes I think we work at it too hard and sometimes we think we're getting closer to it, but I never experience anything physically ecstatic.*

*I am rather hung up when it comes to orgasms. Because I never have them during intercourse, I feel deeply ashamed and inferior. I grew up with that wretched word "frigid"—and I think that a lot of my desire to have orgasms during intercourse comes from this shame and feelings of inadequacy. I think the only thing that will contribute to my having them is when I change the feelings I have mentioned before—when I stop pressuring myself and hating myself because I don't have orgasm—hell, I don't know—I've been in therapy for two years and it has helped me personally a lot, but I'm still no closer to having them during intercourse. I think it will take some radical change in my perception and attitude toward myself.*

Do most of the women in this study orgasm regularly during intercourse (the penis thrusting in the vagina), without additional clitoral stimulation? No. It was found that only approximately 30 percent of the women in this study could orgasm regularly from intercourse—that is, could have an orgasm during intercourse without more direct manual clitoral stimulation being provided at the time of orgasm.

In other words, the majority of women do not experience orgasm regularly as a result of intercourse.

For most women, orgasming during intercourse as a result of intercourse alone is the exceptional experience, not the usual one. Although a small minority of women could orgasm more or less regularly from intercourse itself, since almost all women orgasm from clitoral stimulation (during manual stimulation with a partner or by masturbation), henceforth we will refer to the stimulation necessary for female orgasm as clitoral.

Based on my research, it is clear that intercourse by itself does not regularly lead to orgasm for most women. In fact, for over 70 percent of the women, intercourse—the penis thrusting in the vagina—did not regularly lead to orgasm. What we thought was an individual problem is neither unusual nor a problem. In other words, not to have orgasm from intercourse is the experience of the majority of women.

We shall see later on in this chapter that, often, the ways in which women do orgasm during intercourse have nothing much to do with intercourse itself. In fact, these methods could probably be adopted by other women who wish to orgasm during intercourse—if this were felt to be a desirable goal.

## THE GLORIFICATION OF INTERCOURSE: A REPRODUCTIVE MODEL OF SEXUALITY

Why have we thought women should orgasm from intercourse? There are three basic reasons for this insistence:

A. To ensure reproduction by tying coitus to sexual pleasure.
B. To promote monogamous intercourse and, by it, patrilineal inheritance.
C. The widespread influence of the Freudian model of female psychology.

### A. THE SEXUAL-PLEASURE MODEL OF REPRODUCTION

The sexual-pleasure model of reproduction holds that nature gave us a "sex drive" and the capacity for sexual pleasure in order to ensure reproduction. By logical extension the model holds that coitus is "the real thing" and all other forms of sexual gratification are substitutions for, or perversions of, this primary "natural" activity.

It is important to scrutinize this assumption. Intercourse is necessary for reproduction, and sexual pleasure and orgasm are involved with reproduction. But looking more closely, one sees that only male orgasm during intercourse is necessary for reproduction. It would make sense, in view of the necessity to deposit semen inside the vagina, that intercourse provide almost automatic, perfect stimulation for male orgasm, and of course it does: men orgasm as regularly during intercourse as women (and men) do during masturbation.

However, since female orgasm is not necessary during intercourse for reproduction to occur, why should nature provide stimulation for female orgasm during intercourse? (As a matter of fact, what is the reason for the existence of female orgasm at all?) There are several possibilities:

1. Some researchers claim that female orgasm helps "suck" the sperm up into the uterus. However, Masters and Johnson show that this is doubtful, since the contractions of the uterus progress downward and so are "more likely to have an expulsive action than a sucking action." To check this, they placed a fluid resembling semen, but opaque to x-rays, in a cap covering the cervix, so that if there were any sucking, the fluid would be taken into the cervix. However, x-ray films showed no significant suction at all. Several respondents in this study mentioned that their contractions move downward, or outward. One woman described her orgasm this way: "A clitoral orgasm is a sharp, shuddering, breath-taking pleasure/pain gripping of the muscles in my rectum and vagina. Whatever is in me—a finger, or penis, or dildo—is gripped and pushed outward."

2. Dr. Mary Jane Sherfey writes: "In general, the orgasm in the male is admirably

designed to deposit semen where it will do the most good, and in the female, to remove the largest amount of venous congestion in the most effective manner." But orgasm decongests men, too, and Sherfey herself has made a point of emphasizing that after one orgasm women do not completely decongest but remain in a state of partial arousal, and sometimes after one orgasm arousal can become stronger. Can this be, then, the only function of female orgasm?

Sherfey has also presented a possible reason why, from the point of view of reproduction, women should not have orgasms during intercourse:

> In a woman with a lax perineal body who has borne children, semen easily escapes with premature withdrawal, whereas if the woman does not have an orgasm, the still-swollen lower third acts as a stopper to semen outflow.

Masters and Johnson have also mentioned that there is a greater chance for impregnation for some women if they do not orgasm, for the same reason.

3. Another possibility is that perhaps our orgasmic contractions are for the purpose of ensuring male orgasm, gripping the penis and pulling slightly downward rhythmically. In this model of intercourse, thrusting would not be considered as necessary as it now is, and perhaps intercourse in another culture would be less gymnastic and male-dominated and more a mutual lying together in pleasure, penis-in-vagina, or vagina-covering-penis, with female orgasm providing much of the stimulation necessary for male orgasm.

4. On the other hand, perhaps the function of female orgasm is to provide arousal and "receptivity," or interest in having the woman initiate intercourse. Most female primates have a period of estrus, a specific period of time during which arousal is more or less constant, which guarantees that fertility and intercourse will coincide. Women do not have estrus; they are theoretically capable of becoming aroused at any time. We become aroused in many ways—by kissing, hugging, and even talking. During all these activities, if we find them arousing, a warm, tickling sensation—the desire for clitoral stimulation, perhaps—becomes stronger and stronger. If clitoral stimulation follows, it often leads to a kind of vaginal tickle ("vaginal ache") that feels to many women like a desire to "be penetrated." While continued stimulation brings orgasm and, for many women, a return to arousal, intercourse seems to quiet this feeling. Perhaps one of the functions of our orgasm is continuing arousal—and "receptivity."

It is unclear whether the "vaginal ache" part of the outline just presented holds true for most women, or even for very many women, since most women generally don't use any kind of vaginal entry during masturbation. However, the general idea of our orgasms perhaps serving the function of continuing our arousal and keeping it at just manageable levels for the body is an interesting possibility.

However, none of these theories may be right. For example, if the purpose of arousal and sexuality in general is really connected only with reproduction, why can we have just as much if not stronger arousal and orgasm(s) at times when we are not capable of conception—during pregnancy, after menopause, during menstruation, at other times of the month when conception is not possible, and during childhood?

Perhaps orgasm is basically a release mechanism for the body, as are other bodily reactions, such as laughing, crying, or convulsions. Maybe one function of orgasm is the discharge of all kinds of tensions through this release. Or could it be possible that there is no "reason" for the existence of female orgasm other than pleasure? In any case, whether or not continuing arousal is the function of female orgasm, or whether the function is the release of all kinds of bodily tensions, it is definitely clear that there is no logical reason for insisting that we have our orgasms during intercourse.

## B. PATRIARCHY AND MONOGAMOUS INTERCOURSE

A second reason for insisting that women (and men) should find their greatest sexual pleasure in intercourse, and for seeing intercourse as the basic sexual act, the basic form of sex is that our form of society demands it. With very few isolated exceptions, for the last 3,000 or 4,000 years all societies have been patrilineal or patriarchal. Family name and inheritance have passed through men, and religious and civil laws have given men authority to determine the course of society. In a nonpatriarchal society, where there is either no question of property rights or where lineage goes through the mother, there is no need for institutionalizing intercourse as the basic form of sexual pleasure. In the earliest known societies, families were mostly extended groups of clans, with aunts and brothers sharing equally in the upbringing of the child; the mother did not particularly "own" the child, and there was no concept of "father" at all. In fact, the male role in reproduction was not understood for quite a long time, and intercourse and male orgasm were not connected with pregnancy, which of course only became apparent many months later.

But with changeover to a patrilineal or patriarchal society,[3] it becomes necessary for the man to control the sexuality of the woman. Nancy Marval, in a paper printed by the 1970s organization The Feminists, explains this further:

> In a patriarchal culture like the one we were all brought up in, sexuality is a crucial issue. Beyond all the symbolic aspects of the sexual act (symbolizing the male's dominance, manipulation, and control over the female), it assumes an overwhelming practical importance. This is that men have no direct access to reproduction and the survival of the species. As individuals, their claim to any particular child can never be as clear as that of the mother who demonstrably gave birth to that child. Under normal circumstances it is agreed that a man is needed to provide sperm to the conception of the

baby, but it is practically impossible to determine which man. The only way a man can be absolutely sure that he is the one to have contributed that sperm is to control the sexuality of the woman.[4]

To do this, he had to insist she be a virgin at marriage and monogamous thereafter. As Kinsey put it:

Sexual activities for the female before marriage were proscribed in ancient codes primarily because they threatened the male's property rights in the female whom he was taking as a wife. The demand that the female be a virgin at the time of her marriage was comparable to the demand that cattle or other goods that he bought should be perfect, according to the standards of the culture in which he lived.

In addition to these practical reasons for controlling sexuality (to maintain the form of social organization we know), in the early period of the changeover to patriarchy there were political reasons as well, in that other forms of sexuality represented rival forms of social organization. For example, it is generally accepted by Bible scholars that the earliest Jewish tribes mentioned in the Old Testament accepted cunnilingus and homosexuality as a valid part of life and physical relations, as did the societies around them—which were not, for the most part, totally patriarchal. In fact, prior to the seventh century BC,* homosexual and other sexual activities were associated with Jewish religious rites, just as in the surrounding cultures. But as the small and struggling Jewish tribes sought to build and consolidate their strength, and their patriarchal social order, and to bind all loyalty to the one male god, Yahweh, all forms of sexuality except the one necessary for reproduction were banned by religious code. The Holiness Code, established at the time of their return from the Babylonian exile, sought to fence out the surrounding cultures and set up rules for separating off the Chosen People of God. It was then that non-heterosexual, non-reproductive sexual acts were condemned as the way of the Canaanite, the way of the pagan. But these activities were proscribed as an indication of allegiance to another culture, an adjunct to idolatry—and not as "immoral" or as sexual crimes, as we consider them. They were political crimes.

These codes have continued in our religious and civil law up to this day. Judeo-Christian codes still specifically condemn all sexual activity that does not have reproduction as its ultimate aim. Our civil law is largely derived from these codes, and the laws of most states condemn non-coital forms of sexuality (in and out of marriage) as punishable misdemeanors

---

* Although according to *Jews: Biography of a People* by *Judd Teller*, it was the sixth century BC; recent Israeli archaeological discoveries (1995–2000) have updated and are updating this information.

or crimes. Thus, intercourse has been institutionalized in our culture as the only permissible form of sexual activity.

Forms of sexuality other than intercourse are now also considered psychologically abnormal and unhealthy. However, the full spectrum of physical contact is enjoyed by the other mammals, and their mental health has not been questioned. Furthermore, intercourse is not the main focus of their sexual relations either, but only one activity out of many. They spend more time on mutual grooming than they do on specifically sexual contact, as Jane Goodall and many other primate researchers have described in great detail. They also masturbate and have homosexual relations quite commonly. Among the animals for whom these activities have been recorded are the rat, chinchilla, rabbit, porcupine, squirrel, ferret, horse, cow, elephant, dog, baboon, monkey, chimpanzee, and many others.[5]

Although our culture seems to assume that, since sexual feelings are provided by nature to ensure reproduction, intercourse is or should be the basic form of our sexuality, it is patently obvious that other forms of sexuality are just as natural and basic as intercourse. Women's sexual feelings are often strongest when women are not fertile, and masturbation is perhaps more basic than intercourse, since chimpanzees brought up in isolation (according to Goodall and others) have no idea of how to have intercourse but do masturbate almost from birth.

### C. THE FREUDIAN MODEL OF FEMALE SEXUALITY

The third and final basic reason why women have been expected to orgasm during intercourse is the general acceptance of the Freudian model of female sexuality, the model of female psychology based on it, and in general the acceptance of the concept of "mental health."

Freud was the founding father of the vaginal orgasm. He theorized that the clitoral orgasm (orgasm caused by clitoral stimulation) was adolescent and that upon puberty, when women began having intercourse with men, women should transfer the center of orgasm to the vagina. The vagina, it was assumed, was able to produce a parallel, but more mature, orgasm than the clitoris. Presumably this vaginally produced orgasm would occur, however, only when the woman had mastered important major conflicts and achieved a "well-integrated," "feminine" identity. The woman who could reach orgasm only through clitoral stimulation was said to be "immature" and not to have resolved fundamental "conflicts" about sexual impulses. Of course, once he had laid down this definition of our sexuality, Freud not so strangely discovered a tremendous "problem" of "frigidity" in women.

These theories of Freud's were based on faulty biology. Freud himself did mention that perhaps his biological knowledge was faulty and would turn out, on further study, to be incorrect—and indeed, it has been demolished for some sixty years.

Undoubtedly Freud would have accepted this research by now, but the profession he originated has been unwilling or slow to do so. All too many psychoanalysts and various "authorities" writing in popular women's magazines continue to insist that we should orgasm through intercourse, via thrusting, with no hands, and still see "vaginal primacy" as a crucial criterion of "normal" functioning in women. (The current "g-spot" myth propagates the misconception.) They continue to regard orgasm produced by intercourse as the only "authentic" female sexual response, and climax caused by any other form of stimulation (like "clitorism," as they call it) as a symptom of neurotic conflict.

Freud's theory of female sexuality has also been refuted on psychological grounds. Not only, in Freudian psychology, must a woman orgasm by the movement of the penis in the vagina, but if she doesn't, she is "immature" and psychologically flawed. Her difficulty is supposedly a reflection of her overall maladaptive character structure. She is seen as being significantly disturbed and lacking in "ego integration." It is said that she is struggling with unconscious conflicts that make her anxious and unstable; and her lack of orgasm is only one facet of this general unhappiness.

No major studies in the field of psychology have detected these correlations between personality structure and ability to orgasm during intercourse. If anything, as Seymour Fisher has shown in *Understanding the Female Orgasm*, there is almost an opposite correlation:

> There seems to be good reason for concluding that the more a woman prefers vaginal stimulation, the greater is her level of anxiety. The strongly vaginally oriented woman is tense and has a low threshold for feeling disturbed. This was demonstrated not only in her overt behavior but also her fantasies. As reported, the relatively high anxiety of the vaginally oriented woman was detected by multiple observers who got to know her while she was in the psychology laboratory. It was also revealed in her self-ratings. . . . Obviously, the facts, as they have emerged in the present studies, blatantly contradict existing theories. If these facts receive support from other investigators, a gross revision of such theories will be required.[6]

Despite these demonstrations of the fallacies of Freudian theory about women, "treatment" of women along Freudian lines is still being widely performed, with the large majority of psychiatrists having complete faith in this version of female sexuality and female psychology! Even with all the advances in biological knowledge that make Freud's biology obsolete, and even with the findings of Masters and Johnson, Fisher, and many others, psychoanalytic theory has not changed. As Sherfey, herself a psychiatrist, asks, "The question must be put and answered within the profession. . . . Could many of the sexual neuroses which seem to be almost endemic to women today be, in part, induced by doctors attempting to treat them?"

Probably millions of women could agree with one woman who wrote, "It would give me a great deal of personal pleasure to give Freud a black eye."

## REDEFINING SEXUALITY (CAN WE REDEFINE SEX?)

To try to limit physical relations between humans to intercourse is artificial. But perhaps it was also necessary to channel all forms of physical contact into heterosexual intercourse to increase the rate of population growth. A high rate of reproduction is the key to power and wealth for a small group, and in the early Jewish tribes barrenness was a curse. In fact, children have been the basic form of wealth in almost every society up to the present. From the point of view of the larger society, increase in numbers provides the ability to consolidate more territory and to defeat other tribes. On a personal level, children could inherit one's property and also consolidate the family's holdings, and they could till the fields, hunt, gather food, or tend flocks (and later, work in factories) for their parents.

The desire for maximum population growth was institutionalized in our culture, and out of this grew the definition of women as basically serving this ideal. The glorification of marriage, motherhood, and intercourse is part of a very strong pronatalist bias in our culture, which is discussed in detail in the book *Pronatalism: The Myth of Mom and Apple Pie*, edited by Ellen Peck and Judy Senderowitz.

In summary, since intercourse has been defined as the basic form of sexuality and the only natural, healthy, and moral form of physical contact, it has automatically been assumed that this is when women should orgasm. Heterosexual intercourse has been the definition of sexual expression ever since the beginning of patriarchy and is the only form of sexual pleasure really condoned in our society. The corollary of this institutionalization of heterosexual intercourse is the vilification and suppression of all other forms of sexuality and pleasurable intimate contact—which explains the historic horror of our culture for masturbation and lesbianism/homosexuality, or even kissing and intimate physical contact or caressing between friends.

## "IF YOU DON'T HAVE ORGASMS DURING INTERCOURSE, YOU'RE HUNG UP"

The influence of these psychiatric theories on women has been strong and pervasive. Whether or not a woman has been in analysis, she has heard these unfounded and antiwoman theories endlessly repeated—from women's magazines, popular psychologists, and men during sex. Everyone—of all classes, backgrounds, and ages—"knows" a woman should orgasm during intercourse, and that if she doesn't, she has only herself and her own hangups to blame. As one woman wrote:

*I see my failure to have orgasms during intercourse as my failure largely, i.e., I've had plenty of men who were 1) adept, 2) lasted a long time, 3) were eager for my orgasm to occur, and 4) etc. but none of them were successful. I guess I have a fear of childbearing, a fear of responsibility—I don't know.*

There was a lot of psychiatric jargon in the women's answers. The women may have been in therapy, but it's just as easy to pick up these terms from numerous articles by therapists and others in the women's magazines, and also from male "experts" with whom you may have sex.

The idea that if we would "just relax and let go" during intercourse we would automatically have an orgasm is, of course, based on the fallacious idea that orgasm comes to us automatically by the thrusting penis, and all we have to do is give ourselves over to what our bodies will naturally and automatically do—that is, orgasm. As one woman put it, "It's our fault that we can't be as natural as they are."

I wish we could have back all the time and energy we have spent blaming ourselves and searching our souls about why we didn't have orgasms during intercourse. And all the money we spent "flocking to the psychiatrists" looking for the hidden and terrible repression that kept us from our "vaginal destiny." I would like to have what we would have built with that energy.

## RETHINKING FEMALE SEXUALITY

Insisting that women should have orgasms during intercourse, from intercourse, is to force women to adapt their bodies to inadequate stimulation, and the difficulty of doing this and the frequent failure that is built into the attempt breeds recurring feelings of insecurity and anger. As Anne Koedt[7] put it, in the famous pamphlet *The Myth of the Vaginal Orgasm*:

> Perhaps one of the most infuriating and damaging results of this whole charade has been that women who were perfectly healthy sexually were taught that they were not. So in addition to being sexually deprived, these women were told to blame themselves when they deserved no blame. Looking for a cure to a problem that has none can lead a woman on an endless path of self-hatred and insecurity. For she is told by her analyst that not even in her one role allowed in a male society—the role of a woman— is she successful. She is put on the defensive, with phony data as evidence that she better try to be even more feminine, think more feminine, and reject her envy of men. That is: Shuffle even harder, baby.[8]

Finally, there are two myths about female sexuality that should be specifically cleared up here.

First, supposedly women are less interested in sex and orgasms than men and are more interested in "feelings," are less apt to initiate sex, and generally have to be "talked into it." But the reason for this, when it is true, is obvious: women often don't expect to, can't be sure to, have orgasms:

*I suspect that my tendency to lose interest in sex is related to my having suppressed the desire for orgasms, when it became clear it wasn't that easy and would "ruin" the whole thing for him.*

The other myth involves the mystique of female orgasm, and specifically the idea that women take longer to orgasm than men, mainly because we are more "psychologically delicate" than men and our orgasm is more dependent on feelings. In fact, women do not take longer to orgasm than men. The majority of the women in Kinsey's study masturbated to orgasm within four minutes, similar to the women in this study. It is, obviously, only during inadequate or secondary, insufficient stimulation like intercourse that we take "longer" and need prolonged "foreplay."

### THE MYTH OF WOMEN'S "ABNORMAL GENITALS"

*I really believe my clitoris may not be physically positioned quite right because I almost never can find a position for stimulating it while his penis is in my vagina.*

The truth is that clitoral and labial anatomy are highly variable in size, shape, placement, texture, and other factors.* However, that does not mean that our anatomy is wrong or deformed. It is the cultural pressure on women to orgasm during intercourse that is wrong, along with the stereotyped way in which we define sex.

It is doubtful whether anatomy is an important factor of orgasm during intercourse. Masters and Johnson found no evidence to support the belief that differences in clitoral anatomy can influence sexual response. However, Barbara Seaman, who wrote *Free and Female*, cautions that "this must be viewed as a highly tentative finding since they were unable to observe any clitorises during orgasm." Sherfey also feels that more research should be done in this area. Masters and Johnson have noted that they think certain vaginal conditions can operate to prevent the thrusting penis from exercising traction on the labia and clitoral hood. But it's all animal crackers in the end. The real thing to keep in mind is that it is more unusual than not to orgasm from intercourse, especially without making some kind of special effort to do so by getting additional clitoral stimulation at the same time.

---

* Women of every age fear that their genitals are not "normal"—that is, lips too big, lips too long, clitoris not close enough to the vagina, color variable, and so on. Betty Dodson has documented the various forms, shapes, and textures of the female vulva in much of her work, available on videotape and in her books.

## MASTERS AND JOHNSON ON COITUS

Before describing the methods women in this study used to orgasm during intercourse, it remains to mention how Masters and Johnson have explained the way in which orgasm during intercourse supposedly occurs.

Stressing that all women's orgasms are caused by stimulation of the clitoris, whether direct or indirect, they have sought to explain that orgasm during intercourse comes from the indirect clitoral stimulation caused by thrusting: as the penis moves back and forth, it pulls the labia minora—which are attached to the skin covering the clitoris (the hood)—back and forth with it, so indirectly moving the skin around over the clitoral glands. In Masters and Johnson's own words:

> A mechanical traction develops on both sides of the clitoral hood of the minor labia subsequent to penile distension of the vaginal outlet. With active penile thrusting, the clitoral body is pulled downward toward the pudendum by traction exerted on the wings of the clitoral hood. . . .
>
> When the penile shaft is in the withdrawal phase of active coital stroking, traction on the clitoral hood is somewhat relieved and the body and glans return to the normal pudendal-overhang positioning . . . the rhythmic movement of the clitoral body in conjunction with active penile stroking produces significant indirect or secondary clitoral stimulation.
>
> It should be emphasized that this same type of secondary clitoral stimulation occurs in every coital position when there is a full penetration of the vaginal barrel by the erect penis.[9]

In other words, the clitoris is surrounded by skin known as the "clitoral hood" that is connected, in turn, to the labia minora. Supposedly, during intercourse the thrusting penis (notice the assumption of female passivity) exerts rhythmic mechanical traction on the swollen labia minora, and so provides stimulation for the clitoris via movements of the clitoral hood. Sherfey has termed this the "preputial-glandar mechanism," wherein "the thrusting movement of the penis in the vagina pulls on the labia minora which, via their extension around the clitoris (the clitoral hood or prepuce) is then pulled back and forth over the erect clitoris." That is, the final stimulation is provided to the clitoris by friction against its own hood.

The development of this theory was an advance in that it no longer claimed that friction against the walls of the vagina had anything to do with stimulating female orgasm. However, the existence of this model, and its publicity, has left women with the impression that orgasm during intercourse is still to be expected as part of the automatic "normal" course of things, at least by Masters and Johnson's followers.

But Masters and Johnson selected for study only women who were able to have orgasms during intercourse. It would seem that to analyze what is probably an unusual group of women, and then to generalize from these women, is a mistake. Indeed, the underlying assumption is that orgasm during intercourse is somehow "normal" and not "dysfunctional." (Masters and Johnson have labeled the "inability" to orgasm during intercourse "coital orgasmic inadequacy"; "primary sexual dysfunction" is never having an orgasm in any way.)

Besides the fallacy of generalizing from a special population about just that very thing which makes them special, there is a second problem with this model. There can only be traction between the penis and vagina when the woman is already at a certain stage of arousal, because only then do the labia swell up enough to cause traction (the stage Masters and Johnson call late plateau arousal). So the penis can only pull the labia back and forth if the woman is at the last stage of arousal before orgasm, such that there is sufficient engorgement of the area to cause a tight fit between penis and vaginal opening. (You can check how well this mechanism works for you, by the way, by placing a dildo or similarly sized inanimate object in your vagina when you reach this state of arousal, and then moving it in and out and seeing what you feel.)

Masters and Johnson have not explained how they arrived at the conclusion that this mechanism is the means of orgasm during intercourse. It does seem clear that this "mechanism," if it exists, is indeed the means by which most women orgasm during clitoral stimulation, in that during clitoral stimulation the skin of the clitoral area, or the upper lips, is pulled around or moved around slightly, thus causing the skin to move back and forth over the clitoral glans. As Sherfey puts it: "Mons area friction will have exactly the same effect on the prepuce-glans action as the penile thrusting motion: the prepuce is rhythmically pulled back and forth over the glans."

It seems that penile thrusting activates this mechanism for very few women. Most researchers and sex therapists agree that thrusting is less efficient in causing female orgasm than clitoral area stimulation. Pulling your ear slightly back and forth can also pull the skin on your cheek. Just so, it is possible for thrusting to pull the skin near your clitoris in just the right way to stimulate you to orgasm, and it may happen regularly for a small percentage of women—but not for most women most of the time.

This brings to mind the fact that Masters and Johnson have insisted on treating women, but not men, with their usual sexual partners, whom they must bring with them. (Men were allowed surrogates.) This is usually understood to imply adherence to a moral double standard, but the reason for this rule may in fact have been that, for a woman to orgasm during intercourse, she must adapt her body to inadequate stimulation, and so it is essential that she work out this procedure with a regular partner.

Later, in lectures and private therapy, Masters and Johnson emphasized the specific techniques women can use to orgasm during intercourse, such as being on top of the man or doing most of the moving, as found in this study. Perhaps they, too, have found that the "preputial-glandar mechanism" does not work for most women. However, if this is the case, the message has not reached the general public. The woman-in-the-street (most of us) still has the impression that in their view it is "normal" to orgasm from male thrusting.

There is nothing wrong with saying that the movement of the clitoral hood over the clitoris is what is responsible for orgasm; this is true. What is wrong is to say that thrusting in itself will activate this mechanism in most women. As Alix Shulman has pointedly remarked, Masters and Johnson observe that the clitoris is automatically "stimulated" in intercourse, since the hood covering the clitoris is pulled over the clitoris with each thrust of the penis in the vagina—much, I suppose, as a penis can be automatically "stimulated" by a man's underwear when he takes a step.

But let's apply this same logic to men. As Dr. Sanford Copley put it, when interviewed on the television show *Woman*, this indirect stimulation of women could be compared to the stimulation that would be produced in a man by the rubbing of the scrotal skin (balls), perhaps pulling it back and forth, and so causing the skin of the upper tip of the penis to move, or quiver, and in this way achieving "stimulation." Would it work? Admittedly, this form of stimulation would probably require a good deal more foreplay for the man to have an orgasm! You would have to be patient and "understand" if it did not lead to orgasm "every time."

Masters and Johnson's theory that the thrusting penis pulls the woman's labia, which in turn pull the clitoral hood, thereby causing friction of the clitoral glans, and thereby causing orgasm, sounds more like a Rube Goldberg scheme than a reliable way to orgasm.

It is not that the mechanism doesn't work. It does: if you pull any skin around the area, it can stimulate the clitoris. But the question is, does thrusting do this effectively? For most women, without some special effort or some special set of circumstances, it does not. If this mechanism works so well, why hasn't it been working all along, for centuries? Why is "coital frigidity" the well-known "problem" that it is? And why don't women masturbate this way sometimes? No, having an orgasm during intercourse is an adaptation of our bodies. Intercourse was never meant to stimulate women to orgasm.

### A NEW THEORY OF HOW WOMEN ORGASM DURING INTERCOURSE

Orgasms during intercourse in this study usually seemed to result from a conscious attempt by the woman to obtain some kind of clitoral-area contact for herself during intercourse, often with the man's pubic area. Clitoral stimulation during intercourse could be thought of, then, as basically stimulating yourself while intercourse is in progress. Of course the other person must cooperate. This is essentially the way men get stimulation during intercourse: they rub their penises against our vaginal walls so that the same area they stimulate during masturbation is being stimulated during intercourse. In other words, you have to get the stimulation centered where it feels good.

There are two ways a woman can increase her chances, always remembering that she is adapting her body to less-than-adequate stimulation. First and most important, she must consciously try to apply her masturbation techniques to intercourse or experiment to find out what else may work for her to get clitoral stimulation; or she can work out a sexual relationship with a particular man who can meet her individual needs.

## DO IT YOURSELF

There is an old myth that masturbation causes "clitoral fixation" and "frigidity."

> *Perhaps if you masturbate, you can get a fixation on your clitoris and are thus unable to come during intercourse.*

> *The fact that I've been masturbating since I was ten has made it more difficult for me to orgasm vaginally.*

> *Having been used to masturbating for years as a teenager and repressing my desire for actual intercourse with boys, I feel I developed a conditioned reflex that did not allow me to have a vaginal orgasm with my husband even though I enjoyed the act itself.*

The truth, however, is just the opposite: masturbation increases your ability to orgasm in general, and also your ability to orgasm during intercourse. Why not? It's the same stimulation. Only 19 percent of the women in this study who did not masturbate orgasmed regularly from intercourse—quite a drop from the 30 percent in the overall population. Of course, masturbating to orgasm does not automatically enable you to orgasm during intercourse. There is no mystical connection between the two, just the practical experience with orgasm, how it feels and how to get it.

Finally, was there a correlation between type of masturbation and "ability" to orgasm during intercourse? Were some orgasm types more likely to orgasm during intercourse than others? My impression was that these figures are imprecise because too many women were not counted, including those who did not specify how they had orgasmed during intercourse, those who masturbated in more than one way, and the "questionable-orgasm-definition" group. This left a very small number from which to make correlations.

However, despite all these problems, two definable trends did appear. Most likely to orgasm during intercourse were those who masturbated on their stomachs, especially those who did not use their hands. Least likely were those who held their legs together or crossed.

Still, many women from the first group were not able to orgasm during intercourse. A lot seemed to depend on how interested the individual was in applying her own knowledge of her body to intercourse and actively, unabashedly directing the stimulation to herself.

Of course the question remains whether these body types are made or born. That is, once you learn to orgasm a certain way, does that become a fixed pattern? For example, if you learned with your legs together, could you later learn with them apart? Or are some types of bodies able to orgasm only in certain positions?

This question is, however, important only academically. Women who masturbate with their legs together, for example, can just as well adapt this position to intercourse as other masturbation types. No one type is "better" than another. While a woman who needs to have her legs together to orgasm may have slightly more trouble teaching new lovers ways to have intercourse in which she can orgasm, it is also true that women who hold their legs together are more likely to manage many sequential orgasms, since they do not stimulate their clitorises so directly (the bunched-up skin forms a protective cushion). Whatever type a woman is, she can have fully as much pleasure as every other woman. All she has to do is be active and explore.

## WHY "ORGASM" SHOULD BE A VERB

What is the difference between "to orgasm" and "to have an orgasm"? This idea that we really make our own orgasms, even during intercourse, is in direct contradiction to what we have been taught. Most of us were taught that "you should relax and enjoy it"—or at most help him out with the thrusting—because he would "give" you the orgasm.

It should be mentioned that many of the women who answered in this way were not having orgasms regularly in intercourse. As we saw in the preceding section, orgasm is most likely to come when the woman takes over responsibility for and control of her own stimulation. You always, in essence, create your own orgasm.

> *I create my own orgasm. Sometimes no amount of stimulation will turn me on, because I don't want it. I really resent men who boast of "giving" a woman a good come. I always feel I have created it myself, even if he was doing the stimulating.*

> *My orgasm is my own. I control it, produce it, and dig it.*

> *Although I think mutual pleasure is wonderful, the orgasm is in the end one's own. You have to put in the concentration and physical effort yourself.*

We do give ourselves orgasm, even, in a sense, when someone else is providing us with stimulation, since we must make sure it is on target, by moving or offering suggestions and by tensing our bodies and getting into whatever position(s) we need, and then there is a final step necessary in most cases: we need to focus on the sensation and concentrate, actively desire, and work toward the orgasm.

In conclusion, the two reasons women don't orgasm during intercourse are: they are given false information that the penis thrusting in the vagina will cause orgasm; and they are intimidated about exploring and touching their bodies—they are told that masturbation is bad and that they should not behave "aggressively" during sex with men.

This emphasis on getting your own stimulation does not in any way imply a lack of feeling for the man. One's gratification need not preclude the other's. The female orgasm has been very importantly the focus of this discussion because it is symbolic for women; the ability to orgasm when we want, to be in charge of our stimulation, represents owning our own bodies, being strong, free, and autonomous beings.

## MASTURBATION: THEORY AND PRACTICE

Masturbation is one of the most important subjects discussed in *The Hite Report on Female Sexuality* and a cause for celebration, because it is such an easy source of orgasms for most women. Women in this study said that they could masturbate and orgasm with ease in just a few minutes. Of the 82 percent of women who reported that they masturbated, 95 percent could orgasm easily and regularly, whenever they wanted. Many women used the term "masturbation" synonymously with orgasm: women assumed that masturbation included orgasm.

The ease with which women orgasm during masturbation certainly contradicts the general stereotypes about female sexuality: that women are slow to become aroused and are able to orgasm only irregularly. The truth seems to be that female sexuality is thriving—but, unfortunately, underground.

Masturbation is an important key to understanding female sexuality. Since it is almost always done alone, and since in most cases no one is taught how to do it, masturbation provides almost pure biological feedback. Although some women did not masturbate until after they had had sex with another person, most women discovered it on their own, very early:

> I've never needed anyone to tell me where I have to be touched to have
> an orgasm; I've just been masturbating ever since I can remember.

As Betty Dodson has written in *Liberating Masturbation*,* "Masturbation is our primary sex life. It is the sexual base. Everything we do beyond that is simply how we choose to socialize our sex life." In addition, primates also masturbate more or less instinctively from childhood on.

---

* A pamphlet that later became a book.

Surprisingly, most sexuality researchers have not shown much interest in masturbation. Generally they focus on intercourse since, it is argued, the "sex drive" is fundamentally for purposes of reproduction. However, taking intercourse as the starting point has led to widespread misunderstanding of female sexuality. To assume that intercourse is the basic expression of female sexuality, during which women should orgasm, and then to analyze women's "responses" to intercourse is to look at the issue backwards. What should be done is to look at what women are actually experiencing, what they enjoy, and when they orgasm—and then draw conclusions. In other words, researchers must stop telling women what they should feel sexually and start asking them what they do feel sexually. This is what these questionnaires have attempted to do.

The fact that women can orgasm easily and pleasurably whenever they want (many women several times in a row) shows beyond a doubt that women know how to enjoy their bodies; no one needs to tell them how. It is not female sexuality that has a problem (or "dysfunction"), but society that has a problem in its definition of sex. Sharing our hidden sexuality by telling how we masturbate is a first step toward bringing our sexuality out into the world and a move toward redefining sex and physical relations as we know them.

Masturbation seems to have so much to recommend it—easy and intense orgasms, an unending source of pleasure—but, unfortunately, we are all suffering to some degree from a culture that rules people should not masturbate. This deeply ingrained prejudice is reflected in a quote from a woman who was in other ways very aware of the culture's influences on her:

> *A problem is definitions and usage of words. Probably one of the most offensive statements I've seen in this regard in a long, long time is your question, "Do most men masturbate you?" To some extent, my difficulty with that is that I give a negative connotation to masturbation when compared with intercourse; that is, I would rather have intercourse than masturbation. I take masturbation to mean what I do to myself, alone. Intercourse is what I do with another person, regardless of what takes place. To call vaginal stimulation of the penis intercourse, and to call manual stimulation of the clitoris masturbation, insults me and makes me angry.*

Actually the term "masturbate" had been used (misused actually, to mean someone giving someone else manual clitoral stimulation) in the questionnaire with the express purpose of gauging the reaction to this usage. The meaning was perfectly understood by the overwhelming majority of women, but the implication was hated: sex with a partner legitimizes the activity, whatever it is, and to call it masturbation demeans it.

We as a society have arrived at a point in our thinking where it has become acceptable for women to enjoy sex as long as we are fulfilling our roles as women—that is, giving pleasure to men, participating in mutual activities. Perhaps in the future we will be able to feel that we have the right to enjoy masturbation, too—to touch, explore, and enjoy our own bodies in any way we desire, not only when we are alone but also when we are with another person. "The importance of masturbation," as one woman put it, "is really to love and care for yourself totally, as a natural way of relating to your own body. It is a normal activity that would logically be a part of any woman's life."

## LEG POSITION FOR ORGASM

An interesting and important, but as yet unanswered, puzzle about female orgasm is why some women need to have their legs apart for orgasm while others must have them together; still others prefer to have them bent at the knees or up in the air. Just as different women need different kinds of stimulation for orgasm, they need different leg positions to orgasm.

Unfortunately, many women did not answer this final part of the masturbation question, probably due to the length of the question, and because they assumed their leg position was the same as everyone else's. However, most of the women who did answer usually had their legs apart. Still, a significant number of women in all the masturbation types[10] did hold their legs together.

Reasons women gave for keeping their legs together included the following.

> I like my legs together because then everything (the whole genital area) is tighter and the vibrations travel better.

> If I have my legs apart, I feel almost nothing, no matter what I do!

> Legs together intensifies orgasm—to have everything as tight and tense as possible is best, like a drum.

On the other hand, some women could feel nothing with their legs together. Some women who liked their legs apart also liked their knees bent:

> My legs are apart, either with my knees bent while my feet are flat on the bed, or with my knees at right angles and my feet together. I can masturbate sitting also, and standing, but I prefer lying down in this position.

Some women moved their legs together for orgasm as the feeling intensified, after having them apart during stimulation (and a very small number did the opposite). Most women had only one basic leg position that worked best for them, but a few women found leg position interchangeable:

*I hold my legs together or apart depending on the type of fantasy I am using.*

*My muscles usually tense up, and then right before orgasm my hips start moving back and forth. My legs are the tensest of all, usually bent at the knees, one up and one sideways when I'm by myself. With a partner, there are other considerations that determine what I do with my legs— sometimes they stiffen out straight.*

The reason for the difference in leg positions for different women is still a mystery. Does it depend on how the woman first learned how to orgasm? Or does the anatomy of our genitals (both interior and exterior) vary just enough from woman to woman to make different positions necessary for different individuals? More research in this area is needed.

## THE MEANING OF CLITORAL STIMULATION: ORGASM AND THE SOCIAL CONSTRUCTION OF SEXUALITY

QUESTION:
How have most men had sex with you?

The following answers represent the overwhelming majority. "Foreplay" is followed by "penetration" and "intercourse" (thrusting) followed by orgasm (especially male orgasm), which is the "end" of sex. Answers not falling into this category, not including the lesbian replies, composed less than 5 percent of those in the study.

*In bed with the man above me, in the dark.*

*I've only had sex with my husband. (We were just married for a few months.) He always initiates it. We kiss and he plays with my breasts. He puts one hand down and sticks his finger into my vagina and moves it back and forth like a penis would go. When he's doing this, I lie on my back, and he lies on his side so his body is pressed against my side. He moves his hips back and forth so that his penis rubs against the side of my leg. When he's ready, he has me get on my hands and knees, and he gets in back of me. He sticks his penis into me and moves it back and forth until he finishes.*

*Most of the men I've slept with have had absolutely no idea of what I want or need and no interest in finding out. There have been several men who seemed to care whether I was happy, but they wanted to make me happy according to their conception of what ought to do it (fucking harder or longer or whatever) and acted as if it was damned impertinent of me to suggest that my responses weren't programmed exactly like those of mythical women in the classics of porn. All I can say is, after years of sexual experience that ranged from brutal to trivial to misguided, etc., it's a wonder I didn't just blow off the whole thing a long time ago. I'm glad I stuck with it until I found a partner whose eroticism complements mine so beautifully.*

## ORGASM FROM CLITORAL STIMULATION BY HAND

### DO MOST WOMEN ORGASM REGULARLY FROM CLITORAL STIMULATION BY HAND?

In the reproductive pattern of sex just described, which is far and away the most prevalent in our culture, are women having orgasms during "foreplay" with clitoral stimulation? Those who orgasm regularly (those who answered "yes," always or usually) during clitoral stimulation by hand during sex with a partner represented approximately 44 percent of the total. Although nowhere near the overwhelming majority of women who orgasmed regularly with masturbation, this is a much larger number than those who orgasmed during intercourse (30 percent). But why don't women orgasm as easily during clitoral stimulation with others as they do with themselves?

The first reason is that, more often than not, a partner's clitoral stimulation is not intended to lead to orgasm. The reproductive model of sex has traditionally included just enough clitoral stimulation in "foreplay" for purposes of arousal but not for orgasm—which is perhaps worse than no clitoral stimulation at all, a kind of "cock teasing" in reverse.

### WOMEN'S FEELINGS ABOUT CLITORAL STIMULATION TO ORGASM

QUESTION:
Do you feel guilty about taking time for yourself in sexual play which may not be specifically stimulating to your partner? Which activities are you including in your answer?

Many women interpreted this question to mean, did they feel guilty about needing "foreplay"—rather than interpreting "taking time for yourself" to mean to have an orgasm. This response only underscores the picture already presented, that clitoral stimulation is commonly used for purposes of arousal but not for orgasm. Many women felt guilty for "needing" this kind of "extra" stimulation. As one woman put it, "Women are made to feel sexy women don't require it."

*Yes, I definitely feel guilty about taking time for myself in activities such as clitoral stimulation, erotic massage, and cunnilingus simply because these activities are not specifically stimulating to my partner. I feel selfish, I imagine that my partner is either impatient to "get on with it" or is not enjoying himself very much, or feels uncomfortable because he doesn't quite know what he's doing (which he usually doesn't because he does it so seldom and doesn't ask for any feedback from me, and I'm so reluctant to volunteer it); in other words I can't relax very well when things are being done to me, only, and I don't come very easily as a result.*

*Men think they are really being hip and up front in the vanguard if they do it without your asking. Out of all the information popularized about female sexuality since the "sexual revolution," the idea of clitoral stimulation has really made the heaviest impact. But I still feel my partner is doing something that for him is a mere technical obstacle to deal with before going on to the "main event."*

Remember how beautiful and enthusiastic the language was that was used to describe intercourse and general arousal? But notice how spare and tight, unenthusiastic and secretive the language has become here. Obviously women do not feel proud about clitoral stimulation in any form. Our culture had discouraged clitoral stimulation, even to the point of not giving it a name. "Cunnilingus" at least is a name, even if its meaning is not clear to everyone, but "manual clitoral stimulation" is just a phrase that is used to describe an activity that has no name. Our language, as well as our respect, for clitoral stimulation is almost nonexistent. Our culture is still a long way from understanding, not to mention celebrating, female sexuality.

QUESTION:
Do you ever find it necessary to masturbate to achieve orgasm after "making love"?

The vast majority of women responding to this question wrote that "usually" or "sometimes" they did reach orgasm after "sex" by masturbating. Surely we can create a better, more egalitarian form of sex than this.

Why has clitoral stimulation been left out of the standard pattern of sex?
During "sex" as our society defines it both the man and the woman know what to expect and how to make it possible for the man to orgasm. The whole thing is prearranged, preagreed. But there are not really any patterns or prearrangements for a woman to orgasm—unless she can manage to do so during intercourse. So women are put in the position of asking for something "special," some "extra" stimulation,

or they must somehow try subliminally to send messages to a partner who often is not even aware that he should be listening. If she does get this "extra," "special" stimulation, she feels grateful that he was so unusually "sensitive." So all too often women just do without—or fake it.

But we can change this pattern, and redefine our sexual relations. We can take control over our own orgasms. We know how to have orgasms in masturbation. How strange it is, when you think about it, that we don't use this knowledge during so much of the sex we have with men. Why, in our pattern of sexual relations, does the man have charge of both his stimulation and ours? A man controls his own orgasm in the sense that during intercourse he thrusts his penis against the walls of the vagina in ways that provide the best stimulation for him; this is not considered "selfish" or "infantile" because there is an ideology to back it up.

However, women do not usually, are not supposed to, control their own stimulation:

> I have never tried to stimulate myself clitorally with a partner—I have always been afraid to.

> It seems too aggressive when I act to get the stimulation I want.

> During sex, I must depend on a man's willingness to do an aggressive action for me, while I am passive. (Passive about my own stimulation; moving for his pleasure doesn't count.) Whereas during intercourse a man climaxes through his own aggressiveness.

> I always dreamed of the ecstasy of physical love. I have never been able to reach this kind of feeling with another person. The sensations, the orgasms I can give myself, are more than just in the sex organs, they are feelings of relaxation and pleasure throughout the body, mind, and soul. A sort of sailing feeling, a flowing, rich in colors, rich in well-being, joy. They are "multiple orgasms," each richer than the previous one. A whole, complete feeling. I can have orgasms with a partner, but not these complete intense sensations.

But why can't we touch ourselves? Why can't we do whatever we need to make orgasm happen? Although sharing sex with a man can be wonderful, why does "sharing" for a woman mean that the man must "give" her the orgasm? Why can't a woman use her own hand to bring herself to orgasm? In sex as elsewhere, women are still in the position of waiting for men to "mete out the goodies."

We have the power to make our own orgasms, if we want. You can get control of your own stimulation by moving against the other person, or by stimulating yourself directly in the same way as you do during masturbation. Although this suggestion may sound strange at first, it is important to be able to masturbate with another person, because it will give you power over your own orgasms. There is no reason why making your own orgasms should not be as beautiful or as deeply shared as any other form of sex with another person—perhaps even more so. The taboo against touching yourself teaches essentially that you should not use your own body for your own pleasure, that your body is not your own to enjoy. But we have a right to our own bodies. Controlling your own stimulation symbolizes owning your own body and is a very important step toward freedom.

## CLITORAL ANATOMY

Even after the well-known work of Masters and Johnson has conclusively proved that all orgasms in women are caused by clitoral stimulation (whether direct or indirect), there is still enormous confusion over the terms "clitoral orgasm" and "vaginal orgasm." Why does this confusion continue? There are several reasons: the first is that we lack complete understanding of our anatomy, mainly because most of our sexual organs, unlike those of men, are located inside our bodies. The following description of our sexual anatomy will try to give a fundamental picture of the basic underlying structures.

Mary Jane Sherfey's book *The Nature and Evolution of Female Sexuality* is, although technical, the best and most complete explanation available of our anatomy and worth the time a thorough reading requires. As Edward Brecher paraphrases her main points, in *The Sex Researchers*:

> The truth is . . . that the glans and shaft of the human clitoris are merely the superficially visible or palpable manifestations of an underlying clitoral system which is at least as large, as impressive, and as functionally responsive as the penis—and which responds as a unit to sexual stimulation in much the same way that the penis does.
>
> The penis, for example, has two roots known as crura which play an essential role in its functioning. During sexual excitation these crura become engorged with blood and contribute to erection of the penis. The clitoris, too, has two broad roots, of approximately the same size as in the male. The clitoral crura, too, become engorged with blood early in the woman's sexual excitation.[11]

Again, the penis contains within its shaft two caverns or spaces known as corpora cavernosa, which fill with blood during sexual excitation and contribute to the expanded size of the erect penis. The female clitoral system has a precisely analogous pair of bulbous corpora cavernosa, which similarly fill with blood during sexual excitation. They are not inside the shaft of the clitoris, however. Rather, they are located surrounding the vestibule and outer third of the vagina. The vestibular bulbs and the circumvaginal plexus (a network of nerves, veins, and arteries) constitute the major erectile bodies in women. These underlying structures are homologous to, and about the same size as, the penis of a man. They become engorged in the same way that a penis does. When fully engorged, the clitoral system as a whole is roughly thirty times as large as the external clitoral glans and shaft—what we commonly know as the "clitoris."

Our sex organs, though internal and not as easily visible as men's, expand during arousal to approximately the same volume as an erect penis. The next time you are aroused, notice how swollen your vulva and labia majora become; this change reflects the swelling of the vestibular bulbs and other tissues that lie just below this area.

In short, the only real difference between men's and women's erections is that men's are on the outside of their bodies while women's are on the inside. Think of your clitoris as just the tip of your "penis," the rest of which lies underneath the surface of your vulva—or think of a penis as just the externalization of a woman's interior bulbs and clitoral network. (They are therefore known as the vestibular bulbs.) The spongelike body (corpus spongiosum) inside the penis is paralleled by a similar spongelike structure in the clitoral system, which functions in the same way.

The penis, Sherfey continues, is associated with sets of muscles that help to erect it during sexual excitation. The clitoris is associated with precisely analogous sets of muscles that serve to erect it, too—though, as Masters and Johnson have shown, at a somewhat later stage in the sex act. Other male muscles contract during orgasm, forcing the ejaculation of semen. Precisely homologous muscles function during the female orgasm, causing a rhythmic contraction of the outer third of the vagina. Indeed, as Masters and Johnson have also shown, the male and female sets of muscles respond in the same rhythm—one contraction every four-fifths of a second.

There are also differences, Sherfey concedes, between the penis and the clitoral system—but the differences, astonishing as it may seem to readers brought up in a male-dominated society, are in favor of the clitoral system. That system, for example, includes at least three (and possibly four or five) networks of veins called venous plexi, which extend diffusely throughout the female pelvic area—but especially through the regions immediately to the left and right of the vagina. These networks are also, Sherfey reports, a part of the clitoral system; in addition, they merge with the venous networks of the vaginal system. Together the clitoral and vaginal networks become engorged with blood during female sexual excitation.[*]

---

[*] Ruth Herschberger has made some pointed comments about terminology in the essay "Society Writes Biology" in Adam's Rib: "The patriarchal biologist employs erection in regard to male organs and congestion for female. Erection of tissue is equivalent to the filling of the local blood vessels, or congestion; but erection is too aggressive-sounding for women. Congestion, being associated with the rushing of blood to areas that have been infected or injured, appears to scientists to be a more adequate characterization of female response."

Thus the clitoris itself is merely the visible portion of a vast anatomical array of sexually responsive female tissue. The total blood-vessel engorgement of the clitoral system during sexual excitation may actually exceed the more obvious engorgement of the male.

As Barbara Seaman has explained in *Free and Female*, our sexual structures expand as much or more during arousal as men's; the only difference is that male erection (engorgement) takes place outside the body and is therefore more visible, while ours takes place underneath the surface, under the vaginal lips. The total size of our engorgement is no smaller than the size of an erect penis.

Helen Kaplan, in *The New Sex Therapy*, explains a further anatomical cause of the continuing confusion between "clitoral" and "vaginal" orgasm:

> Apparently, it is this dichotomy—on the one hand, the location of orgasmic spasms in and around the vagina and concomitant perception of orgasmic sensation in the general vaginal and deep pelvic region; on the other hand, the location of the primary area of stimulation in the clitoris—which has served to perpetuate the myth that the female is capable of two distinct types of orgasms, and has also given rise to the incredibly stupid controversy surrounding female orgasm. The orgasm is, after all, a reflex and as such has a sensory and a motor component. There is little argument over the fact that the motor expression of this reflex is "vaginal."
>
> The entire argument really only revolves around the location of the sensory arm of the reflex. Is orgasm normally triggered by stimulating the vagina with the penis? Or is it produced by tactile friction applied to the clitoris? The clinical evidence reviewed clearly points to the clitoris.[12]

In other words, clitoral stimulation precipitates female orgasm, which takes place deeper in the body, around the vagina and other structures, just as stimulation of the tip of the male penis evokes male orgasm, which takes place at a lower level, adjacent to the interior base of the penis and testicles.

Despite the seeming contradictions, both of these groups of women seem to be describing the same thing. While one group terms clitoral orgasm "more intense and focused," the other group calls it more "localized" and therefore more "limited." While some women found orgasm during intercourse "more diffused" and more "whole-body," and therefore not as exciting as the locally intense clitoral orgasm, other women found the "whole-body" feeling during intercourse more fulfilling than the "locally intense" and "limited" clitoral orgasm.

Which way you interpret these feelings is a question of your own individual situation, your relationship with a partner or yourself, and of course the cultural pressures to find intercourse more fulfilling. Whichever way you interpret the physical feelings, however, there is no argument that the sensations differ: a clitorally stimulated orgasm without intercourse feels more locally intense, while an orgasm with intercourse feels more diffused.*

Thus it can be concluded that the presence of a penis seems to diffuse and generalize the sensation of orgasm. This is not to say that orgasm without intercourse is "better" or to make any other value judgment, since only individuals can make those. The sole purpose here is to define the actual physical feelings as most women experience them.

The fact is that clitorally stimulated, nonintercourse orgasms—especially in masturbation—are physically stronger than orgasms during intercourse. Masters and Johnson have also reported not only that contraction patterns were stronger in masturbation orgasms than in intercourse orgasms, but also that their study subjects gave the same subjective opinions. As a matter of fact, the highest cardiac rates of all the orgasms they studied occurred during female masturbation.

Is the feeling of orgasm weaker during intercourse because of the presence of the penis or because of other factors?

There may, for some women, be an increased intensity in orgasm during masturbation because alone they are not self-conscious. But other women felt just the opposite; intercourse is more acceptable than masturbation, and therefore one can "let go" more. Perhaps orgasm during masturbation is stronger because you can get the stimulation more perfectly centered and coordinated, including your leg position.

> For me, the intensity seems to depend on 1) not rushing the orgasm but trying to hold on as long as possible, when the peak excited stage has been reached. The longer I hold on (I can't wait longer than about one minute at that stage) the more intense the orgasm. The second factor is 2) letting go at just the right moment. This leads to very intense orgasms. If I let go too soon, or a little too late, I have a less intense orgasm.

### THE PLEASURES OF INTERCOURSE: "VAGINAL ACHE" AND EMOTIONAL ORGASM

Orgasms during intercourse may feel stronger psychologically because of very real feelings for the man or because we are culturally conditioned to feel that intercourse is the highest expression of our sexuality.

Orgasms during intercourse may feel more whole-body because there is usually a longer buildup period than during masturbation. However, none of the factors just

---

* These findings are quite similar to Seymour Fisher's in his study of 300 women. Fisher wrote: "Scanning the comments the women offered, I was struck by how often clitoral stimulation is described with words like 'warm,' 'ticklish,' 'electrical,' and 'sharp,' whereas vaginal stimulation is more often referred to as 'throbbing,' 'deep,' 'soothing,' and 'comfortable.'"

mentioned changes the basic conclusion that the physical intensity of orgasm is greater for most women when intercourse is not in progress, and especially during self-stimulation.

Despite this finding, a majority of women stated flatly that, no matter what the difference in feeling might be, they would always prefer orgasm during intercourse because of the psychological factor of sharing with and being loved by another person, the warmth of touching all over, body to body.

*Love of another is what makes intercourse orgasm better, in its way, and self-manipulation is more intense in its way.*

*Orgasm during intercourse is less intense, but more emotionally satisfying.*

*With penetration I feel more whole and loved.*

*I feel the contractions less during intercourse, but I enjoy the feeling of fullness, and psychologically, being seen as complete.*

There is an important question that has been saved until last: the phenomenon of "vaginal ache," which is often perceived as the desire for vaginal penetration. It is part of the question just discussed—that is, the difference between orgasm with intercourse and without. This feeling of intense desire, or "ache" (desire to be filled), comes during the buildup to orgasm, very near the moment of orgasm itself, and then spills over into the orgasmic contractions.

What happens is this: sometimes building up to and just at the moment of orgasm there is an intense pleasure/pain feeling deep inside the vagina, something like a desire to be entered or touched inside, or just an exquisite sensation of pleasure, or "vaginal ache." It is an almost hollow feeling, and is caused because the upper end, the deeper portion of the vagina, is ballooning out, expanding into what has been thought of as a little reservoir for the semen.

Some women perceive this feeling as hollow, empty, and unpleasant, while others find it intensely pleasurable. For most women, the pleasant sensation of "vaginal ache" is not felt so intensely with a penis present; the penis seems to "soothe" and diffuse the feeling. Others prefer not to diffuse what is for them a feeling of pleasure.

Without intercourse the sensation of "vaginal ache" was described like this:

*I feel an urgent yearning way deep inside to envelop and take him inside me.*

*During arousal, there is a craving in my vagina—which is, by the way, disappointed if satisfied.*

*Sometimes while masturbating, I'll feel the urge to push something up me—usually always I am disappointed with the result.*

*After cunnilingus, just at the moment she reaches orgasm, she likes me to place my tongue in her vagina, as it seems to soothe the ache.*

*Just at the moment when I orgasm, there is a beautiful, painful feeling in the vagina.*

## CONCLUSION: WHICH FEELS BETTER, ORGASM DURING COITUS OR WITHOUT COITUS?

We have seen in this section that with the presence of a penis, the orgasm and contractions are felt less concretely and that the "vaginal ache" (which is an exquisitely pleasurable feeling—not pain) is either soothed or not felt during intercourse. In general, then, vaginal penetration or the presence of a penis seems to have a soothing, diffusing, or blanketing effect.

There are two ways of interpreting this phenomenon. You could say either:

1. During intercourse the penis works as a pacifier—the touching and rubbing kills feeling, allows less intense contractions and sensations, and disperses and diffuses the focus of orgasm, making it less intense and less pleasurable.

2. During intercourse the penis, by soothing or quieting arousal, gives more of a feeling of peace and completeness, relaxation and satisfaction, than nonintercourse orgasm, which in many cases only leaves you a second later with continued arousal. Thus, intercourse (actually, with or without orgasm) is more "fulfilling" than orgasm without intercourse.

Whichever you prefer on any given occasion is personal and a matter of temperament—whether you define pleasure as desire or its satisfaction. Is the greater pleasure desire (arousal), or its fulfilment?

You could prefer either sensation at different times:

*I cannot describe the difference, it is neither better nor worse, just different. Sometimes I want penetration, and other times I am happier engaging in other activities. It depends on my mood.*

### EMOTIONAL ORGASM

Some women who mentioned that they have a different type of orgasm during clitoral stimulation or masturbation than during intercourse meant that they have "real" orgasms during clitoral stimulation and something else during intercourse— what has often been called "vaginal orgasm." By this they did not mean they felt vaginal contractions, or intense clitoral or vaginal sensations, but that they felt an intense emotional peak (sometimes an extreme opening sensation both in the vagina and the throat) accompanied by strong feelings of closeness, yearning, or exaltation. We will call this "emotional orgasm":

*Clitoral orgasm gives me a full-blown climax. During intercourse, none of the flash sensations occur, but there is a tremendous calm and loving feeling that makes me cry—kind of like having an emotional (rather than physical) orgasm.*

*It's difficult not to use clichés I've heard or read, but some of them are so accurate. It is a full, warm sensation in the vagina lips, and surrounding pubic area, that spreads out, plus a feeling of tremendous exhilaration in my chest. If the man is an important part of my life, I find myself wishing his penis could reach clear up to my neck, that he would just crawl inside of me. He can't seem to get deep enough or close enough.*

*First all feeling seems centered in the genital area and it spreads through my entire body in great waves of sensation and sensitivity. Sometimes I feel as though I want to sing, as though the sensation has traveled to my vocal cords and has set them vibrating in a key yet to be discovered.*

*This kind of orgasm for me is metaphysical immersion in another world, religious, ascending a mountain. It happens mostly in my mind, which is flushed with sensation, and sends me very close emotionally to the person I am with.*

*Orgasm: a compelling sensation of light. My vision dissolves into brilliance behind my eyes, blinding me; my body dissolves into pure light. I see nothing but light, hear nothing at all, feel nothing that can be named— but every blood cell is dancing and every pore outpouring radiance— and the spiders in the closets and the ants on the floor must be full of joy at receiving the overflow of love.*

Emotional orgasm is a feeling of love and communion with another human being that reaches a peak, a great welling-up of intensity of feeling, which may be felt physically in the chest, or as a lump in the throat, or as a general opening-up sensation, a feeling of wanting deeper and deeper penetration, wanting to merge and become one person. It could be described as a complete release of emotions, what one woman called "a piercing feeling of love," or an orgasm of the heart.

## THE SUPPRESSION OF FEMALE SEXUALITY AND ORGASM

We have seen that the basic value of sex and intercourse for women is closeness and affection. Women liked sex more for the feelings involved than for the purely physical sensations of intercourse. As most women's answers reflected, the emotional warmth shared at this time, and the feeling of being wanted and needed—not the plain physical act—are the chief pleasures of sex and intercourse.

Sex in our society is an extremely important way of being close, almost the only way we can be really physically or even spiritually intimate with another human being. And sex is one of the few times that we tangibly feel that we are being loved and can demonstrate our love for another person. And yet, in another, as yet unborn society, it would not be necessary to define "sex" in such a closed and rigid way. It would not be necessary for women to accept an oppressive situation in order to get closeness and affection.

It is not that women don't want or don't like intercourse. What makes them sexual slaves is the fact that they have few or no alternative choices for their own satisfaction.

> *I have wanted to have orgasms with a man for years—about twelve. Seems like the impossible dream. I can be a loving eunuch with him, but only a full sexual person by myself.*

Why does this woman say this? Why, if she can be "a full sexual person" by herself, can she be only "a loving eunuch" with a man? This woman's comment points to a dilemma that has become clearer and clearer. We have seen that heterosexual sex usually involves a pattern of foreplay, penetration, and intercourse, ending with male ejaculation—and that all too often the woman does not orgasm. But women know very well how to orgasm during masturbation, whenever they want. If they know how to have orgasms whenever they want, why don't they feel free to use this knowledge during sex with men?

The fact is that the role of women in sex, as in every other aspect of life, has been to serve the needs of others—men and children. And just as women did not recognize their oppression in a general sense until recently, so sexual slavery has been an almost unconscious way of life for most women, based on what was said to be an eternally unchanging biological impulse. We have seen, however, that our model of sex and physical relations is culturally (not biologically) defined, and can be redefined—or remain undefined. We need not continue to have only one model of physical relations—foreplay, penetration, intercourse, and male ejaculation.

Women are sexual slaves insofar as they are afraid to "come out" with their own sexuality and are forced to satisfy others' needs and ignore their own. As one woman put it, "sex can be political in the sense that it can involve a power structure where the woman is unwilling or unable to get what she really needs for her fullest amount of pleasure, but the man is getting what he wants, and the woman, like an unquestioning and unsuspecting lackey, is gratefully supplying it." The truth is that almost everything in our society pushes women toward defining their sexuality only as intercourse with men, and toward not defining themselves as full persons in sex with men. Lack of sexual satisfaction is another sign of the oppression of women.

This, of course, is not to say that women don't like sex, or that they don't enjoy intercourse in many ways. When asked if they enjoyed sex, almost all women replied yes, they did. Furthermore, there was no correlation with orgasm; women who did not orgasm with their partners were just as likely to say they enjoyed sex as women who did. However, the important question is, "What is it that women enjoy about sex/intercourse, and what do women mean when they say they like it?"

To repeat: If women know how to have orgasms, why don't they use this knowledge during sex with men? Why don't they break out of the pattern? There is no reason why using this knowledge and taking the initiative in new directions would diminish the warmth and closeness of sex. Or is there?

## A. HABIT

It could be said that we think of "sex" as we do—as foreplay, "penetration," and intercourse, culminating in male ejaculation—because we are taught that this is what sex is, that this is what you are "supposed" to do. Our idea of sexual relations is structured around reproductive activity, which is defined as "instinctual." Although sexual feelings are instinctual, intercourse is not strictly so. One of our society's myths is that it is "nature" or our "instincts" that make us have "sex" as we do. Actually, most of the time we do it the way we do because we have learned to do it that way. Even chimpanzees and other animals must learn to have intercourse.[13] Sex and all physical relations are something we create; they are cultural forms, not biological forms. However, we do not think of ourselves as free to explore and discover the varied physical relations that we might want or that might seem natural to our individual feelings and needs. Instead, we tend to act as if there were one set formula for having intimate physical contact with other people (who "must" be of the opposite sex).

From this point of view, the answers women gave when asked if they like "sex" can be seen as socially constructed: If intercourse is instinctive, and if the way we have sex is nature itself, how can anyone (who is not "neurotic") claim they don't like it? Or how can anyone state they would like to change it? Sex is sex, either you like it or you don't. However, as we have seen, the more specific questions did bring out all kinds of satisfactions and dissatisfactions with sex as we know it.

There is great pressure on women to say they like "sex." As one woman put it, "With the current spotlight on sex, the knowledge that I have a good sex life protects me from damaging doubts about myself every time I read an article about sex." Women must "do it right" and especially they must enjoy it. Any woman who admits she does not like sex is labeled "neurotic," "hung up," "weird," or "sick" by the psychiatric profession and others. Women, for all kinds of reasons, must like "sex." This means, essentially, that women must like heterosexual intercourse.

In fact, to even hint at questioning the glory and importance of intercourse is like questioning the American flag or apple pie. One cannot even discuss feelings about intercourse, whether one likes it, and so on, without arousing a strong emotional reaction in many people, who feel that one is attacking "men." But this is not true. The strong reaction is merely another indication of how stereotyped our ideas about physical relations are, and how emotionally and politically sensitive a topic sex is.

To reinforce these ideas of what sex is we have all kinds of people—from physicians to clergymen to self-styled sex experts in books and women's magazines to our own male lovers—instructing us in the proper ways of having it. But how can there be a "proper" way of touching another human being? Sex manuals tell us with mechanical precision where to touch, how to touch, when to Orgasm, that it is Bad not to Orgasm, and so on. Especially we learn that, no matter what else, intercourse and male orgasm must take place. Although this subject will be pursued further in a later chapter, it is important to stress here that, although sex manuals can be helpful, only we know what we want at any given time, and we can create sex in whatever image we want. There is no need to follow any one mechanical pattern to be close to another human being.

### B. LOVE AND SEXUAL SLAVERY: CAN LOVE CAUSE "VAGINAL ORGASM"?

Somehow, the truth is more complicated than the simple idea that women are oppressed in bed as elsewhere out of "habit"—"just as women are used to serving men their coffee, so they are used to serving them their orgasms." It is remarkable how easily we bring ourselves to orgasm during masturbation, and how totally we can ignore this knowledge during sex with men. It seems clear that we are often afraid to use our knowledge during sex with men because to do so would be to challenge male authority. Somehow it is all right for a woman to demand equal pay, but to demand equality in sex is not considered valid.

Why are women afraid to challenge men in bed? First, they fear losing men's "love." The question of what love is, of course, is very complicated, but it is clear, as seen throughout this chapter, that the importance of sex for women is inextricably bound up with love:

> *Sex for me is a very private and almost sacred thing. To me sex means the supreme proof of love.*

> *In my own case, I desire happiness, togetherness, love, etc., and I know that if for no apparent reason I kept refusing sex, I would lose some of the happiness in my life, and I might lose the love my man has for me. He*

*would assume that something was wrong and make changes, perhaps excluding me from his life.*

*It's a trade. Like my mother says, men give love for sex, women give sex for love.*

It does seem to many sex researchers and therapists that fear of losing a man's love is holding many women back from having orgasms with men. As Seymour Fisher writes:

> The psychological factors—for example, fear of object loss—which my work suggests may interfere with orgasm attainment in many women may exemplify at another level the general cultural feeling transmitted to woman that her place is uncertain and that she survives only because the male protects her. The apparent importance of fear of object loss in inhibiting orgasm can probably be traced to the fact that the little girl gets innumerable messages which tell her that the female cannot survive alone and is likely to get into serious trouble if she is not supported by a strong and capable male. It does not seem too radical to predict that when women are able to grow up in a culture in which they are less pressured to obedience by threats of potential desertion, the so-called orgasm problem will fade away.[14]

Although Fisher, as a psychologist, tends to see these fears of loss of love as emanating from childhood experiences, it is obvious that they also can stem from adult concerns such as the fear that as you get older the man you love will stop loving you, that he needs you less than you need him, and so forth.

### C. ECONOMICS

Not only may a woman be afraid of losing a man's love if she asserts herself or "challenges" him sexually, she may also be afraid of losing her economic security. All too often economic intimidation is involved. It can take many forms, some subtle, some overt. The most obvious form of economic intimidation is when a woman is totally dependent on the man with whom she has sex for food and shelter, with no economic alternatives, such as being able to get a job herself. We have all seen the connection between affection and economics in a mild form on *I Love Lucy*, where affectionate words and embraces were always a standard part of talking Ricky into a new sofa, a new hat, or a vacation. Some of the women in this study mentioned the connection between sex and economics in their lives, as answers to the following illustrates.

QUESTION:
Do you feel that having sex is in any way political?

> *I'm not sure if it's political, but it's economic. I really felt I was earning my room and board in bed for years, and if I wanted anything, my husband was more likely to give it to me after sex. Now that I am self-supporting, I don't need to play that game any more. What a relief!*

> *I think it is used for "horse trading." I know I have used it that way, and I think most women have been forced to use it that way (for bargaining purposes and to gain economic support) at one time or another, although this is gradually changing as jobs become open to us.*

Anyone who is economically and legally dependent on another person, as women traditionally have been, and in the majority of cases still are, is put in a vulnerable and precarious position when that provider expects or demands sex or affection. Although the woman may genuinely want to please the man, the fact that she does not feel free *not* to please him, and that she puts his satisfaction before her own and keeps secret her knowledge of her own body, reveals the presence of an element of fear and intimidation. If a woman is financially dependent on a man, she is not in a good position to demand equality in bed. Economic dependency, even where love is present, is a subtle and corrosive force.

Women who are not married can be economically intimidated in other, more subtle ways. Even a woman who is only on a "date" with a man can be made to feel that she "owes" him sex:

> *Sex can be political, when the woman is made to feel obligated, for instance, to pay for a date with sex in exchange for anything.*

> *I hate Disneyland dating—the old "I-took-you-here-and-spent-$$$-so-now-you-go-to-bed-with-me."*

As Dr. Pepper Schwartz, of the University of Washington, has pointed out:

> Even when the situation arises that makes them independent of such considerations (personal wealth, a successful career, and a bevy of admirers, etc.) they are so used to having other exigencies define their sexual and marital structure that they do not reevaluate their life style. They believe the myths they have heard about their emotional and sexual needs.[15]

There are also economic pressures on single women to get married—leading to the same financial and legal dependency discussed earlier. As one woman, age twenty-seven, explained her situation: "Even with the jobs I can get—and I'm a good secretary—I still can't afford to pay my rent. I'm forced to move in with a man, or else have roommates. Roommates do not give you any privacy, and living with some guy—first one guy and then, after a year or two, another guy, and so on—is a horrible way to live. You feel like an itinerant worker, moving all your belongings from place to place. It's humiliating. So you have the pressure to get married and settle down and forget it. And—(!!) if you are just living with a man on a supposedly equal share-the-rent basis, guess who still gets to clean house and cook? And be loving and affectionate and always ready for sex? And if, God forbid, you just don't feel like it for a while—out you go! So—you wind up thinking you'd be better off married."

As the feminist group the Redstockings put it in the 1970s, "For many women marriage is one of the few forms of employment that is readily available." To advocate that women "liberate themselves" by giving up marriage reflects a strong class bias, automatically excluding the mass of women who have no other means of support but a husband.*

Of course this is not to say that love (for husband and children) cannot also be involved. Unfortunately, however, economic dependency can eventually corrode and subtly undermine the most beautiful feelings, or even go hand in hand with those feelings, in a kind of love-hate situation. But marriage could become even more a real love contract (either heterosexual or homosexual) if women had more chances for top-notch economic autonomy.

The negative effect of economics on women's freedom, both sexual and otherwise, have been widespread. According to the U.S. Department of Labor, in 1975 women who worked full-time year-round (40 percent of American women) still earned only about 60 percent of the wages of similarly employed men. At the turn of the century the number was 80 percent. When will this gap disappear? Women, despite their education and qualifications, are still largely absent from management and nontraditional professional positions. Federal subsidies of child day-care centers have been cut back, and job layoffs have affected women more frequently, as they traditionally have more peripheral jobs. This means that most women—whether single or married—still find it hard going to achieve financial independence.

In other words, as Ellen DuBois, of the State University of New York at Buffalo, has written me,

---

* Dorothy Tennov, in *Prime Time* (a journal "for the liberation of women in the prime of life"), has looked at it another way: "Those who recognize that wives who remain in marriage for economic reasons are, in fact, selling sexual services may condemn the practice on the basis of the male-serving edict that there is something wrong with selling sexual services. The thing that is wrong with the wife's situation is not that she gets paid for her services—sexual and others—but that she receives so little for what she provides that she remains dependent."

An erroneous and dangerous assumption is that the only thing that stands between a woman and "satisfactory" sex is her realization of her own physical needs. As an oppressed people, what we women lack is not knowledge . . . but power, social power, economic power, physical power. To put it another way, it is not our ignorance that has condemned us to sexual exploitation and dissatisfaction, but our powerlessness.

## WOMEN REBEL AGAINST THE SEXUAL REVOLUTION

*If the Sexual Revolution implies the attitude that now women are "free" too, and they can fuck strangers and fuck over the opposite sex, just the way men can, I think it's revolting. Women don't want to be free to adopt the male model of sexuality; they want to be free to find their own.*

The "sexual revolution" of the 1960s was a response to long-term social changes that affected the structure of the family and women's role in it. (Contrary to popular opinion, the birth-control pill was a technological response to these same social changes rather than their cause.) Up until the second half of the twentieth century, and throughout most periods of history, a high birth rate had been considered of primary importance. In social terms, it was thought that the larger the population, the wealthier the society would be, and the stronger the army. Modern technology, however, has ended the need for huge work forces, and nuclear power and technology are far more significant militarily than massive human armies. Large populations are still valuable principally as consumers.

In terms of the individual, large families are no longer the social or economic asset they once were. Children used to add to the family income by working, and they assured the parents of support and protection in their old age. Male children continued the family name and increased the family's social prestige. Today these assets are considered negligible. Furthermore, children cost a great deal, since their education is prolonged, and after the second or third child a couple's standing in the community diminishes rather than rises. In addition, most men no longer feel that carrying on the family line is a matter of primary importance—although they may very well enjoy having children and being fathers. Marriage (in its original form as a property right) had been created so that the father could be sure of his paternity of the child; now that paternity was no longer so important, the marriage contract could be loosened and women could be "allowed" sexual "freedom."

This change in the woman's role was double-edged. Insofar as having many children had become less important, the status of women declined. That is, since women had traditionally been seen almost completely in terms of their childbearing role, as a class they became less important, and less respected, when that role was no longer so important. At the same time it was said that, now that women were "free" from their old role, they could be "sexually free like men." There was some truth to this idea that new possibilities for female independence had opened up. However, as with the slaves after emancipation, becoming independent was more easily said than done. In fact women did not have equal opportunities for education or employment, and so they were stuck in their traditional role of being dependent on men. In spite of the so-called sexual revolution, women (feeling how peripheral, decorative, and expendable they had become to the overall scheme of things) became more submissive to men than ever. This was even more the case outside of marriage than in, since marriage did offer some forms of protection in traditional terms. This increased submissiveness and insecurity was reflected in the childlike baby-doll fashions of the 1960s—short little-girl dresses, long straight (blond) hair, big innocent (blue) eyes, and of course always looking as young and pretty as possible. The change in men's attitude toward women (from mother to sex object) is summed up in Molly Haskell's title to her book about women in the movies, *From Reverence to Rape*. This situation eventually led to the women's movement of the late 1960s and 1970s, which tried to implement some positive changes to make women truly independent and free.

Insofar as the importance of childbearing has diminished, women are, so to speak, out of a job. This change has come about over a long period of time. As women we can improve our status only by going forward and reintegrating ourselves into the world and perhaps, if we find it necessary, changing that world.

In conclusion, what we think of as "sexual freedom"—giving women the "right" to have sex without marriage and decreasing the emphasis on monogamy—is a function of the decreased importance of childbearing to society and of paternity to men. Although this change has been labeled "sexual freedom," in fact it has not so far allowed much real freedom for women (or men) to explore their own sexuality; it has merely put pressure on them to have more of the same kind of sex. Finally, it is important to remember that you cannot decree women to be "sexually free" when they are not economically free; to do so is to put them into a more vulnerable position than ever and make them into a form of easily available common property.

## PRESSURE ON WOMEN TO HAVE SEX: A CRITIQUE OF THE CONCEPT OF "SEX DRIVE"

*I went to a New Year's party with one guy once and crashed there. I said I didn't want to sleep with him and he said I could have the sofa. I felt I should be more relaxed, and I said no, I'd sleep on the floor too. Then he talked me into a corner: Why was I so afraid of touching? Afraid of sex? We didn't have to ball after all, we could just hug and touch. I felt raped even though we never had intercourse; we had oral sex. He didn't know my cunt from a hole in the wall. If this happened to me now I would have acted totally opposite but this was two years ago and I didn't really know that I could actually say no, and not have to prove that I was a "woman."*

> *Only with my husband. It was a condition of our marriage as it developed, that if I refused him sexually he was insufferable. I think this is a common degradation of women in marriage. But rape is too strong a word, as force was not involved. I felt I was prostituted, being used as a whore, with no regard for my desires. I think it is a barbaric tradition, that men cannot be refused by women in marriage, and this led to my finding my husband sexually repugnant.*

How strong is the male "sex drive"? These quotes graphically illustrate the pressure that is on women to have intercourse, both in and outside of marriage. One of the worst forms of this pressure comes from the idea that a man's "need" for "sex" is a strong and urgent "drive" that, if not satisfied, can lead to terrible consequences. As one woman phrased it, "Men being sexual animals, at least to my way of thinking, their bodies drive them to the culmination of sex, the climax, ejaculation, and depositing of their seed. I feel that most of them could gladly do without foreplay. At times I have felt guilty, especially if waiting for me has robbed my partner of some of the intensity of his climax."

This particular stereotype of male sexuality is commonplace, frequently presented by sex manuals, psychologists, psychiatrists, physicians, men's magazines, and many other sources. Typically, the male "sex drive" is seen as a constantly surfacing and demanding feeling; Theodor Reik has expressed it in *The Psychology of Sex Relations*:

> [T]he crude sex drive is a biological need which represents the instinct and is conditioned by chemical changes within the organism. The urge is dependent on inner secretions and its aim is the relieving of a physical tension.
>
> The crude sex-urge is entirely incapable of being sublimated. If it is strongly excited, it needs, in its urgency, an immediate release. It cannot be deflected from its one aim to different aims, or at most can be as little diverted as the need to urinate or as hunger and thirst. It insists on gratification in its original realms.[16]

This glorification of the male "sex drive" and male orgasm amounts to justifying men in whatever they have to do to get intercourse—even rape—and defines the "normal" male as one who is "hungry" for intercourse. On the other hand, the definition of female sexuality as "passive and receptive" (but, since the sexual revolution, also necessary for a "healthy woman") amounts to telling women to submit to this aggressive male "sex drive." Especially since the 1940s the glorification of male sexuality has often been justified as a kind of natural law of the jungle (the product, we are led to believe, of caveman hormones), even by some of the most serious social scientists. Actually the information available does not warrant such conclusions. This idea of male sexual "right" (via biology) is not much more scientifically based than the old idea that kings were monarchs by the grace of god and natural law. Just as kings insisted that any other political model (like democracy) would be unnatural and would not work, so men say that if women are aggressive sexually (that is, anything but passive), sex will be unnatural, they will become "impotent," and sex for them will be impossible.

What is "sex drive"? Lester A. Kirkendall, in "Towards a Clarification of the Concept of Male Sex Drive," writes:

> As the term "sex drive" is now used, it has become a blanket term which obscures the components with which we are actually dealing. We should distinguish between sexual capacity, sexual performance, and sexual drive ... that is, what you can do, what you do do, and what you *want* to do.[17]

Kirkendall explains that although capacity ("what you can do") has a biological base, sex drive ("what you want to do") "seems to be largely a psychologically conditioned component. Sex drive seems to vary considerably from individual to individual, and from time to time in each individual, and these variations seem related to psychological factors." In other words, sex drive (not capacity) is more a function of desires than "needs."[18]

A further point along this line is that even if a man has a strong physical desire for orgasm—an erection, for example—there is nothing in nature, nothing physical, that impels him to have that orgasm in a vagina. The stimulation he feels is linked to the desire for orgasm and not to any desire for intercourse per se. There is no "beeper" or sensory device on his penis that makes him seek a vagina in which to put his penis. This pleasurable connection is learned, not innate; as mentioned earlier, even chimpanzees must learn to have intercourse, although they masturbate on their own from early childhood.

Finally, there is not even a medical term for the colloquial "blue balls." Contrary to popular opinion, it is no harder on a man not to have an orgasm than on a woman. Men feel no more "pain" than we do. Kinsey gets right to the point:

> There is a popular opinion that the testes are the sources of the semen which the male ejaculates. The testes are supposed to become swollen with accumulated secretions between the times of sexual activity, and periodic ejaculation is supposed to be necessary in order to relieve these pressures. Many males claim that their testes ache if they do not find regular sources of outlet, and throughout the history of erotic literature and in some psychoanalytic literature the satisfactions of orgasm are considered to depend upon the release of pressures in the "glands"—meaning the testes. Most of these opinions are, however, quite unfounded. The prostate, seminal vesides, and Cowper's are the only glands which contribute any quantity

of material to the semen, and they are the only structures which accumulate secretions which could create pressures that would need to be relieved. Although there is some evidence that the testes may secrete a bit of liquid when the male is erotically aroused, the amount of their secretion is too small to create any pressure. The testes may seem to hurt when there is unrelieved erotic arousal (the so-called stoneache* of the vernacular), but the pain probably comes from the muscular tensions in the perineal area, and possibly from the tensions in the sperm ducts, especially at the lower ends (the epididymis) where they are wrapped about the testes. Such aches are usually relieved in orgasm because the muscular tensions are relieved—but not because of the release of any pressures which have accumulated in the testes. Exactly similar pains may develop in the groins of the female when sexual arousal is prolonged for some time before there is any release in orgasm.[19]

If a man's desire for intercourse is not shared by a woman, there is no reason why masturbation or other stimulation will not provide him with an equally strong or stronger orgasm, although the psychological satisfaction may not be the same. Or there is no overriding reason why he must have an orgasm at all. The point is that there is no physical necessity for a man to have intercourse. Women need no longer be intimidated by this argument. As one woman answered, when asked, "Have you ever been afraid to say 'no'?", "No. This is my body, my breasts, and my cunt, and they are my territory and if anyone, even my husband, tries to take what I do not wish to give, it's WAR, baby."

## THE DOUBLE STANDARD

Women who did try to be open and share with men, having sex in the new, free way, in all too many cases wound up being disrespected and often hurt—because the double standard still operated.

> I think the sexual revolution is very male-oriented and anti-woman. The idea is that men are telling women they're free to fuck around with whomever they want. But the catch is that the double standard is still employed. A man who has many lovers is "sowing his oats"; a woman who has many lovers is a "prostitute" or "nymphomaniac."

> Usually after they know they "have" me, I get the feeling I am a piece of ass. I feel their hostility and their contempt. The double standard is alive and well.

---

* "Blue balls."

*Although I live at a college campus which is considered nationwide as a place of avant-garde sexual and intellectual ideas, it is not. Men here still disrespect women who have sex with those they're not "in love with," and if a woman cares about her esteem, it is only safe to have sex with either a male who cares about her so he won't make her feel bad and talk about her to other men so they disrespect her—or else with a person no one finds out about (like flings at ski resorts or vacations, etc.). One male, considered a leading radical here, was talking to a supposed female friend of his the day before Halloween. They were invited to a costume party and she, having trouble deciding what to wear, asked him, "What do you think I should go as?" Very cruelly, he replied, "Why don't you go as a virgin? I'm sure nobody will recognize you!"*

## BE A "GOOD GIRL"!

Almost all the women who answered these questionnaires had been brought up to be "good girls." Girls are still being kept from finding out about, exploring, and discovering, their own sexuality. At puberty girls are given information about their reproductive organs and menstruation, but rarely told about the clitoris!

The sexual-revolution ideology stated that it was old-fashioned to want to connect sex with feelings—it meant you weren't "hip." Not only marriage but also monogamy and love, or even tender feelings, were often considered to be something only "neurotic" women wanted. The idea was that "people should spontaneously have sex and not worry about hurting each other, just behave freely and have sex, no strings, anytime with anybody, just for pure physical pleasure." But few women in this study wanted that kind of sexual relationship.

To be told that we should have a regular "appetite" for intercourse does not coincide with how most women feel: periods of greater interest in sex, for most women, fluctuate according to attraction to the partner and, to a lesser extent, the menstrual cycle. What causes the awakening of intense desire or love for another, specific person is personal and often mysterious, as one woman described:

*Leaving out love and even commitment for the moment, good sex has to be more than anatomy or even "psyching" yourself into it. It has to involve a certain amount of chemistry between two people. After a singularly disastrous experience trying to make a sexual relationship work when there was no attraction (just affection), I don't want to try to add sex to my friendships (unless I feel attraction too). I don't understand it in any way but Chemistry, but there certainly is such a thing as sexual attraction, which can't be forced into existence.*

## THE RIGHT NOT TO HAVE SEX

Finally, since the 1960s sexual revolution and its tenet that sex is no longer "serious" (you don't have to fear pregnancy, and marriage is no longer a requirement), it became "hip" to have a lot of "sex" (intercourse). In fact, we are often told that the sex "drive" must be regularly expressed to maintain "healthy functioning." Many women resent this commercialization and vulgarization of sex—"beds on the sidewalks, pills in the vending machines, and 'hot babes' everywhere to be had":

> We are taught that every little twinge is a big sex urge and we must attend to it or we'll be an old maid. I'm getting sick to death of sexuality—everywhere sex sex sex! So what? Sex is not the end-all and be-all of life. It's very nice but it's not everything!

> I wish there wouldn't be as much of a "hype" about sex as there is now. I hate the media's exploitation of sex and women. I would hope that women wouldn't be looked upon as things to look nice and to have sex with. For the most part, women are judged by their potential sexual worth. I would like sex to become more matter-of-fact, and more personal. In a way, I'd almost like to have back the hush-hush good old days when you just didn't talk about sex. It would not be hidden because it was dirty, but because it was a sweet, private thing.

Unfortunately the idea that sex is necessary for health has become big business. Magazines, books, television ads using sex (or the happy couple) to sell their product, some psychiatrists, counselors, sex clinics, films, and massage parlors—all have a vested interest in the idea. Makers of Viagra and other drugs are certain they are increasing "pleasure." We are constantly being reminded of sex in one way or another and subtly coerced into doing it: "Why aren't you doing it? Everybody else is. Get on the bandwagon! You're missing all the fun if you don't!" (And you're probably neurotic and mentally unhealthy.) Many women commented on this or felt defensive that they did not want to have sex more often:

> I think our culture has made sex over-important. Everyone thinks that everyone else is having a great time fucking all the time and so we all compete against the American myth. Given this, I think that sex in my life has assumed a correct proportion, that is, an expression of love between us; yet, I still feel hung up about the myth sometimes—maybe having sex is less important to me than to others.

> The thing I enjoy most is making love with people I have that "special" feeling for—this is when it's most satisfying totally, even if it never gets

*down to real sex—it's still beautiful just holding them and feeling warmth and love with them.*

Of course not all sexual activity or physical relations are based on this kind of attraction; most women do not feel that their sexuality is purely a mechanical need for "release."

In fact, there is nothing unusual about spending various periods of one's life without sex:

*I am currently celibate. I enjoy it but the society makes it hard to be partnerless sometimes. There are activities I avoid because they will be "couple-y." People often think there's something wrong with you if you're not part of a couple, but being independent is worth it.*

*Periods of celibacy can be useful for re-evaluating your life and rediscovering your sexuality—the fallow period before new things can grow. I did it for five years on and off once. By not having to please anyone else, I was able to get really deeply in touch with myself, and develop my understanding of the world—whereas before, always having boyfriends had kept me so narrowly focused on them that I hadn't had time to think about my relationship to the larger scheme of things. I found that giving up physical sex was a small price to pay.*

However, other women felt cut off and isolated during periods of celibacy, since sex is almost the only activity in which our society allows us to be close to another human being—since all forms of physical contact are channeled into heterosexual intercourse.

*When I go without sex for a while, I begin to crave affection and reaffirmation. I feel closed off from others, and begin to notice an intense need for affection, warmth, and any form of contact with another human being.*

*It doesn't seem to bother me physically, but emotionally I tense up. I miss body contact and find it extremely frustrating. There is a special kind of loneliness in being one in a culture that seems to think in terms of pairs.*

*I miss feeling wanted and needed, and the body warmth when I wake up. I usually start feeling unattractive and undesirable too—mentally depressed, bored, low-energy. I lose my sense of humor.*

Physical contact, "flesh to flesh, warm and tight," is tremendously important, and sex is almost the only way to get it in our culture, after we are grown up. As one woman explained, "If I was deeply depressed, cold, lonely, even with a stranger sex could be regeneration to me. The closeness gives me a sense that I am not alone, and that life is not all rough edges after all. It makes me feel loved and special." Another woman reported that what she liked best about sex was "the feeling of crazy friendliness it gives, sometimes falsely. And the reassurance, however momentary, of being held. The closeness, intimacy, honesty—and after, when you feel alive and happy in a way you never do at any other time."

## WOMEN, POWER, AND THE SEXUAL REVOLUTION

Finally, what was the ultimate significance of the "sexual revolution" of the 1960s?

Although sexuality is very important, it is questionable whether it is important in and of itself, apart from its meaning in life as a whole. The increasing emphasis on sex and personal relations as the basic source of happiness and fulfillment could be a function of the lessening probability of finding even partial fulfillment through work.

Sexuality and sexual relationships can be surrogates (or obscure our need) for a more satisfying relationship with the larger world. But as long as we accept a compartmentalization of public and private life, we are abrogating our moral obligation to take an active part in the direction of the larger world and accepting an ethic of powerlessness. Meanwhile the commercialization and trivialization of sex advances further and further into our private lives and obscures their deeper personal meaning for us. In fact, we haven't had a sexual revolution yet, but we need one.

## THE FUTURE OF INTERCOURSE

It must have been clear throughout *The Hite Report on Female Sexuality* how tired women are of the old mechanical pattern of sexual relations, which revolves around male erection, male penetration, and male orgasm. As one woman said:

> *Cutting an orgasm short doesn't leave me frustrated if I'm masturbating, but I am becoming more and more short-tempered about cutting sex with my husband short just because he is satisfied. Continuing along the same unsatisfying sexual patterns expresses to me a lack of care and concern for me that I am finding unacceptable. It isn't so much cutting an orgasm short and the biological tension that results that hurts—it is an emotional hurt that frustrates me.*

In answers to many different questions women mentioned their frustration and annoyance with this pattern, and many wished for something different.

QUESTION:

What would you like to do more often? How would you like to see the usual "bedroom scene" changed?

Answers like the following came up over and over again:

> *I wish men would be more sensitive rather than acting like a big penis, having an orgasm and that's all. I would say that seventy-five percent of the men I have known knew nothing about a woman except that they had an orgasm and that should be a big treat to me.*

> *I'd like to change the whole kiss-feel-eat-eat me-fuck routine.*

Many women felt that this mechanical approach on the part of most men reflected not only a general lack of feeling for them, but also a lack of development of the man's own sensuality and ability to enjoy his own body:

> *Yes, they enjoy intercourse more, but I think that's conditioning, because men feel that sex play is undignified and revealing. Actually, they can enjoy it as much as we do.*

> *If a man feels that way, I think of him as childish and undeveloped—he doesn't appreciate the subtleties of sex.*

> *Yes, men often don't know how to get into play, or just touching, and get hung up on orgasm. But they can learn.*

### DO WOMEN ALWAYS WANT INTERCOURSE?

Not only were women tired of the old mechanical pattern of "foreplay," penetration, intercourse, and ejaculation, but many also found that always having to have intercourse, knowing you will have intercourse, is mechanical and boring. If you know in advance that intercourse has to be a part of every heterosexual sexual encounter, there is almost no way the old mechanical pattern of sexual relations can be avoided, since intercourse usually leads to male orgasm, which usually signals the end of "sex." (It would be very interesting to explore whether this needs to be so.) If heterosexual relations are to be deinstitutionalized, intercourse must not be a foregone conclusion, or male orgasm during intercourse must not necessarily signal the conclusion of "sex." Women must claim the right not to have intercourse, unless they want it, even when having physical relations with a man. After all, why is it "natural" for a man to expect intercourse to orgasm with or without clitoral stimulation, but treasonable for a woman to expect clitoral stimulation to orgasm without intercourse?

In addition, the kind of change we are talking about here is much deeper than just the idea that "a woman needs an orgasm too."

## "FOREPLAY" AND OTHER PLEASURES

*The term foreplay is a very strange one. What is foreplay? For me to have an orgasm, intercourse must be preceded by foreplay. But I don't like that word because it makes it sound more subordinate than it is.*

Well, it is common knowledge that "foreplay" is all of the body stimulation prior to, before, intercourse. There is no "before-play" to speak of in masturbation for most women. "Be-fore" has been retained here because its meaning is so clear, but in general it is important to emphasize that there is no reason why "be-foreplay" must come before anything.

The question of what else these activities could be called is interesting. The lack of an appropriate word for them in our language reflects the way our culture has narrowly defined sexuality: only activities surrounding intercourse have been considered legitimate. Thus clitoral stimulation and general touching is referred to only as "foreplay," which everyone "knows" precedes intercourse and which everyone also "knows" will end in male ejaculation. In short, all our terms are geared to a linear progression: "foreplay" is to be followed by "penetration" of the penis into the vagina, and then intercourse (thrusting in and out), followed by male orgasm, and then "rest." If one does not accept this pattern as being what "sex" is, one is left with almost no vocabulary to describe what could be alternatives. Of course the possibility does exist for many different patterns of sexuality, and many different kinds of physical contact between people that are sensual/sexual and that do not necessarily have orgasm (or anything else) as their goal.

Would women still want intercourse if they didn't feel obligated to have it? The point is not whether women in general would still want to have intercourse, but that it would become a choice, an option, for each individual woman. Whether she wanted to have intercourse or not would become her own choice, not something she had to do to have physical relations with a man.

Intercourse, as a pleasurable form of physical contact, will always be one of the ways people choose to relate. However, it will not continue to be the only way. It will become deemphasized, one of many alternative possibilities in a whole spectrum of possible physical relations. Heterosexual intercourse is too narrow a definition to remain the only definition of sex for most people most of the time.

Of course, it can only be surmised how much of what we feel during intercourse is real physical pleasure and how much is a product of the glorification of intercourse. Most women, living a new sexuality, would probably still want intercourse sometimes—especially with men for whom they had strong feelings. Some women might like intercourse almost always, while others would almost never want it.

Perhaps it could be said that many women might be rather indifferent to intercourse if it were not for feelings toward a particular man.

Three women had stopped having intercourse but continued sleeping with their partners, for various reasons and with varied results:

*I used to like intercourse but my lovers' insistence on the pattern foreplay/fuck/sleep turned me off to intercourse. I always felt/feel pressured to fuck (are you ready yet?). I started to resent it and now I don't like fucking and I've fucked only once or twice in the past year. I like putting my foot down and trying new ways to get what I want from my lover, but it's created another block, because I've had to stop fucking out of stubbornness and not anything co-operative and mutual, and it seems like communication around this is hard for both of us. However, since I've stopped letting myself be fucked, it's been hard for my lover to ignore my sexual dissatisfaction—which was real easy for him to ignore as long as he was happy. At least now he's started to look for solutions too.*

*With my boyfriend of four years, we pretty much stopped fucking, because it just wasn't worth it for me, and he doesn't want me to do it if I don't like it. What with the problems of contraception and no orgasms, it's a waste. We fucked about twice in the past four months. I feel a little guilty about not fucking my boyfriend, but I know I'm right. He still comes, and I do too, and I don't have to worry about pregnancy. It's good this way. I get mad if we fuck and I don't come (and I never have)—I feel "frigid" and "out of it" when my partner is ecstatic. I feel silly. I feel like a punching bag.*

*I've just come home from vacation all geared up and enthusiastic about being sexually honest, and I ran into a difficulty with my boyfriend. He's been pressing me to go and get a diaphragm, and I have some kind of stigma about it. I thought it over and decided that I didn't want to make an "official" promotion of sexual intercourse by getting something to make it always possible because I really don't like sexual intercourse. I told this to my boyfriend and he felt very highly insulted and made a scene and told me we'd discuss it later. We haven't discussed it yet (two days later) but I have the feeling that in order to continue seeing him there is a prerequisite that I have to have intercourse with him. This is terribly upsetting to me.*

Not only are intercourse and male orgasm not necessary in every heterosexual contact, but in addition the manner in which intercourse is practiced can change to be more mutually satisfying and more varied. It is not necessary for intercourse to be a male-dominated activity. Intercourse can become a varied and personalized practice, done in any way you might create. For example, there are many ways of joining and having intercourse besides male "penetration" and thrusting. Intercourse need not be as gymnastic as we have usually thought, and it is probable that what we think of as the "natural," physical movements of intercourse are nothing more than "learned" responses. Isn't it possible that men have been told that "mounting and thrusting" is the "right" thing to do, but that they too, if allowed to experiment, would find many other ways they liked to have intercourse?

Although the most common position used for intercourse is the man-above-woman ("missionary") position, there is no physical reason why it should be better for men. As a matter of fact, Masters and Johnson have pointed out that if a man is on the bottom he can receive more orgasmic pleasure, since he is not at the same time physically supporting his body. There is, of course, the "behind" position, with advantages for both partners. Furthermore, to call male "mounting and thrusting" natural or instinctive is questionable. Most men masturbate not by thrusting but by moving their hands on their penises. What is natural?

In fact, a few women felt the man-on-top position was more political than natural.

However, once again, the point is not to reverse the situation but to expand our ideas of what physical relations can be; there is no reason to believe that being on the top is always better than being on the bottom for all women.

## DO MEN NEED INTERCOURSE?

Before we automatically react to the previous section with, "Well, what about men? Don't they need intercourse? Won't less intercourse mean less pleasure for men?"— let's reexamine briefly what little we know about male sexuality. There is no basis for saying that men are getting the greatest pleasure they can get from our current model of physical relations, although they are at least having orgasm. Isn't it possible that male sexuality is capable of more, and more in the way of individual variety, than men's sex magazines would have us believe? Are we sure we know what male sexuality is? Books and articles by men have started to appear that question these old stereotypes, and many men—though far too few at present—are beginning to take a fresh look at what they are getting out of their sexual relationships.

Rollo May and Marc Feigen Fasteau, among others, have written that they feel men, by concentrating on achieving orgasm and the satisfaction of desire, are in a way missing the whole point of sexual pleasure—which is to prolong the pleasure and the feeling of desire, to build it higher and higher. Rollo May writes:

> The pleasure in sex is described by Freud and others as the reduction of tension; in eros, on the contrary, we wish not to be released from the excitement but rather to hang onto it, to bask in it, and even to increase [it].[20]

If the importance of female orgasm has been underemphasized, to say the very least, the importance of male orgasm has been greatly overexaggerated. Although orgasm is wonderful, a very large part of the pleasure is building up to the orgasm, as Fasteau wrote:

> What the masculine disdain for feeling makes it hard for men to grasp is that the state of desire . . . is one of the best, perhaps the best, part of the experience of love.[21]

A woman in this study said something similar: "My sexuality has more to do with the desire than with satisfaction. I am not interested in 'satisfaction.' I don't know what it is or why it is considered valuable. I like to be hungry for a person, to desire intimacy and understanding, to be inspired to be loving and to find reciprocation." The real pleasure of sexual relations, in this sense, then, is the prolonging and increasing of desire, not ending it or getting released from it as quickly as possible.

It was recommended in ancient Sanskrit and Hindu literature (and was actually practiced in the New York Oneida Colony in the nineteenth century) that men could achieve the greatest pleasure by the continual maintenance of high levels of arousal and refraining from orgasm for long periods of time.

There is no reason why the reintegration of intercourse into the whole spectrum of physical relations should threaten men. Men too can profit by opening up and reexamining their conception of what sexuality is.

### RESISTING THE MYTH OF MALE "NEED"

Suppose men won't cooperate in redefining intercourse, or in leaving it out sometimes? What if they still try to follow the same old mechanical pattern of sexual relations? There is no reason why women must help men during intercourse. The fact is, we usually cooperate quite extensively during intercourse in order for the man to be able to orgasm. We move along with his rhythm, keep our legs apart and our bodies in positions that make penetration and thrusting possible, and almost never stop intercourse in midstream unless the man has had his orgasm. We do not have to cooperate in these ways with a man if he will not cooperate with us.

Although we do not have to, we are taught that if we are anything but helpful (or at least non-interfering) during intercourse, it is tantamount to castrating the man. This is nonsense. Our noncooperation with men in sex is no worse than their non-cooperation with us—for example, their using clitoral stimulation as a "foreplay" technique and withdrawing the stimulation just before orgasm. It is perfectly all right for us to follow the example of one woman who said, "I feel quite confident about ending sexual activity in midstream if it is not working out, or if I begin to drift or feel disinterested." As another woman advised, "Try to get what you want and do what you feel. (Don't be afraid to act on your most basic, secret, and ultra-secret desires.) If you are not enjoying it in the midst of sex, say so. Ladies, you don't have to do anything you don't feel like doing!"

And another woman: "I spent most of my adult life doing what I 'ought'—and having an awful time. it was only when I broke out of that, fairly recently, that sex began to mean anything to me, or feel like anything. And I got no help from the popular culture, or from psychoanalysis, or indeed from anything except something a friend chanced to say, and the women's movement. I would advise women to look to their own hearts and bodies, and follow them wherever they lead."

## TOUCHING IS SEX TOO

### STEPPING OUTSIDE PATRIARCHAL CULTURE TO SEE HOW SEXUALITY COULD BE DIFFERENT

Besides changing the inevitability and manner of intercourse, what other changes did women emphasize they would like to see in physical relations? One of the most basic changes involves valuing touching and closeness for their own sakes—rather than as prelude to intercourse or orgasm.

> In the best of all possible worlds, sex would be a way of being close, of communing with another person. This would not necessarily mean that we would all have sexual experiences with more people or that I, for example, would be running around bedding down with all our male acquaintances. It might even make it possible for me to have the closeness and affection I need without having it lead, inevitably, to sexual intercourse. Perhaps if we all had more people we related to with physical affection and touching, we'd have a generally more loving atmosphere in which to dwell; we wouldn't necessarily feel that every contact points in the direction of intercourse . . . a warning and yet somehow commanding finger . . . so that you don't feel free to take Step A unless you are willing to take Step B, C, D, etc.

QUESTION:
Does having good sex have anything to do with having orgasms?

Women often said, in answer to this and to many other questions, how much more important body contact and closeness were to them than orgasms in sex with a partner. This response could be accepted purely at face value; however, since women do masturbate for orgasms, it is clear that orgasms are also very important to women. The truth is that both orgasm and close body contact or touching are extremely important to women,* but they have often been forced to seek them separately. The important point to realize in reading the answers below is how important touching and body contact are and how undervalued they have been in our model of physical relations.

*I have intense orgasms during masturbation, but intercourse involves a sort of emotional as well as physical satisfaction being with the man I love. Just from the point of view of having an orgasm, masturbation can be just as satisfying, but the rest of my body isn't always satisfied. I still want the rest of my body to be touched and kissed and to feel a warm man next to me.*

*Closeness with another person is more important to me than orgasm (which I can have by myself, if necessary). If I had to choose between the two, I'd choose touching. I really dig kissing, hugging, fondling, looking at, and feeling the other person.*

*Best are the long tender hours of stimulating each other and relaxing before orgasm, then starting again, talking, petting. It is extremely important to me to have this much body contact, and I also like sensual touch games—wrestling is great, and dancing nude and sexy, and also just "immature cuddling." A previous lover told me I'd taught him lovemaking was seventy-five percent touching and twenty-five percent intercourse.*

*I like to neck on the floor, fully clothed, to music—and play silly games pretending this and that, feeling utterly abandoned!*

*There's something very warm and intimate and very beautiful about lying in the dark with someone, holding them close and talking softly. Frankly, I enjoy it more right now than genital sex, but that could be due to my rather limited experience.*

*Sex itself is not terribly important to me, but physical contact in the form of touching, hugs, embraces, caresses, etc. is most important. I am more interested in having that kind of physical contact than sex.*

*I do feel very strongly that keeping in physical, real physical touch, flesh to flesh, with another, or with other human beings, is absolutely*

---

* Many other answers to this question did reflect a militancy about getting orgasm, not represented in these quotes. For example: "Having fabulously outrageous sex has to do with having orgasms for me. I can have a wonderful sexual experience without orgasm if I am very high emotionally. But sooner or later I feel that I am missing out unless my partner learns to bring me to orgasm."

*necessary to keeping healthy: sane. I know that for me it is. That's why I do feel that "there's more to sex than that," only nobody's found ways (no biological stain, or recording device) yet to see what the effects are of sex, mating, fucking, touching, all that physical stuff—on the people who do it together. I feel that there may be subtle neural and chemical interactions set in motion in each partner's body by direct physical contact with the other partner.*

The overwhelming number of answers received to this question were just like these; desire for more touching and body contact was more or less universal.

Sometimes it has been implied that petting is "immature," something people do only when they aren't able to "go all the way." This is not true. Petting has been a major form of sexuality from time immemorial, but once again, it was condemned in the Judeo-Christian codes unless it was an adjunct to intercourse, and it continues in this status up to the present.

Other mammals also engage in a lot of petting and "making out," as Kinsey pointed out:

> Among most species of mammals there is, in actuality, a great deal of sex play which never leads to coitus. Most mammals, when sexually aroused, crowd together and nuzzle and explore with their noses, mouths, and feet over each other's bodies. They make lip-to-lip contacts and tongue-to-tongue contacts, and use their mouths to manipulate every part of the companion's body, including the genitalia. . . . The student of mammalian mating behavior, interested in observing coitus in his animal stocks, sometimes may have to wait through hours and days of sex play before he has an opportunity to observe actual coitus, if, indeed, the animals do not finally separate without ever attempting a genital union.[22]

There is no reason why we should not create as many different degrees and kinds of sex as we want—whether or not they lead to orgasm, and whether or not they are genital. If the definition of sexual pleasure is sustaining desire and building arousal higher and higher—not ending it—many possibilities for physical pleasure and for exciting another person open up. The truth is that "sex" is bigger than orgasm and involves any kind of deep physical intimacy one shares with another person. Intense physical contact is one of the most satisfying activities possible.

QUESTION:
In the best of all possible worlds, what would sexuality be like?

*Sexuality would become just a simple joy and recognition of one's sexual feelings and from there letting all humans define their sexuality as is most comfortable for them at any given time, in any given situation. "Sexuality" would become an integral part of being, greatly varied and personalized, part of life as a whole.*

*Sex would be more nourishing. Self to self, self to others—lots of warmth and involvement and love and touching on all possible levels as a natural expression of body and emotions. Babies, children, pets, old, young, everyone would be cuddled and fondled, touched and encouraged to do so to and for each other and themselves. There would be public rejoicing in the pleasure of affection and the human body.*

## WHAT KINDS OF TOUCHING DO WOMEN LIKE?

### SLEEPING TOGETHER

*My lover and I are very physical with each other although we don't have sex very often. We sleep naked and intertwined together every night, we shower together and kiss and hug, pat and touch, bite, etc. all the time.*

*I really like touching, sleeping next to, and waking up the next morning with the person still there. Holding them. I have slept with two of my close friends like this, and it was wonderful.*

*Touching is very important. I sleep cuddled up with my best friend and have for six years, although we do not participate in sexual behavior. (That is her decision, not mine.)*

*I love to embrace and touch completely. I love to curl up back to front together in bed. I intensely enjoy sleeping with my little girl, cuddling with her, stroking her back or her mine.*

### PRESSING TOGETHER*

*Lying pressed together is a wonderful feeling—a kind of body-to-body embrace. I like to lie in this position, bodies touching all around, kind of mushing.*

*My favorite: deep kissing and pressing of bodies together full length with*

---

* Why isn't there any word for this, when it is one of the most important physical activities there is? Full-length body-to-body contact, so important to over-all gratification.

*arms holding tight. Opening my whole mouth to the other person and vice versa.*

*I get this kind of swelling feeling in my chest, a feeling like I will burst with emotion and feeling—and a desire to press them to me and myself to them so tightly—*

*I love it when my husband presses me up against him real tight, squeezing me all against him. I like to wrap him up in my body, bury my nose in him, wrestle, kiss, and fuck.*

*Until a few years ago, I experienced desire separate from sexual desire: it was an intolerable burning sensation in my chest rather than in my genitals.*

*What is most stimulating to me is the closeness of the entire other person. If I can feel any separateness or separation of us, it reduces the excitement. Pressure is the single most important arousal element— generalized, dull (i.e., not sharp), rhythmic pressure. This gets me really excited, and my nipples, clitoris, and genital area go crazy for it. If it keeps up like that, I will have an orgasm.*

*Merely lying on top of a desired person will bring me extremely close to orgasm. The only thing required is body movement.*

*I like the total immersion of body and mind—if it were possible for the entire surface of my body to be simultaneously very lightly stroked, slow probing kisses all over, tender yet firm—hugging our bodies together and rubbing.*

*I like to get in bed and hold each other, flesh to flesh, warm and tight.*

*The embrace, which involves the whole body, is important to me. Having my naked body lying against the naked body of my partner—especially my full front touching my partner's full front.*

## TOWARD A NEW THEORY OF FEMALE SEXUALITY

Our definition of sex belongs to a world view that is past—or passing. Sexuality and sexual relations no longer define the important property right they once did; children are no longer central to the power either of the state or the individual. Although all of our social institutions are still totally based on hierarchical and patriarchal forms, patriarchy per se is really dead, as is the sexuality that defined it.

We are currently in a period of transition, although it is unclear as yet to what. The challenge for us now is to devise a more humane society, one that will implement the best of the old values, like kindness and understanding, cooperation, equality, and justice throughout every layer of public and private life—a metamorphosis to a more personal and humanized society.

Specifically in sexual relations—which we should perhaps begin calling simply physical relations—we can again reopen many options. All the kinds of physical intimacy, including simple forms of touching and warm body contact, that were channeled into our one mechanical definition of sex can now be reallowed and rediffused throughout our lives. There need not be a sharp distinction between sexual touching and friendship. Just as women described "arousal" as one of the best parts of sex, and just as they described closeness as the most pleasurable aspect of intercourse, so intense physical intimacy, apart from intercourse, can be one of the most satisfying activities possible.

Although we tend to think of "sex" as one set pattern, one group of activities (in essence, reproductive activity), there is no need to limit ourselves in this way. There is no reason why physical intimacy with men, for example, should always consist of "foreplay" followed by intercourse and male orgasm; and there is no reason why intercourse must always be a part of heterosexual sex. Sex is intimate physical contact for pleasure, to share pleasure with another person (or just alone). You can have sex to orgasm or not to orgasm, genital sex, or just physical intimacy—whatever seems right to you. There is never any reason to think the "goal" must be intercourse and to try to make what you feel fit that context. There is no standard of sexual performance "out there" against which you must measure yourself; you aren't ruled by "hormones" or "biology." You are free to explore and discover your own sexuality, to learn or unlearn anything you want, and to make physical relations with other people, of either sex, anything you like.

## FEMALE EROTICISM: WHAT WAS WOMEN'S SEXUALITY ORIGINALLY LIKE?

What would women's sexuality be like without a society to shape it? Do we know? Women in my research asserted that women have a right to "undefine" sexuality, to redesign it individually; that we have a complete right to say "no" to sex; and that we may not really know yet what "female sexuality" is.

Is sex basically intercourse—or a personal vocabulary of activities? Sex could become a personal vocabulary of activities, chosen to show how we want to express ourselves at a given time, with a specific feeling and meaning: an individual choice of activities, not necessarily "foreplay" followed by "vaginal penetration" (why not call it "penile covering"?) or intercourse, ending with male orgasm.

The Judeo-Christian tradition, for one, has had a very narrow idea of what "sexuality" should be, focusing on reproductive activity. It spells out, in the Bible and in rabbinical and papal encyclicals, how often one should have coitus, with whom, when, and so on—giving the impression that coitus is the central act of "sex," and that it is, furthermore, the central connecting point, the nexus, of the two genders. Interestingly, the Bible does not speak of female orgasm, only male orgasm. Is this because it is only male orgasm that is necessary for pregnancy and reproduction?

## UNDEFINING SEX: AN INDIVIDUAL VOCABULARY

As long as the "male" ideology persists that sees women as either "scores" or mothers, the atmosphere around physical pleasure will not change. We will not be free to discover and feel, and to design new types of sexuality that celebrate the richness of the whole spectrum of what "female sexuality" and "male sexuality" can be all about.

We still haven't undefined sex enough to permit such personal redefinitions of sexuality. Or is it that we haven't changed society enough yet to feel free to do this?

Can women, even now, define sex on their own terms?

If understanding our own bodies well enough to know how we have orgasms and not to be inhibited from telling this to men is a "sexual revolution"—and in fact it is a profound change from the days when, after sex, a woman would go into the bathroom and close the door and masturbate, thinking something was wrong with her—the fact remains, according to women in my latest research, that almost every man with whom a woman has sex continues to expect that sex will center on intercourse/penetration, almost as his automatic "right." Although many more men now understand most women's need for clitoral stimulation to orgasm, most men continue to see intercourse/coitus as the only "real" definition of sex. This is not to say that women don't enjoy that activity, but that the focus on it, the glorification over all others, by the society is as much a matter of ideology as of physical desire. Coitus, without all this propaganda, might not be the primary sex act.

## DO MEN REALLY ENJOY THEIR DEFINITION OF SEXUALITY SO FULLY?

Although it seems obvious, do we know what male sexuality really is? After all, it is impossible for us to know exactly how much of what we see men do is natural and how much is learned or reinforced behavior.

The current definition of "male sexuality" (as a driving desire for "penetration") is clearly a cultural exaggeration. Male sexuality comprises a much larger, more varied group of physical feelings than what we call "male sexuality."

Surprisingly, when looked at more closely, the definition of "sexuality" put forth by the "male" ideology is actually quite negative. This is surprising because it is often thought that men are very prosex, while women are antisex. In fact, women are more prosensuality; most women think in terms of a much broader concept of sexuality than the reproductive model we have come to believe is "natural." The basic "male" ideology refers to sexuality as a "body function," an instinct, an "animal feeling" of pleasure—the opposite of spiritual feeling.

The "male" ideology (and the life cycle it creates) robs men of the chance to enjoy love by warning them against "confusing" a passionate attraction with "love," warning them against real closeness, urging, "You can't trust women," "Don't let your sex drive confuse you," and so on—stating that a "real man" should be "independent," remain "free" and unmarried for as long as possible, watch out for being "tied down." "Real men" should go after/want to have sex with as many women as possible, as often as possible. "Real men" don't fall head over heels in love. The result of all this training of men to control their feelings is that many men become alienated from their deeper feelings.[23]

The reinvention of "male sexuality" was discussed in *The Hite Report on Men and Male Sexuality*, with many men seeming to feel on a gut level that somehow they were missing out—that no matter how much sex they had, they were left feeling unsatisfied on some level. And yet our culture's lessons to men have been so strong that few men have been able to go past them, to create their own personal sexuality, or to transcend the double standard. But a new sexuality and identity is certainly possible for men.

This is by no means to downgrade men's traditional "lust," but to redefine it. Passion is one of the most beautiful parts of all sensuality—the desire to possess, to take, to ravish and be ravished, to penetrate and be penetrated. But is physical love real love? While love is caring, love is also passion and desire, the desire to belong to, to mingle with, be inside of another. Part of love is a sheer physical feeling—a desire not only to have orgasm and "sex," but to lie close while sleeping together, to inhale the breath of the other, to press chests (and souls) together, so tightly, as tightly as possible; to lie feeling the other breathe as they sleep, their breath grazing your cheek and mingling with your own breath; to smell their body, caress their mouth with your tongue as if it were your own mouth, know the smell and taste of their genitals—to feel with your finger inside them, to caress the opening of their buttocks. What is love? Love is talking and understanding and counting on and being counted on, but love is also the deepest intermingling of bodies. In a way, body memory of a loved one is stronger and lasts longer than all the other memories.

## CONTINUING CONTROVERSIES OVER THE NATURE OF FEMALE ORGASM: THE POLITICS OF COITUS

But haven't women made profound changes in their sexuality over the past years? In terms of orgasm, yes. The idea that most women need some form of clitoral or exterior (nonvaginal) stimulation in order to orgasm has now been accepted by women (and by gynecologists and counselors) on a large scale, both in the United States and in many other countries.

As early as the 1950s, questions were raised about whether vaginal intercourse alone leads to orgasm for most women, notably in Albert Ellis's 1953 essay "Is the Vaginal Orgasm a Myth?"[24] Another pioneer was Anne Koedt, whose influential

1970 essay "The Myth of the Vaginal Orgasm" was later published in the anthology *Radical Feminism*.[25] In Germany in 1975 Alice Schwarzer published *Der kleine Unterschied*, also attacking the idea that women should be expected to orgasm from simple vaginal penetration. In 1973 Dr. Leah Schaefer published, as part of an earlier Ph.D. thesis done at Columbia with Margaret Mead and others, in-depth interviews with thirty women about their sexual feelings which demonstrated that it was more "normal" for women not to orgasm from simple coitus than it was "abnormal."[26] In a psychological study published in 1972, Seymour Fisher, although not describing this as "normal," stated that two-thirds of the women in his study stated that they could not orgasm during coitus per se (although they could in other ways), while one-third of them could. Dr. Fisher tried to connect this "ability" to orgasm with whether or not the women had been encouraged to achieve in general by their fathers—since, among all the variables, this was the only correlation he found.[27] Finally, in 1974 Helen Singer Kaplan, in *The New Sex Therapy*, also questioned whether it is correct to label the large number of women who do not orgasm from coitus alone (but do orgasm in other ways) "abnormal."[28]

In 1976 *The Hite Report on Female Sexuality*, based on research extending from 1971 to 1976 and including 3,500 women, found that two-thirds of women do not orgasm from intercourse (matching Fisher's proportion) but orgasm easily in other ways. On the basis of women's statements, the book went on to call into question the definition of "sex" our culture had considered a biological given. *The Hite Report* also documented the many ways women have of reaching orgasm easily during self-stimulation (masturbation), suggesting that these stimulations should be included as part of what we call "sex" and considered as important and exciting as the activities that lead to male orgasms.

## REINTEGRATING SEXUALITY AND SPIRITUALITY: TOWARD A NEW SEXUALITY

In traditional Western philosophy and religion the body has been seen as separate from the mind and soul. In consequence, sex has been seen as "lower" or "lesser." For most women in my research, however, this body/mind split hardly exists; for women the body and spirit are united, and sex is inseparable from emotion. As one woman describes her feelings, "Love is a longed-for feeling of unity, bliss, fulfillment. A strong feeling you feel for someone right from the beginning—a feeling of well-being all over. Sexual passion and the desire for a relationship are indistinguishable." And another:

> *I usually feel the closest after we make love, because it is an expression of all the wonderful and closest feelings I have towards her. When we make love, I feel as though we are a total entity—I can't tell where she leaves off and where I begin. It seems to be a "complete" feeling, capturing my emotions, my intellect, and my physical awareness.*

Thus passion includes not only the body but also the mind and the emotions; a "passionate connection" is not simply a feeling of lust. As one woman puts it, "There are more passionate and less passionate relationships. The passion is involved in every part of knowing the person, not just the sex. And many women, referring to a deeply passionate attraction when speaking of 'falling in love,' also include transcendent or spiritual feelings."

To try to downgrade sexuality to mere lust again presents a problem of language.[29] The phrases we have to work with in English are "lust," "loving," "caring," and "being in love." But are these really the categories women feel? Many women in my research described passion as an intensity of the mind and body felt at the same time.

The evidence from my research of 1978–1986[30] is that the majority of women—although they recognize the distinction—do not feel such a split, in spite of the fact that conventions reinforcing the "male" ideology's separation of sexual and motherly love are all around us, particularly in the Eve/Mary split—the "good" woman and "bad" woman of Judeo-Christian tradition. "Good women" are mothers, asexual (like Mary, who bore a child without having sex), while "bad women" are sexual and pleasure-seeking (those who "eat the apple of carnal knowledge" and "lead men astray").

Such stereotypes pervade popular culture and can cause women and even girls in high school to fight their effects, as boys treat them with disrespect during and after sex. And girls and women themselves may interiorize these images and face a split identity, wondering which "type" they are before they are even old enough to know that they need not choose.

As seen in my study *Women and Love*, the dominant "male" ideology holds that the way men do things is somehow "reality," "the real world," whereas how women do things is a "role." In this way of thinking, if women connect sex and feelings it is because of a "role" they have been taught, a "romanticism" about sex, a form of inhibition and prudery that they should drop, not "reality" or part of "nature." "Natural" sex is what men do. "Natural" sex means seeing no need to connect sex with emotional life. However, most people (men as well as women) probably experience a passionate attraction to someone, falling "in love," as both physical and emotional. Indeed, almost all women in my research hold that early feelings of attraction include both physical and emotional elements, they are not separate.

Actually, in the earliest civilizations, before the "Garden of Eden," sexuality may have been not only an individual behavior but also part of spirituality, and religion, sometimes even part of religious rites; back then reproduction and the feelings leading up to reproduction were seen, rightly, as part of the mystery of rebirth. In other words, some of the meanings of sexuality were probably once religious, related to the worship of reproduction, the sacredness of the re-creation of life.[31] Thus seen, women's resistance to separating sex and feelings may have an entirely different cast to it, as something with roots in the distant past—in a different philosophy. And it may presage a very different future.

## REQUIEM FOR THE G-SPOT, HELLO TO THE C-SPOT!
## (ARE WE REALLY MODERN?)

My research indicates that it is the "c-spot"(as I propose to call it) or clitoris, rather than the "g-spot," that is most important for women.

Yet the "vaginal orgasm" tried to make a comeback under a trendy-sounding new name; in the 1980s the idea was floated in the media that women have an interior "g-spot" inside the vagina, which causes orgasm if stimulated in the proper way—a new version of the old "vaginal orgasm" idea. Thus women should not need "extra clitoral stimulation." How convenient-sounding! Yet has it worked?

If the so-called g-spot were so effective, rather than being just a contemporary apology for the status quo, why haven't more women been having orgasms for centuries during coitus when the spot was contacted? Why don't more women masturbate by insertion, trying to touch themselves "there" inside the vagina, instead of caressing their pubic and clitoral areas, as they do? Clearly women are voting with their actions.

As has been mentioned earlier, the notion of a g-spot has now been debunked by researchers in several countries from Australia to Canada to Italy. However, although there has been much talk in the media of this g-spot, so that people have had ample time to try finding and contacting this "point" to cause orgasm during intercourse, no research shows an increase in the rate of orgasm during intercourse without the use of stimulation of the mons/clitoral area; indeed, various 2004 research continues to show that approximately two-thirds of women "have difficulty" having orgasm with their partners. (This supposed difficulty could be avoided if new thinking about sex and orgasm was allowed to flourish.) Of course, common knowledge for at least a century has been that women have "difficulty" reaching orgasm during simple coitus ("the act"); why would this have been true if an interior spot was capable of causing orgasm in women? If there had been a physiological g-spot, it would have proved effective for female orgasm all along. During 1999–2001, medical and anatomical research in several countries found that no such spot exists.

My research and others'indicates that it is the "c-spot" or clitoris, rather than the "g-spot," that is most important for women. In fact, most women need separate stimulation or massage of this area (external to the vagina) in order to fully orgasm—thus implying that sex should develop a new focus. Why don't more women masturbate by insertion to touch themselves inside the vagina, aiming for this spot, instead of caressing their pubic and clitoral areas as they do?

For many, hasn't looking for a theoretical spot inside the vagina simply been a way of putting off making the changes in sexual relations being called for by women? Isn't insisting that there is a mysterious "spot" inside the vagina only a way of continuing an outworn definition of sex, pushing women, as in the past, to "find their vaginal destiny"?

Again, women are clearly voting with their actions. Women have a right to clitoral or exterior pubic stimulation to orgasm during sex with a partner. This is part of the broader movement for women's rights and part of the changing society around us. This is not to say that the vagina is not highly erotic and sensitive or that, with the right partner, it cannot bring intense satisfaction to a woman: there is something very symbolic about being "penetrated" by another (as men, too, can experience). Women do feel highly charged sexual sensations during coitus, though the stimulation is usually not the kind that leads to orgasm.

The vast majority of women can masturbate easily to one or more orgasms by simply placing their hand or fingers externally on their bodies, caressing the clitoris and mons area of their vulva, sometimes lower down. This type of stimulation can be built into the sexual scenario between two people, as it already is between women who have sex together. Though certainly some men—especially during the last two decades—have learned to appreciate this circumstance, no such type of activity to orgasm has ever been shown in a Hollywood films (films often imply a couple will have or is having intercourse).

The constant glamorization of the vagina (and feelings inside the vagina) as opposed to "the clitoris" means that many people want to believe there is a "g-spot"—probably so that they won't have to change.

For almost every woman, masturbation (the stimulation chosen by women themselves to use in private as the most effective means to orgasm) is clitoral/exterior. Women (not having been taught by society how to masturbate, and thus simply discovering their bodies' feelings and needs, usually as girls) indicate with their choice of stimulation during masturbation how they most easily orgasm. The definition of sex that is now evolving—"normal practice"—should reflect this reality.

If the g-spot were an important reality for most women, at least some women would masturbate by contacting it, or would at least use this internal stimulation (touching or stroking this part of their vagina with their finger or an object) to enhance stimulation during clitoral masturbation. Neither is the case for the overwhelming majority of women.

This does not mean that women do not enjoy or seek intercourse and "vaginal penetration"(or "penile covering"). This is one of the complexities of sexual desire: for many women, coitus or "vaginal penetration" is an extremely pleasurable part of foreplay, bringing them to a high pitch of arousal, though they then want clitoral stimulation to orgasm to follow this "coital foreplay."

The trendy sound of the catch-phrase "g-spot" should not fool people into believing that coitus—a practice that didn't bring women to orgasm for decades—suddenly will do the trick. Women need stimulation of the c-spot all the way to orgasm!

It is the definition of sex that should change, not women's bodies.

## A MISSING NAME

### THE FEMALE ORGASM: HOW DOES IT USUALLY HAPPEN WITH A PARTNER?

The female orgasm usually happens via an activity that has no name.

It is not a tragedy or "sexual inadequacy" if a woman does not orgasm during intercourse, either for the woman or man. Though movies, videos and pornography all imply frequently that a "real woman," a truly sexy woman, just "loves to have it stuck into her" and that this is what brings on those roaring multiple orgasms, this procedure is not the reality most of the time.

Why do such stereotypes and clichés persist, not only in pornography but also in mainstream films? These depictions mislead men, including younger men, who by now should be getting better information, and women are put in the position of having to "explain." The mystification surrounding female orgasm lingers to this day.

Clitoral stimulation is very erotic and exciting when two people share it, and should be a cherished and normal part of sex. Women today want their partners to understand the beauty and functioning of the clitoris. Only one stumbling block remains: there is no name for clitoral stimulation by hand to orgasm! There is a missing name in our sexual vocabulary. How is anyone to speak of this stimulation or ask for it if it doesn't have a name? It is stranger than fiction that the way in which most women actually orgasm *has no name*.

Sex should regularly include "clitoral stimulation" to orgasm. "Sex" doesn't have to be centered around intercourse or "the act." Sex is an individual vocabulary of ways to touch another person, to express a multitude of feelings. Our feelings are much more subtle and interesting than the body vocabularies currently given to us.

Men who are curious about how a woman has an orgasm should ask their partner to help them, show them how she masturbates, or move her hand on top of theirs to touch in the right place and with the best rhythm. Although many men feel quite nervous the first time they try to stimulate a woman in this way to orgasm, in fact most men can learn to do it and enjoy it.

### FEMALE SEXUAL IDENTITY: WHAT IS A WOMAN'S "SEXUAL NATURE"?

If the traditional definition of sex means that there is no equality in sex in terms of orgasm (and the stimulation necessary for orgasm to occur), shouldn't the definition of "sex" change—or is it "just nature," "the way it is"? Should women and men accept this inequality, "live with it"?

No one has ever, it seems, asked this question. Nor has any previous research shown evidence of what a "female sexual nature" could be—nor perhaps could it: since all human beings grow up in society, their "nature" is inevitably culturally influenced.

The assumption that there is a "sexual nature" (in men or women) is simplistic. In reality, all humans have a desire for body contact, to hold the body of another at full length, to kiss with lips and mouth, to feel alive and aroused, to be physically connected. Humans also have a desire for orgasm, evidenced by the fact that almost all human beings masturbate to orgasm (some more than others), without social pressure telling them to do so. People who think that because of the physiology of men and women (the penis protrudes, while the vagina is internal) men are destined to have a "thrusting nature" and women "an accepting nature" are fooling themselves. Yet opposite clichés—"women really have a desire to be as sexually aggressive as men"—are also wrongheaded.

In fact we hardly know what women's "sexual nature" is, since the "modern woman" is now pressured to express her sexuality "like a man": she is urged to be "gutsy, tough, realistic," and so on. (On the other hand, men's "sexual nature" may be much less orgasm-focused than most men have learned.)

Women's natures have simply been assumed to be "like men's." It has been thought that "women are sexual animals underneath it all, animals who crave satisfaction—and the satisfaction they crave is 'penetration' by a penis." My research, however, shows a different picture.

Women often say that they are not getting enough "foreplay" with men. As one explains,

> I loved it before we lived together, because we would kiss for hours and he would put his hands all over me, we would feel each other everywhere for hours. There wasn't such an automatic procedure to sex. All that touching got me really high, I felt beautiful inside and out. By the time we had sex, I really wanted it.

Another woman wrote:

> My favorite activities during sex with my boyfriend are when he takes me in his arms, then after awhile, he lies with his whole body on top of mine—in bed, or on a sofa—and I can feel his whole body against mine. I can feel him breathing, feel his face and his strong shoulders, his legs and his hard cock against me—we embrace together like that until I run out of breath, usually. I find it exciting to feel him covering all of me, especially when he tells me at the same time that he's crazy about me, whispering in my ear and moaning. It's heaven.

Another part of sexual expression or "foreplay" that women find exciting is "exhibitionism": dressing up, displaying the body. Though the word has negative connotations, it is an ancient form of sensuality. People like to watch entertainers like Madonna, fashion models, film stars, and other performers display themselves. Exhibitionism is wrongly believed to be a psychological problem, even a sin allied to narcissism instead of a simple pleasure.

Why is it that many of the most important sensual activities women like to pursue have no names, in most languages? For example, the pleasure most seek sexually in the full-length extension of their body pressing against the full-length body of another person has no name, generally being assumed to be part of the vague category "foreplay."

An activity that has no name is undervalued and difficult to access. The most glaring example of this nameless state is the stimulation most women find necessary for orgasm. Can you imagine a woman having to ask her partner, "Can you please stimulate my clitoris with your hand and don't stop until I have an orgasm?"

For the record, female sexual "nature" is neither specifically heterosexual nor lesbian. Eroticism is a vast area that includes dressing up, playing, talking, making up stories, posing—all ways of inviting someone else to be involved sensually with you. Passion and desire are the objective, feeling one's body come alive with another person. Women want men to rethink their idea of sex, to include much more of this sensuality. Most now think sex with a man should mean forging a new definition of sexuality between them, rethinking the question of who orgasms when and how, the questions of which activities are included, experimenting together.

NOTES

1   MacMillan, 1976; Dell Books, 1977; Pandora/Harper Collins, 1988,; Simon & Schuster, 1996; Hamlyn 2001, as well as a new edition published by Seven Stories Press in 2005.

2   See the Appendix for the Hite Report questionnaire on female sexuality, as well as discussions of how this study was conducted and its new methodology.

3   Books related to this subject include *The First Sex* by Elizabeth Gould Davis, *The Mothers* by Robert Briffauit, *The White Goddess* by Robert Graves, *The Cult of the Mother Goddess* by E. 0. James, *Woman's Evolution* by Evelyn Reed, and *Prehistory and the Beginning of Civilization* by Jacquetta Hawkes and Sir Leonard Woolley.

4   Marval, Nancy, "The Case for Feminist Celibacy," New York: The Feminists, 1971 (pamphlet).

5   Kinsey, Alfred C., et al., *Sexual Behavior in the Human Female* (New York: Pocket Books, 1965), p. 322–24.

6   Fisher, Seymour, *Understanding the Female Orgasm* (New York: Bantam Books, 1973), pp. 113–14.

7   Ti-Grace Atkinson has also written about this in *Amazon Odyssey* (Links Books, 1974).

8   Koedt, Anne, *The Myth of the Vaginal Orgasm* (Boston: New England Free Press, 1970).

9   Masters, William, and Virginia Johnson, *Human Sexual Response* (Boston: Little, Brown and Company, 1966), p. 59.

10   See the masturbation typology in *The Hite Report: A Nationwide Study of Female Sexuality*.

11   Brecher, Edward M., *The Sex Researchers* (New York: Signet Books, 1969), p. 156.

12   Kaplan, Helen Singer, *The New Sex Therapy* (New York: Brunner/Mazel, 1974), p. 29.

13   See Yerkes, Harlow and Harlow, H. C. Bingham.

14   Fisher, Seymour, *Understanding the Female Orgasm* (New York: Bantam Books, 1973), p. 258.

15   Schwartz, Pepper, "Female Sexuality and Monogamy," University of Washington, Department of Sociology; also appearing in *Renovating Marriage: Toward New Sexual Life Styles*, eds. Roger W. Libby and Robert Whitehurst (San Ramon, California; Consensus Publishers, 1973).

16   Reik, Theodor, *Psychology of Sex Relations* (New York: Farrar and Rinehart, Inc., 1945), p. 11.

17   Kirkendall, Lester, "Towards a Clarification of the Concept of Male Sex Drive," Journal of Marriage and Family Living, Vol. 20, 1958, pp. 367–72.

18   For a discussion of possible hormonal influences, see John Money and Anke Ehrhardt's *Man & Woman, Boy & Girl* (Baltimore: Johns Hopkins Press, 1972).

19   Kinsey, et al., *Sexual Behavior in the Human Female* (New York: Pocket Books, 1965), p. 612.

20   May, Rollo, *Love and Will* (New York: Laurel/Dell Publishing, 1974), pp. 71–72.

21   Fasteau, Marc Feigen, *The Male Machine* (New York: McGraw Hill, 1974), p. 31.

22   Kinsey, et al., *Sexual Behavior in the Human Female* (New York: Pocket Books, 1965), p. 229.

23   See material from *The Hite Report on Men and Male Sexuality* in Part Two.

24   Albert Ellis and A.P. Pillay, eds., "Sex, Society, and the Individual," *International Journal of Sexology* (1953), pp. 337–49.

25   Ellen Levine and Anita Rapone, eds., *Radical Feminism* (New York: Quadrangle, 1973).

26   Leah Cahan/Schaefer, *Women and Sex: Sexual Experiences and Reactions of a Group of Thirty Women As Told to a Female Psychotherapist* (New York: Pantheon, 1973).

27   Seymour Fisher, *The Female Orgasm* (New York: Basic Books, 1972).

28   Helen Singer Kaplan, *The New Sex Therapy* (Boston: Little, Brown, 1971).

29   See Alisson Jaggar, *Feminist Politics and Human Nature* (Roman and Allantold, 1983), and unpublished papers presented before the Society of Women in Philosophy.

30   See the third Hite Report, *Women and Love* (Knopf, 1987).

31   See Marija Gimbutas, *Goddesses and Gods of Old Europe* (Los Angeles: University of California Press, 1982). See also Colin Renfrew, ed., (London: Thames and Hudson, 1981).

# Part 2

# Male Sexuality and Love
# Described by Men
## (1981)

*This section contains excerpts of work done during the 1970s and 1980s, much of which was originally published in 1981 as* The Hite Report on Men and Male Sexuality. *With over 7,000 men in the U.S. participating,[1] of all ages (13–97) and backgrounds, it shows the truly diverse nature of men's feelings about sex—as opposed to the clichéd version, which holds that the "real" man is the young man who lusts for vaginal penetration and orgasm. Featuring testimonies ranging from teenage men talking about their earliest orgasms and experiences to those of men in their sixties, seventies, and eighties (who are, for the most part, not in fact desperate to have their sexuality returned to an earlier state, as ads for penis stimulants now imply) talking about how sex has changed for them, this section also contains later essays based on Hite's reflections on this material.*

# Origins of Male
# Psychosexual Identity

Oedipus Revisited:[2] Growing Up Male (The Part Freud Left Out)

Male psychosexual identity is one of the most important bases of the culture. Therefore, how boys are taught to think about "maleness" is one of the most revealing areas we can study; this psychology—often considered to be "based on biology" rather than on cultural precepts—is creating the situation we live with today; examining this mind-set, especially as it is revealed in sex (one of the key definers of "masculinity"), has a lot to tell us.

## SEXUAL VIOLENCE AND BETRAYAL OF THE MOTHER:
## A LIFETIME PROBLEM WITH LOVE

Lurid stories of sexual violence scream at us every day from newspapers, films and videos, TV, magazines, the lives of friends, even our own lives. Statistics suggest high rates of sexual violence toward women. During the more recent wars in Bosnia, Serbia, Rwanda, Sierra Leone, and elsewhere, rape was used as a common tool of war. Sadism toward women is a leitmotif of pornography.

But where does it come from, the male ambivalence toward women, the impulse towards sexual humiliation or violence? In my research for *The Hite Report on Men and Male Sexuality*, most men responded, surprisingly, that they do not marry the women they most passionately love and that they are proud of this fact. They believe that they did the right thing by "choosing rationally," remaining "in control of their feelings" even when they lamented their tragic "lost love." This, the most profound and important finding of that seven-year research study, seems to indicate that many men feel that "true love" is doomed from the start, that it cannot last. Women do not generally share such cynical feelings about love; they believe that problems can be worked out. Why don't men? Where did they learn their point of view?

Through my research on love, sexuality, and childhood I have developed a picture of men's psychosexual identity and its development that differs radically from established theory.

Earlier research tells us that boys reach puberty—that is, experience a sexual "awakening"—between the ages of ten to twelve, when the changes in their bodies make orgasm with ejaculation possible for the first time and when most boys begin a very active masturbatory sex life. What has not been previously noted in psychological theory is that, while sexual feelings are becoming strong for boys, they also go through a moral crisis—a dark night of the soul—regarding their emotional identity, and especially their relationship with their mothers.

Most boys' early sex lives are subliminally yet powerfully associated with feelings for their mothers. They love their mothers; their mother is the woman with whom they are most intimate. They have been kissed by her, have seen her body, felt her arms around them, know her personal habits in the bath, watched her combing her hair—and they know that sex is part of her life or part of the hidden things they cannot know about her life.

"I remember it as a time of secrets," one boy relates. "It seemed a whole and complete second world was opening up around me. My father started explaining about sex, and my mother told me about menstruation, how girls sometimes bled between their legs. I began using pornographic pictures and magazines."

Another remembers lying in bed in his room, masturbating while listening to his mother in the kitchen making dinner.

Many boys feel especially close to their mothers, often preferring to spend more time with them than with their fathers. But then, around puberty, they learn that they must reject their mothers. They are pressured by the prevailing culture (especially at school) to change their behavior, with taunts like, "Don't hang onto your mothers apron strings," "Don't be a wimp," "Get out of the kitchen and hang out with the boys," and so on. Most of all, they are expected to demonstrate their new identity, showing that, "She can't tell me what to do," distancing themselves from their mothers and sometimes even ridiculing them publicly in front of male friends, fathers, and brothers.

Boys learn that, in order to enter the "male" world—to be respected by other males, to get a job and find a place for themselves—they must put aside everything that is called "feminine" ("gushy," "childish" behavior) and "grow up" to "be a man." They must repudiate and betray the person for whom they have felt the most love.

## BREAKING UP WITH THE MOTHER: MUST LOVE ALWAYS END?[3]

The "breaking up" with the mother puts boys under severe mental and emotional stress. In many, it creates a lifelong pattern of believing that love cannot last, cannot be counted on. Most boys feel guilty for adopting these new behaviors; they simultaneously feel that they are being disloyal to a person they love and who loves them and that they have little choice but to do so. Others, in a familiar reversal of psychological logic, come to feel that their mothers deserted *them*. And thus they take away the idea that women are not to be trusted. Others take with them a lifelong belief that strong, passionate feelings cause terrible suffering and are to be avoided.

To sum up, at the same time that boys experience a sudden flowering of sexual feelings, they are hit by a traumatic change in their psychological and emotional landscape: they go through a period of emotional turmoil that culminates in the "desertion" of the mother. This crisis can affect their relationships with every other woman in later years: they may feel irritated by what they perceive as women's unspoken "demands"—which are their own buried memories of their mothers' hurt and pain. This can make it hard for them to love and accept love, because a woman's love brings up feelings of guilt and fear which are displaced onto the "evil" woman who is "provoking" and "seducing" them.

This confusion carries over into many men's sexual feelings. At puberty, many learn to mix up sex and violence. Dissociating themselves from their mothers while simultaneously experiencing the beginnings of strong sexual feelings causes a peculiar love-hate response to develop in many boys in relation to women: a sexuality connected to guilt and anxiety. Many learn to associate eroticism with hurting women. And when mothers, even as they are being rejected and ridiculed, keep coming back and offering more "love" and "understanding," the more hostile and difficult the boy becomes, so the pattern is reinforced. The mother's continuing nurturing is seen as a form of self-humiliation that affects how the boy will learn to define the "love" that comes from a woman.

Too many boys construct a sexuality toward women that combines desire and contempt. To show desire is to show contempt; it's all part of the same thing during sex. This is how it was with their mothers; they must love and want them, while at the same time distancing and disrespecting them.

Thus men's physical and emotional relationships with women contain elements of "love" and "hate," desire and repulsion. It can seem normal and erotic for men to want to humiliate women at the same time that they want to kiss them.

A man's sexual identity can be so dangerously distorted that, loving and hating the mother (and by extension all women), he can feel perfectly justified, when sexually challenged, in striking out, engaging in emotional resistance, exploding in psychological or physical attack. It feels "right" sexually to combine intense desire, even love, with pain and aggression, domination and humiliation.

This is not to say that it is politically incorrect to have sex and include ideas of power—growing up in the culture we do, we cannot avoid them. But we should at least know what it is we are doing, and why, as opposed to stupidly calling this response "hormones" and glorifying it, claiming that we have no choice but to live as we do.

It is not the inevitable "male nature" to be ambivalent or even hostile during relationships with women—though obviously not all men feel this way. These attitudes are part of an ideology that society endlessly reiterates to boys, especially at puberty. Pressure on boys to express disdain and contempt for their mothers, at the same time that there is pressure to begin to be "sexual" toward women—these messages together cause a traffic jam in boys' minds and short-circuit their brains (trauma), fusing the two commands together forever. The block becomes so completely built into structures in the mind that we can't "see" it anymore.

Clearly, men do fall in love with women; still, they usually continue to put "masculinity" before love (often hiding their true feelings outside of the house). It is more important to them to be "one of the boys" than to work out a relationship with a woman, no matter how wonderful it makes them feel.

If there is a crisis today in masculinity—an identity crisis in the male soul, of which the recent widespread "return to traditionalism" is only a symptom—the dilemma cannot be solved by appealing to war or "traditional family values," since that is where the syndrome has been perpetuated (see Part 4), with women considered "lesser" or "helpmates" and men emotionally irritable and distant.

The solution to the Oedipus dilemma is a change in the male codes, in men's "value system"—that is, "masculinity" as currently structured. (This can happen, male psychology is not "as it always was and always will be"; simply because a sixth century BC playwright in Athens wrote about Oedipus in a way that we interpret as "contemporary" does not prove that "male psychology" has always been as it is now, nor that men are doomed to have a tragic conflict with women—neither the women they love nor their mothers.) The socially created "male" way of thinking leads to the I-must-conquer-things (such as the environment, love and relationships, work and politics) mind-set; changing it would have a positive effect internationally. At the moment, a new kind of male heroism is required, a reinvention of the male psyche, a fresh identity for contemporary culture to reflect.

## FATHER, BEHOLD THY SON[4]

Sons crave their fathers' approval but often find an emotional chasm between them.

Participating in sports is one of the few ways fathers and sons spend time together. Bonding together against an opposing team is the only way most men are allowed to achieve emotional contact with their father in the traditional family system.

Being on a team, men (fathers and sons or male friends) are allowed to feel excitement together; sharing emotions in a "team" makes emotional sharing "legitimate," since the emotions are directed (ostensibly) at something other than each other. Thus, the men have an emotional interchange, an emotional climax, that is sanctioned by the society because it is channeled through an abstract "third party."

Watching team sports together is part of boys' socialization process, especially at puberty and after. Through seeing "the game," men learn about "what men do" in groups. The appropriate etiquette to use with other men is crucially important for men in their business and work lives, as well as in their social relationships with other men. Which emotions and facial expressions should they show? The players show little emotion (except for outbursts of anger); "staying in control" while still "showing power" is everything. Through sports viewing, men can enjoy the feeling of being part of a group of men.

In this way "male psychology" is learned through sports. Being able to form a team with other men is an essential element of the male genderizing process—learning the proper way of behaving to fit into the world of men. Boys learn quite early that there is no masculinity, one cannot be truly "male," without joining and conforming to a male group—unless one is a heroic loner, a rebel. Examples of this "alternative role" are Shane (the hero of the 1950s western), Marlon Brando, most male rock stars, even Jesus. Yet this role does not truly offer an alternative; since the "rebel" is in fact almost the mirror image of the father, he is simply challenging the father for power, setting up a different power center. The symbolism of the son's struggle with the father is always central in this psychological schema; all ethical battles take place within this inner circle.

The father (or the heavenly archetype of the Father) is the only one the son must "fear." Alienation of father and son is common. Boys describe enormous distance in their relationships with their fathers, but also a feeling of longing, wanting to reach the father, somehow to communicate emotionally with him.

Relationships with women are in another sphere, with different rules. Oddly, most men in my research report that they look to women when they need someone to talk to and for emotional support. Most married men respond that it is their wives who are their best friends (although women do not say this about their husbands).

This distance from the father, combined with the pressure to be with men, puts men in an odd, uncomfortable position that sometimes takes unusual forms, as this man describes: "During adolescence I had erotic fantasies of being caressed and approved of by my father. I was well into my 20s before I began to work on these feelings. What I realized was that I had very powerful urges of wanting love and confirmation to flow between us. It makes sense to me, now, that I wanted some reinforcement for puberty's confusions."

Some men today believe that the traditional male genderizing process not only hurts women (when men grow up and can't talk to them), but also hurts men themselves, and they are engaged in an inner debate about their tradition and power. They have come to believe that male dominance is not a matter of biological inevitability or superiority but a historical circumstance that should be changed.

On the other hand, the movement now to "return to traditional values" rejects such self-questioning, even labeling men who "think like that" as "wimps"! Maintaining the traditional family hierarchy—women in the home and men "in power"—is, however, a futile attempt to turn the clock back.

This does not mean that "the new man" should be "soft and cuddly" or that "the new woman" must show her "true sexy animal nature" in order to be part of the "progressive movement." It means that the way forward is to create a new blend of traditional and current values, a solid sexual morality for the future, based on equality. Stop bashing boys.

## BOYS AND THEIR FATHERS

*I used to go hunting with my dad during my boyhood. Unfortunately, I have always been a very poor marksman (my hands shake too much). I gave up hunting after an incident in which my dad and I were duck hunting in a boat with some other men. I had just brought down a duck, and we paddled the boat over to pick it up. As we reached it, I was astonished and delighted to find it still alive and looking well. It seemed so cute and attractive I envisioned taking it home with me, nursing it back to health, and keeping it for a pet. One of the men picked it up and proceeded to beat its brains out over the side of the boat.*

The tragedy of the father/son relationship is explained by one man:

*All the time I was growing up, it was funny—I was closer to my mother than my father, she was the one who was more loving—but I knew it was my father's opinion of me that counted, it was his approval that I really wanted. Why? I don't know. But I'm still that way, in a sense: I love my wife, very much, and we are happy together—but to be really happy, I want more than anything to be part of the world of men and to be recognized by other men as a man and successful.*

In a patriarchal society relationships between men are what matters to men, even more so than male-female relations. Men look to other men for approval, acceptance, validation, and respect. Men see other men as the arbiters of what is real, the guardians of wisdom, and the holders and wielders of power.

But are men able to be close to one another in our society? What do men learn from their fathers about being men? Paradoxically, even though men regard one another as "who is important," most are afraid to become too close. "Feelings" for other men are supposed to be expressed only casually and should not go beyond admiration and respect. Thus, men's relationships with men tend to be based on an acceptance of mutually understood roles and positions, a belonging to the group, rather than on intimate personal discussions of the details of their individual lives and feelings. As one man put it, "We are comrades more than friends." Our culture simultaneously glorifies and severely limits men's relationships, even relationships between fathers and sons. Still, men often feel a deep sense of affinity and camaraderie with other men.

When asked, "Are you or were you close to your father? When you were a child, were you physically close (affectionate)?" almost no men replied that they had been or were close to their fathers:

*He was always busy. He was a quiet man of few words, though extremely witty, and articulate—and very loving and affectionate, which slowly disappeared as I got older to eventually become a formal, stiff, cold relationship.*

*Not particularly. We played sports, talked politics. I can talk to him about nonpersonal subjects, but we are not personally close.*

Most men were not able to talk to their fathers: "He is a very quiet and simple man, I guess the fact that he is quiet never allowed me to talk to him as much as I would have liked. As a child we were pretty close because he did things with me that I enjoyed, like baseball, football, etc. We would pass time together rather than talk."

Or, as another puts it: "I've never said anything important to my father."

Physical relationships with their fathers, even early on, seemed to have been off limits for many men; when asked whether they had been physically close to their fathers as children, very few could remember being carried or cuddled by their fathers—although they often remembered being spanked or punished.

Some men wanted more affection: "During my childhood, my relationships with my parents were unpredictable and insecure. I always felt that my father wanted me continually to prove my feelings and loyalty, but I felt that I couldn't rely on my parents to come through for me. I think that I learned early that boys don't show affection, and hence stopped being affectionate with my mother also at an early age. Now I see physical affection as a sign of assurance, trust, etc.—the opposite of unreliability. But I feel uncomfortable with it, I'm afraid to reach out and give it— I think it looks inappropriate, too feminine, silly. Maybe this is why I don't connect sex with feelings much—it seems too nerve-wracking and I don't feel comfortable with it."

These were some of the saddest stories in my research with men: the poignant tone of missing something, longing for something—a deeply lonely feeling— emerged in man after man. Surprisingly most said that there had been no father-son talks; they had learned from their fathers only through example and from disapproval or condemnation and ridicule when they did something "wrong." As one man puts it, "We didn't do much together, he said I played baseball like a girl."

Most boys did not spend a lot of time doing things with their fathers: "I discovered the male role more from watching James Cagney, Humphrey Bogart, and James Bond than from my father. At least, a male as I would like to be." And another: "We did not really attend sports events together or play much except to kick a soccer ball around occasionally. Because of the nature of his business, we were not able to spend much time together except when we were on vacation . . . I don't remember much about those trips."

Thus, the testing grounds for masculine identity, according to men in the study, are as follows:

SPORTS: most men said there had been great pressure on them as boys to be interested in and participate in sports, to compete with other boys in sports involving physical strength. SEX: there was pressure to have "made it" sexually—to have penetrated a girl! FRIENDSHIPS: there was pressure not to play or associate with girls, not to have girls as friends. THE OUTDOORS: hunting was another testing ground of "masculinity" or toughness. HAZING: fraternities and clubs also often involved initiation ceremonies designed to test "manhood"—to see if the applicant could withstand humiliation or teasing.

As men describe their childhoods, they often speak of the distress they felt while trying to learn the stressful male role, which demands complete obedience, strength (or the appearance of it), a competitive attitude, success, and control. Mothers are usually blamed for "bringing their sons up like that," but in my research men describe feeling or having felt these pressures coming from the older men around them (older boys at school, their fathers and older brothers, uncles and so on, as well as television messages and the like). Most men described their father as demanding these characteristics and behaviors, although most also described their fathers as very distant (often because of the father's being caught in his own attempt to comply with the stereotypical fatherly role, in which the father is always stable, never shows feelings or "weakness," nor "burdens" his family with his worries). As one man put it, "My father told me: Work hard, never complain, and don't spend all your time with your mother. If I cried, he was humiliated and told me to be a man—or to go to my room and stay there until I got control of myself. Other than that, I hardly knew him."

Another man probably articulated what many men had missed and longed for when he reported, "I think a relationship between a father and son is one of the most, if not THE most, important in society today. Yet it is probably the most troubled. A father/son relationship must not be fraught with hatred and a tense tyrant-subject relationship; this will ultimately destroy one or the other or both. It must be a wide-open relationship, in which the man will give of himself so that his son will become the man he wants to become."

## HOW BOYS LEARN TO "BE LIKE THE OTHER GUYS": GENDER CONFORMITY

Prominent among the gender lessons boys learn is that they must stay in control, especially of their emotions, but also of information and of friendliness. Boys are taught not to be too effusive, to keep a cynical eye peeled for others' motives, to look out for number one. A man should look, act and behave like other men—but be on top.

The unstated subtext boys learn is gender conformity.

Most men report that they do cover over feelings—especially of pain or frustration, but even of great happiness and enthusiasm—lest they be teased:

> I was raised to conceal my actual emotions and to display whatever emotion I believed was most appropriate, to maintain or achieve control of

*a social situation. Now I hope I can kick the habit, even though other men may laugh at me.*

*Men are trained at an early age to disregard any and every emotion, and be strong. You take someone like that and they wonder why they don't and can't express feelings. Not only that, they are supposed to be a cross between John Wayne, the Chase Manhattan Bank, and Hugh Hefner. We are only human, for christsake.*

Strangely (or perhaps not so strangely) most men never quite feel they live up to all the rules. The majority of men, when asked their opinion on any topic, will soon respond, "But don't ask me, I'm not really typical, so my opinion may not be valuable or valid." Although on one level most men accept traditional definitions of masculinity, on another they doubt whether they can ever completely "measure up."

In most cases, underneath the outward conformity necessary for personal survival, there lurks a man who feels he is not quite "what a man should be."

Teaching men to deny their feelings has roots in biblical tradition. The ultimate story of denial, and the need to follow laws, rules, and orders unflinchingly, is the story of Abraham on the mountain preparing to sacrifice Isaac, his own son, in order to follow the will of God the Father. This story also exists in the Muslim religion. No more wrenching story of a man learning to kill his own feelings can be found.

Some men, when asked how they would define masculinity, expressed a kind of rebellion against the rules: "They say masculinity is someone who thinks he is superior to the opposite sex. That masculinity is easily defined by muscle, or masculinity is someone who never cries, is always tough. Let's face it, I'm so full of the 'masculinity' crap, it is sickening. I consider myself 1/4 masculine, 1/4 feminine (oh, if those jocks could hear me now), and 1/2 fighting for something in between. I cry when I feel like it, yet there is pressure to not cry ('Young men don't cry'), but then I tell myself, the hell with everyone else, I feel sad and crying is the only way. The other part of me says, 'Boy, you are a real sissy crying, you are showing a weak character.' The other part (feminine) says, 'Who ever claimed that if a man cries, he is weak? It takes a stronger person (man) to cry, you know.' That's the kind of thing I'm fighting. The answers, I am trying to find them."

Learning to be "tough" and to stay in control of emotions puts men in a difficult situation when trying to express love or negotiate a relationship with a woman. The whole "male" value system is antithetical to the role a person needs to fill in a warm and generous, emotive and empathetic relationship—a relationship in which the Number One rule is, Don't try to dominate the other person. Men would usually not try to dominate in a friendship with another man. But not dominating a woman could seem "unmasculine." And therein lies the rub—the dilemma for a man in love with a woman.

## TWO MEN SPEAK ABOUT THEIR PRIVATE LIVES

Many men wrote lengthy descriptions of their sexuality and relationships. Thirty were reproduced in *The Hite Report on Men and Male Sexuality*, two of which are reproduced here.

### MAN #1

I am a twenty-nine-year-old white male, living off and on with my lover. I work as an electrician. Every day is a real struggle, both with work and with our relationship together, but I love her and we have the best sex life I've ever had—the greatest. I've been thinking a lot about my life lately, being together so intensely with my lover has made me have a lot of thoughts, but none of the men I know ever talk about these things. That's why I'm answering this questionnaire. I would really like to know how other men feel, and I want to tell about myself.

For me, being in love is not exactly the fairy-tale sugar-coated happily-ever-after story of the movies, novels, and "great" moments in history. At times it has been painful, and a lot of times I have felt unsure of what was going on and my role in it.

When I was in my teens I thought love always implied settling down, getting married, having children, and me getting a job and supporting the lot of them, like my father and grandfather before me. It meant sacrificing one's true feelings to put on the appearance of being happy all the time. I also believed that marriage was inevitable, as everyone just gets married finally, and forgets about what they really want to do. This idea of marriage is security-oriented rather than passion-oriented. I guess I really disliked the idea of traditional marriage on many levels, but felt like a weirdo for not liking it. I thought there was something wrong with me for not liking the "normal" way of life for couples.

However . . . !!! I found myself feeling lots of new feelings when I got my lover.

When we first met I had decided never to go out with or get involved with anybody again, as it was always such a nightmare in the past, including one very difficult relationship which ended in disaster. But I felt this unbelievable sexual, physical, and personality attraction to this woman as soon as I met her. We did not get involved physically for a couple of months, although I fantasized about her since the day we met. I was extremely afraid of getting involved, because I thought it would be painful, complicated, and wouldn't last. However, she was so irresistible and sexy I couldn't control myself. I have never desired someone's body as much as I desire hers. I can never believe how exciting it is when we make love. I've never felt so many emotions before.

When I fell in love with her I felt as if I had discovered my emotions—but immediately I was also in turmoil. Although she made me feel alive and exhilarated and more sexually excited than I ever thought I could get, and made me experience all kinds of feelings that I didn't know I had, this "great love" also made me fear obligations. I was afraid. When my lover told me she needed me, I got scared, because

I thought a lot was expected of me. (Now I understand that "I need you" just means "I love you" to my lover. She means "I need to love you." It doesn't mean she expects anything from me at all—it means "Let me love you, loving you makes me feel good.") I thought that now I would have to be a "husband" like my father and tied to her. The result was the relationship was very rocky because I felt so torn between my lover and my ideas of obligation, duty, etc. I felt that I was getting into something really serious, something that demanded a great deal of sacrifice from me. At times it seemed burdensome, so I would rebel against this feeling of restriction by saying or doing something to hurt her, since I thought she was the cause of my tension. Really it was not her expectations of me but my idea of her expectations of me that was burdensome. I assumed she needed me and me only—that only I could fulfill her needs, and that I was trapped, because she said she loved me.

I also assumed she couldn't hurt me, or wouldn't hurt me, even if I hurt her. I refused to believe she was in control of her life and could solve her problems without me or that she could leave me if I made her unhappy. It's funny I thought this way because she is independent and successful, more than I am. I didn't want to believe that she could hurt me if she wanted to, or could break up with me, or could reject me. I didn't want to accept that she could do this—I didn't want to accept her as an equal (emotionally), and I didn't want to be vulnerable. (But I wanted her to be vulnerable.) But if you want to really feel close to somebody you must become vulnerable. It's the chance you have to take.

It's funny how men have these stereotypes of what women need. The men who have the most rigid stereotypes are the ones who have never really been close to a woman. Some of them are married to women they don't even know—they only know who they want to believe she is—they know their image of her, not her— they never ask her who she is.

Men think they please women by just being around and letting the woman please them. They can't really love a woman because they either put her on a pedestal or treat her like a mommy or a child. Very condescending no matter how you look at it. The way I was raised and brought up to be really arrogant, I thought I was God's gift to women. Men think of themselves as being really interesting—everyone is interested in what they have to say—people want to listen to them. But who wants to listen to a woman?

Most men's mothers treated them like kings, and so men feel like any other woman should too. Certainly it's not worth fighting very much with a woman to make the relationship better, since another woman will be glad to please me—at least that's the way I used to think. But fighting with my lover helped me develop as a person. Even though the fights were terrible, really, I felt I was growing in an important way. It's really precious to know someone so closely.

Every time I decided to give up my lover, I became physically ill, and couldn't eat, my stomach felt like it had been stomped on, and I had tension headaches. Finally I realized that I need her love—she makes me feel happy, warm, alive—like living and doing positive things rather than negative things. I need her, and I need her love, and I want to show her that I love her any way I can because the thought of being alone again is the worst thing I can imagine right now. It's funny, because before I met her I thought I was happy alone.

One thing I never knew about before her was clitoral stimulation. I used to think that my role was to have an orgasm. I thought I should fuck until I had an orgasm, or my performance would not be up to par—I thought she could feel my orgasm. I thought it would disappoint her if I didn't have an orgasm. I thought I wasn't a man if I didn't have orgasms. Fucking would make me sweat, and make my beard grow faster! Furthermore, I thought the very best possible thing was to orgasm simultaneously—and I would time my orgasm till she had hers (during coitus) and try to come at the same time she did. I thought any vaginal spasms were the contractions of female orgasms—they felt great to me. I was sure (at the time—this is with an ex-lover) that I knew when she was orgasming, and thought she knew when I was (she could feel the hot sperm, I thought), even though we didn't ask each other very often. I never masturbated her to orgasm—I didn't know how to, didn't ask, I thought sticking a finger in her vagina was masturbating her. Sometimes during intercourse I realized she didn't orgasm. I would feel that I didn't fuck as good that day (or long enough), but I believed that intercourse was the only way to achieve female orgasm—the only right way! So I felt I had let her down, but we never discussed it, we just went to sleep. The thing I have worried about since we broke up is whether or not she had orgasms as often as I assumed she did, and also whether she liked them regularly, as some of the women in *The Hite Report* said they did. At the time my masculinity and ego would have been miniaturized beyond comprehension and I'm sure I would have developed a huge complex if I thought I wasn't giving her orgasms.

When I read that women usually didn't orgasm from intercourse, my face fell—imagine that—I believed all this time that I could give women an orgasm by fucking them—suddenly this fundamental belief of mine was shattered, and I wondered if women had been faking it all along or what. I felt helpless and really embarrassed upon learning this. I had been taking this huge credit for giving women orgasms, when I didn't even know how to! It seems so funny now, but it was really a crisis when I found this out. A complete ego crisis. Not only was my ego shot, but now I had to face the problem of how to give my lover an orgasm.

The first time my lover asked me to give her an orgasm, she told me to hold my hand in a fist and put it on her pubic mound and to move it. I wasn't in a real comfortable position. But I had read *The Hite Report* at that point, so I wanted to try. Even though if you read the book you think you know a lot, but, still, to actually do it is really interesting because I'd never felt anyone's body that way before. She had shown me exactly what to do, which was so straightforward, all of a sudden I felt really enlightened.

But I also felt nervous because I kept changing the rhythm, and wasn't doing it the same way all the time. I'd speed it up and slow it down and move in different directions. Then she told me not to do it like that. I started feeling kind of insecure, because I thought, well, I don't know if I'm really doing this right, plus I couldn't anticipate when she was going to have an orgasm—I didn't know how long I was going to have to keep doing this. I didn't know if I was doing it right, I didn't know if someone else could do it better than me, or what. My confidence was on the line. I felt if I didn't do it good, if I failed . . . if I couldn't do it, she could easily humiliate me for not knowing how to do it—by criticizing me, like "Hey, man, haven't you ever done this before?" or "You're not doing it right at all!" She didn't say anything. She just moved my hand back down there and told me to just do one thing, don't move around. Even though I was getting kind of worried, don't get me wrong, I really loved it! Since it was the very first time I was doing it, I was trying to make sure I was doing it right. But the thing that was really exciting was that she showed me exactly what to do—that meant she was very excited too, excited enough to want me to do it to her. It made me feel really close to her and special since nobody ever did that before—really intimate, because I always thought of masturbation as a very private thing. If she wanted me to masturbate her, that seemed really private. I felt, how could we be any closer?

Men never talk about masturbating women, at least I've never heard them talk about it. They talk about women masturbating them a lot, but they never talk about themselves masturbating women, or there being thirty-two different ways women masturbate! And I didn't even know one. I thought women masturbated by putting something inside. Masturbation had still for me a real pejorative context, like it's not the real thing, or that's just what women would do when they don't have a man. A frustrated woman would want to stick something in her, I thought, but it could never be as good as a cock. I guess that's why men think that a woman needs a man, that she could never masturbate herself as well as a man could—I've heard that said so many times. But really, a woman can just put a vibrator or her hand on her mons and just come and come and come.

Anyway, getting back to the first time I gave her clitoral stimulation, after a while when I kept trying, she was really excited and breathing heavy, her whole body was tensing up with her legs tight together and straight out—and then she got really tense and tight and moaned and held herself like that for a few minutes. Then she told me she came. It was a revelation for me.

Of all the things we had done before that—like when we were kissing and I could hear her moaning, her head is right by my ear sometimes, and I'm listening and I can feel her breathing—never was it that exciting, it was so thrilling during her orgasm. I felt like she was really strong! That was my first reaction to the whole thing—that she had a tremendous strength—a really powerful energy that was inside her. Also I felt really small next to her when she had an orgasm and I didn't!

I also felt like—well, I used to believe that the idea was to fuck until you both had orgasms together, but all of a sudden I realized it was a really good feeling to enjoy someone else's orgasm, even if I didn't have one. Plus, to discover that she could have one that made me envious—plus I think she had another one about a minute later—well, I was really amazed! Later, after we did it a lot, I really got to enjoy it. She feels energetic and powerful and independent when she orgasms, and it makes me feel good to be next to someone so strong and active and alive.

Do you know the difference between being next to a really passive person and someone that's really excited? It makes me feel great, it makes me feel really excited, aroused, like having orgasms, really strong, it makes me feel like an animal. I just want to hop on and screw her at that point, and I often do.

But I consider my masturbating her one of the major things that we do. I don't consider it as a warm-up thing. Sometimes when we don't do it I miss doing it. Sometimes she's said things to me while I'm doing it that make me feel really good, or really hot. I get sweaty when I'm doing it, and I like that feeling a lot. I'll usually be really close against her body while I'm doing it, so I'll rub myself on her or I'll rub myself on the bed, or if my arm is in the right position I can rub it on my arm. I feel really wild when she's having the orgasm—she feels really wild to me, like she's breaking away from all physical restraints of any kind.

I've never told my friends or anybody else any of this. I never tell the guys much of anything I do. I don't know what their reactions would be. But, since most of the guys I know are always boasting about their exploits and I never do, then they boast all the more because they think I'm a prude, because I don't talk about my sex life.

But if I told them about this whole clitoral stimulation thing, they'd probably just say it's "kinky." Or couldn't she make it any other way? They'd probably be really freaked out because I've never heard anybody tell a story like that. I don't think most men know how to do it, and then the ones who do would be afraid to be ridiculed for talking about it. It seems like all men ever talk about is how they fuck. It would make me very nervous to talk about clitoral stimulation to the guys. When you're working with other men, for example, the first topic that comes up during the lunch break is "Wow, I really fucked a lot last night!" Somebody will start boasting about what he's done, and then they expect you to come up with an equally macho story—the more graphic, the better, of course. And I never do come up with any stories. Then they think you can't get laid, or you're too sensitive or whatever. They don't like to talk about it in emotional terms. Of course, mostly they're not talking about their wives—sometimes they are, but usually they're trying to say they are having affairs with somebody. Most of the time they are bragging, they are also bragging that they are seeing more than one person. But sometimes people will say, "I'm going home to fuck my wife!" I've heard that. I thought it was really nice when I heard it. It was somebody that I didn't know very well, and he said, "I'm going home and fuck my wife!" (He was really drunk.) It sounded like a great thing to do. I should have wished him a happy time. But most men seem to think that anything outside of intercourse is a deviation from the norm, or it's not the "real thing." All I know is, that seems to me now like a really limited way of seeing things.

Another thing I've always heard was that you weren't supposed to have sex when the woman was having her period. Women are always supposed to hide it, and not let anyone know they're having it, and men aren't supposed to know about it, and everyone is supposed to pretend like it doesn't happen.

One time we were making out, lying in bed, she didn't have any clothes on, and we were thinking about intercourse, but she still had the Tampax in. I said I wanted to take it out for her. She was going to take it out herself in the bathroom, and then wash herself, but I wanted to take it out. And it was really sexy to take it out. I wanted to look at it while it was coming out—not just reach around and pull it out—I wanted to watch it, I wanted to see the colors on it. I thought it would be really great to look at it and watch the thing come out. It seemed really beautiful to watch it come out. It was part of her on the Tampax—I just wanted to watch it, I don't know why. It was really sexy. When I took it out I had it and I didn't want to throw it away. I wanted to keep it. It smelled good. So I put it in my mouth. It was great to be chewing on it, tasting it.

It smelled strong but it smelled really good, it was really sexy the way it smelled, plus it was part of her. It smelled sweaty, kind of, a sharp and kind of sweaty smell, just like regular blood and mucus together, but also with some kind of a sharp, strong odor—the more, the better.

It is very exciting to just mess around sometimes. I like kissing, squeezing, my cock fondled and stroked, I like to be licked, and stroked on the neck and back, and be bitten on the chest. I like to be sucked. We both make advances, because we both love to mess around. If I want to get her excited, I make an advance. When she makes an advance, it gets me very excited.

I love to masturbate my lover to orgasm and feel her tremble when she orgasms. But also just caring for her is lots of fun. I like to give massages to my lover and bathe her. I wasn't raised to do this—quite the contrary—I was raised to keep distant from others physically.

If I'm with my lover I sometimes have orgasms, sometimes not. Making love doesn't require having orgasm to be beautiful. I like to get more and more excited, and to stay like that. Why end it? The building up of feelings is much more exciting than having an orgasm and going to sleep. My lover often drives me crazy, to the point that my desires get very strong and uncontrollable. I love her for making me feel that excited. I crave her, need her, and it feels great to really want someone like that—it makes me feel real, alive. I like to get my desire built up to a frenzy. It gets painful, it's such a gnawing, craving desire. As the excitement builds up, we get rougher. Orgasms that come from frenzy are the best—they are uncontrollable. This is very different from "timing my orgasm with hers"—what a conceited practice—and boring! My lover doesn't orgasm from intercourse, but she is a great fuck, because she makes me crave her. I want to fuck her in every part of her body, and cream all over her. To feel this way is the best feeling in the world.

I love intercourse. It feels great physically. Emotionally it is very satisfying and soothing. We have intercourse several times a week. Sometimes I come very soon upon entering, and it feels good when this happens involuntarily. But I'd rather build up the excitement. Knowing that I don't have to make her orgasm from intercourse makes intercourse less traumatic, and I don't feel obligated to orgasm myself. I can enjoy being inside her for various lengths of time, and go back in later, and do other things meanwhile.

I have only orgasmed once from fellatio. It is very pleasant but too gentle to orgasm. I need harder pressure to orgasm, or a huge amount of penis stimulation beforehand to orgasm this way. I love it when my lover masturbates me, but it takes a long time to bring me to orgasm. I like my balls rubbed, and a finger up my ass sometimes.

The first time my lover stuck a finger up my ass, it hurt and felt good simultaneously. I didn't really like it; it made me feel like a little baby being punished, and brought tears to my eyes. But it also felt sort of like an orgasm—a continuous orgasm, not like a regular quick, pleasurable, painless ejaculation. Sometimes it feels like I am regressing to childhood—I feel like I am unlearning sphincter control, because sphincter discipline is the definition of being an individual, a responsible person. With a finger up my ass, I feel utterly helpless, like a child, like I can't control my shitting, like my partner has complete control over me. Ironically it is very pleasurable. I feel completely out of control, compared to intercourse, where I feel in control, powerful, like a man, an adult, in control of my body. And penetration makes me feel free and like I am being filled.

I usually have at least two orgasms a day from masturbation if I'm alone. Sometimes I masturbate one to five times a day, usually two to three. I like to do it, but I don't talk about it much. It relieves tension, but it makes me a little depressed later. I like it because it is a quick way to have an orgasm. I don't like it because it doesn't really satisfy me or make me happy, the way making love does.

To be a man means to come out on top. Or like my mother used to say, "I don't care what you are, just be the best at whatever you do." Competition begins at an early age—kindergarten, where kids try to outdo each other in everything they do. Of course, the boys have boy games and girls have girl games. The emphasis is on excelling: who can run fastest, play harder, play rougher. I always felt insecure about it, because I wasn't very aggressive and didn't want to be—on the physical level, that is. I was deathly afraid of getting into a fight. I was paranoid all the time that somebody would pick a fight with me. In order to survive, I had to develop and excel somehow. So in grade school I excelled in my classes. At least people respected me from being smart in class.

It seems like people love to take out their frustration and hatred for the system on an individual who doesn't succeed. Especially in high school, where individuals are outright ostracized for dressing "funny," being slow, being quiet, introverted, "square," "prudish," "ugly," fat, you name it, the group can tease someone to death. I survived a lot of this somehow, and now I've even learned to get the group's respect—

but I feel really bad that this harassment and pressure is so prevalent. I've seen guys actually drop out of school because the rest of the class teased them so much.

This cruel quality in men seems to be a big part of masculinity—to be able to inflict pain on weaker, slower individuals is the tough, macho way to show your superiority. Men justify cruelty by emphasizing that the victim is a "weak" person, who deserves it. And this mentality also says, "Why not? I deserve everything I got, I earned it—the slobs deserve everything they get too (punishment)." I don't understand this competition fully, except I do know it is prevalent in every aspect of my life, and I do it myself too. But I hate it—I feel "on guard" all the time around other men.

Only men work where I work—lately we are repairing dangerous telephone wires and lines that have been cut, etc., and other electrical wiring. The most macho ones are the meanest, sweatiest, most foulmouthed, drink more beer, smoke bigger cigars, and tell the "dirtiest" jokes, very abusive towards women. When a woman passes by where we are working, every man becomes self-conscious of his macho image. They light up a cigarette, stop working and stare at her, undress her mentally, very aware that the others are doing the same thing, and will nod to each other if she is sexy, or make a face if they don't think she is. Men in groups are hostile, edgy, and like to show that they don't have feelings—feelings of tenderness, caring, or friendship (except under the rules of bonding), or feelings of pain, be it emotional or physical. Men pride themselves among each other on their ability to not flinch while in pain. Many jobs we do involve exposure to dangerous live wires, or require us to work at dangerous heights, but most macho men won't wear safety equipment unless it is required or the situation is extremely dangerous, because macho men like to show each other that they don't feel any pain.

Macho men comment to each other about female passersby, and if you don't have a comment to support the group's opinion you are considered (1) a fag, (2) a mama's boy, (3) a prude, (4) a real jerk, (5) a jerk-off. Then you draw the next round of insults from the group, and become the victim of their further abuses and hostile comments. It's very childlike, the way children ostracize and tease the kid with glasses or a stutter or any physical weakness. The thing is, this whole macho group-bonding thing is actually taught in the high schools and trade schools, as the students who are studying skilled trades like plumbing and electricity and carpentry must also withstand the nonstop group harassment and teasing that goes on in the classroom. Even the instructors do it, and humiliate or abuse slow or weak students. "You gotta be a real man to get into the Brotherhood of the Plumbers Union!" To keep a job one must deal with this horrible social system. The foreman is typically the very most macho, grouchy, cursing, angry-looking person on the site. There is never any positive reinforcement for good work, only criticism for bad or slow work. One never admits ignorance in one's job just as one never does about women, because that would bring the roof down on your own head and all the humiliation that goes with it.

Most of the men I work with get paid very well for their work, and resent women who try to break in as equals. They really don't want women as equals, only as a fuck, or a "mommy," or a cute daughter. They want to protect the "poor things," be a big hero all the time, and bring home more money than the women. Men act very different among themselves than they do in groups with women. They don't talk about women among themselves as equals or humans—they say stuff like "She likes cock," "She's frigid," and especially "She loves my ass." They don't say, "I love her," "I respect her," "I need her," or "I hope she is feeling good." The worst part of it is that I don't do anything to change this really. I just put up with their attitudes because I want the money. And to be perfectly honest, I also want to be accepted.

My father always expected the women of the family to do certain daily things, like clean the house, cook, take care of the children, and the boys and men to do other, more special things, like shovel snow, fix cars, clean the garage and basement. I'm sure he expects me to know more about the world than my wife and to make more money than her. He believes his role is to support the family and wife. He's worked seven days a week, fourteen hours a day (as a plant maintenance supervisor) to do this since I can remember. He doesn't spend time with his family. I never got to know my father till I began working with him. He is a workaholic, and doesn't understand how anyone feels about anything. I hate him but I also love him very much. My mother always listened to me, and trusted me to make my own decisions, even though we never talked heart to heart or were never really physically close.

It was my sister I was really close to (one year older). She was my "best friend" in second, third, and fourth grades. We did things together as equals with no sexual (role) barriers. We were friends. As a child I remember that boys were supposed to play with boys' toys and girls with girls' toys. Girls played "house," "dolls," and "shopping," and boys played army men, fort games, snowball fights, and more strenuous games. But there were some games that boys and girls could play together, like cards and table games, ride bikes. There were times when I felt torn between playing with my sister, who was my best friend, and playing with the boys. Especially skating—the girls did figure skating, and the boys played hockey. Of course, it was an honor to be accepted into the group of boys as a hockey player; I remember feeling like I had betrayed my sister when I went to the rink with her but didn't play with her once we got there. I didn't want to be a sissy, so I let her play with her girlfriends and I played with the boys.

It was never the same after that. We took off on our respective masculine and feminine roles. As an adult, it is almost impossible for a man to be "friends" with a woman or "best friends." The roles we are assigned don't allow it. Men have their wives, and their friends (other men). Men don't see women as equals; perhaps they did as children, but when they follow their roles, they begin to feel guilt for leaving women behind, and later feel contempt for women who are not their equals, since they didn't let them be. Men show contempt for women because they are not able to treat them with respect and honesty, because they consider themselves superior.

My lover is a feminist—and I respect her for it. She is honest and courageous. She won't stand to be treated like a second-class person. She is very strong. But I used to think that the women's movement was a minority of women radicals who were very bitter people, who were overly critical of society, and generally too extreme to be taken seriously. I never thought of it as if I were a woman, nor did I ever experience what it's like to be a woman, to be stared at by men, discriminated against on the job level, the educational level, and even in conversation. Feminists made me nervous: I felt I was innocent—I never intentionally was unfair to women—I was nice to them—why should they be mad at me?

Of course, I didn't understand. The weird thing is that even though I wasn't satisfied with society's definition of me as a "man," I was not inspired by the group of women who were rebelling against the society's definition of them as women.

I have discovered that the most important thing for keeping our relationship on an even keel is a daily sharing of feelings, how we feel. I never grew up thinking this was important. I thought I was always supposed to be objective, and that I should suppress any other feelings, to express them would be weak. One result of this was that, sometimes she would get very angry and upset because I didn't express my feelings to her. Other times, too, she would tell me her feelings about something that had happened, but I just sat silently and she would get mad. When she got upset at me I felt very nervous, upset, afraid, angry, mean, and confused. But I never expressed this either, nor did I ask her why she felt so angry. My basic impulse was just to get out of that situation; I wanted to avoid situations in which I felt anything other than loved, confident, wanted, happy, and stable. I thought her anger was just a waste of time. I thought to myself, "I love her—doesn't she understand that? Why doesn't she let me love her?"

It really helped when I finally realized that communication about feelings and moods is something that has to be kept up every day. Even now, if we are not really communicating and keeping in touch and sharing with each other how we feel, I get confused, estranged, and insecure about where I stand. Then I get paranoid and pretend that everything is O.K., instead of saying the truth, like "I feel weird, we're drifting apart. Why? Aren't I communicating, or aren't you?"

I answered this because I want to know how other men feel about these things. I haven't been able to talk these things over with anybody, and they are very important to me. And at the same time, I also found it a relief to say I find some of my friends' behavior really revolting sometimes. But I could never say this to their faces. It's really crazy, but at the same time I like them.

## MAN #2

At age seventy, with the awareness that death and oblivion are much closer now than ever before, I have become much more conscious of the essential loneliness of the human condition and of an increasing desire for a warm, close, and loving relationship with another person, and, for me as of now, sex is an essential component of such a relationship. The physiological aspects of sex and achievement of orgasm, while still very enjoyable, are not as strong or compelling a part of my sex life as formerly, while the psychological components as expressed in hugging, kissing, and caressing are now much more important. In retirement, with the interests and challenges of my work no longer demanding my concern, my need for this latter type of sex seems to have greatly increased.

My wife and I have been married thirty-nine years, during most of which we struggled to overcome a sexual incompatibility deriving from our mutual ignorance of female sexuality.

From adolescence on my wife has been obsessed with the conviction, probably derived from the many romantic novels that she has read, that the highest peak of sexual ecstasy that a woman can reach is in experiencing a vaginal orgasm, and any woman who goes through life without having them has only half lived. She has also long been convinced that the main obstacle to her achievement of this blissful experience was my inability to maintain an erection and continue "pumping" indefinitely. Having a smaller than average penis, I was preconditioned to feelings of inadequacy, and with no basis for disputing her faith in vaginal orgasms (*The Hite Report on Female Sexuality* came thirty-five years too late to salvage our sex life!), our sexual encounters became sessions of frustration, bitter recriminations, and mutual hostility so distasteful that I eventually became impotent and we stopped having sex altogether.

I am white, in good health, and the father of three grown children. My parents were of the lower middle class with only grade school educations. They were loving and moderately religious. I have an M.A. in chemistry, worked thirty-six years for a major oil company doing technical work that I enjoyed, retired, taught chemistry in school for a few years, and again retired. In religion I am humanist. I had no sexual experiences until around age twenty-two, when I finally rejected the brainwashing of my parents regarding the terrible effects of "playing with oneself," and began to masturbate regularly.

After marriage to my wife, a sexually quite inhibited woman, the sequence of operations gradually evolved to include (1) imbibing two or three cocktails to relax my wife's inhibitions, (2) insertion of a diaphragm by my wife, (3) preplay in the form of kisses and caresses applied to various supposedly sensitive areas of my wife's head and body, (4) finger or tongue massage (usually the former with which she felt less embarrassment) of the clitoris to near or incipient orgasm, (5) hasty mounting "missionary" style, and thrusting in and out with the penis in a consistently unsuccessful effort to convert the near-orgasm to what my wife has always firmly believed must be the epitome of ecstasy for any woman, but after thirty-nine years of trying has not yet achieved: a vaginal orgasm, (6) rapid fading of my wife's sexual excitement of the near-orgasm to a feeling of bitter disappointment and frustration while I pumped away and eventually had my orgasm, the pleasure of which, however, was tempered by the knowledge that I had somehow again failed to achieve for my wife the one thing that she felt was essential for a woman's happiness, (7) finger massage of the clitoris to complete (though sometimes only simulated) orgasm, and (8) a "post-mortem" of the operation which usually constituted the final scene of this little comedy-tragedy, with my wife, sometimes in tears, agonizing over her failure once again to attain vaginal orgasm and ascribing the failure at times to some lack within herself, at times to my inability to continue the in-and-out thrusting indefinitely on the chance that her sexual excitement might eventually again be stimulated to the desired orgasm. Gradually these always disappointing and, for me, guilt-laden sexual encounters acquired such consistently negative associations that they became distasteful to me, I had increasing difficulty obtaining erections, and eventually, after thirty-nine years of married life, became impotent.

Although my sex life with my wife has always been very unsatisfactory to both of us, in other respects we enjoy a good, even if unexciting relationship. In fact, aside from our sexual difficulties, our married life has been surprisingly harmonious, and it is especially so now that we are no longer fighting "the battle of the sexes." I think I can truly say that we still respect and love each other in a nonsexual way.

I am quite sure that, although I was in love several times before marriage and a few times (at a distance) since, I have never been as deeply in love as I am right now with my lover. Not too long ago, at my suggestion, we adopted open marriage and now my wife at age sixty-five has a "young" lover in his forties with whom she can continue to pursue her will-o'-the-wisp, the vaginal orgasm, and I have found a warm, hugging, kissing, caressing, oral-sex-oriented woman who has revitalized my sex life and with whom I have fallen deeply in love. Although of very different backgrounds and with a sixteen-year difference in our ages, we seem to be made for each other in the unprecedented degree to which our tastes, interests, likes and dislikes, coincide. I'm in seventh heaven while we're together and miss her terribly when we're apart. I certainly never expected to fall so deeply in love at this age! It's a moot question whether the delights of being together outweigh the pain of separation and the near-hopelessness of our ever being able to get together permanently. However, I find our relationship very deeply satisfying emotionally, and it adds a whole new dimension to my life. Also, as she says, the delightful periods that we do spend together are like a permanent honeymoon taken on the installment plan, with the periods of separation ensuring the permanence of our enchantment with each other. My relationship with my lover is essentially a monogamous one on my part, although not on hers, since she still has sex with her husband.

As I grow older, I find that the greatest pleasure in sex, for me, is the feeling of closeness or "oneness" with my loved one that it gives me. I enjoy being touched and kissed because the sensual pleasure and feeling of intimacy is more prolonged. Still, although having orgasms is not as important to me now at age seventy as when I was younger, they are important. I certainly would feel deprived if my partner did not help me to an orgasm every other day or so of our lovemaking, if only as a demonstration of her concern that I should get as much pleasure as possible.

I enjoy masturbation when I am separated from my loved one and feel "in the mood." When we are separated, I may masturbate from one to three times per week. Masturbation with me always leads to orgasm. I usually masturbate in the shower, with a hard jet of hot water hitting against the underside of my penis. I usually fantasize variations of cunnilingus.

I enjoy cunnilingus with any woman sexually attractive enough that I could enjoy kissing her on the mouth, but even more with the woman I deeply love. The pleasure is both physical in the warmth and softness of her parts and the stimulating "femaleness" of the taste and odor, and psychological in that cunnilingus comes closer than anything else to satisfying the strong desire I have for attaining the greatest possible intimacy with her. Another important and pleasurable aspect of cunnilingus is the intense satisfaction I feel when my partner achieves orgasm, as she normally does.

I also very much enjoy fellatio and always orgasm this way. Even at age seventy I'm sure that I could orgasm every day this way if I had the opportunity. However, since my lover and I are only able to get together for two or three days at a time and only in the daytime, these occurrences are limited to two or three times every week or so. With my lover's fellatio, I never have difficulty having an orgasm.

With a new partner whom I love, ejaculation is just one episode in an extended period of loving and caressing. In a shallow, physical sense I feel momentarily satisfied, but in a much deeper sense I have the feeling that I could never really be fully satisfied unless our bodies could somehow be melted and fused together into a single unified being. For me kissing, hugging, and caressing seem to bring me closer to this ideal state than simply ejaculating. This life is a very lonely place when one has no one with whom to share human closeness and warmth and love, and for me the sense of mutual caring and concern are much more important than a mere orgasm.

## THE VARIED SEXUAL PLEASURES OF BEING MALE: SEEING IN A NEW WAY

### WHAT IS A MAN'S "SEXUAL NATURE?"

Most men have been taught to think of their bodies as sexual tools of reproductive activity. The canon goes like this: "You must get an erection, you must insert it into the vagina, and you must have an orgasm—but not too soon!" Starting in the James Bond 1960s, a man was thought odd if he did not want sex with a young (reproductive-age) woman at the drop of a hat; a "real man" should always have a hard penis, "have it ready," gun loaded. Today the many articles and emails praising Viagra and other drugs make the same point.

There is an assumption that men are sexual "beasts" with "raging hormones" and that we are all "natural creatures" underneath society's "varnish," that our sexual nature is biologically structured. Male sexuality especially is understood in terms of its being animal or bestial.

According to this popular hypothesis, a man is a beast who can't help himself.

Certain things turn him on and he gets going and just can't stop, it's nature's way of making him deposit his seed here, there, and everywhere.

In recent years, have men become less focused on erection of the penis or on the drive for coitus à la James Bond? Or are most men still basically worried about how big their erection is?

Our culture's lessons to men have been so strong that few are able to get past them, to create their own personal sexuality. We live in a culture that has taught us that sex is a reproductive activity; that other activities (such as masturbation or oral sex without coitus) are less valuable, even evil. Men are thus focused on achieving erection—even though many women make it clear that erection is not the key to their sexual satisfaction.

Fashionable drugs, such as Viagra and Cialis, offer men a "miracle pill," an erection on demand, reinforcing the idea that erection is the be-all and end-all of male sexuality—the only way a man can be sexual—and reinforcing the belief that erection is mechanical, more related to bodily functions than to a relationship or emotions. In fact, if a man does not have an erection, the problem may very well be with his relationship or his situation, not with his hormones or penis. However, though emotions and the erection are clearly connected, many men would rather believe anything else, such as, "Well, I guess when you get middle-aged, this is bound to happen."

Thus men often see the penis as connected to a self-generating set of hormones or body mechanisms that should operate independently of what a man is (or is not) experiencing, as if the penis were a foreign object between the legs, not a part of a man's overall "being"—not his "self," but just a rude "piece of meat," "down there." The admonition, "He thinks with his penis" is further damaging, since it implies that when men have erections and desire sexual connection, they are not thinking but being "stupid" or animalistic. "He's a jerk" is another insult with sexual connotations. The word jerk comes from *jerk-off*, meaning someone who masturbates or "plays with himself."

The truth is that the penis is a delicate part of the male being, one that responds with exquisite sensitivity to every nuance of emotion a man can feel. However, society has tried to insist that a "real man" should "get hard" at will, whenever he decides (in his brain?) that such a course is "appropriate." But it is impossible to will an erection into being. Trying to do so has caused a great deal of psychological pain and self-hate in many men—and often in their partners, too, as both take "lack" of erection as a sign of lack of love.

Erections come and go in men, during sex and during sleep. A man who is kissing a loved one may stop, worrying that "I can't get an erection now, so I'd better not keep on with this." In fact, he could continue being physically intimate with his partner. Many men stimulate themselves during sex, masturbate for a minute or two to make sure that their penis is hard at the very time they want it to be. This approach works perfectly for most men.

On the other hand, a man can enjoy "sex" even without having an erection—

though, of course, erection itself is pleasurable for men and no one wants to deny this fact. But since orgasm in women is generally not caused by "penetration" or coitus, in most cases there should be no pressure on a man to have an erection "to please the woman." The definition of sex has centered on the reproductive act to the detriment of other activities because we have evolved from a culture that wanted to increase reproduction. Now, however, most of us use birth control.

Our sexual behavior has been channeled into a limited form of expression; sex could be more interesting if it were not always focused on one scenario: "foreplay" followed by "penetration" (insertion), the high point being "fucking" (coitus). Sex should comprise a varied, individual vocabulary of ways of touching, caressing, and exciting oneself and one's partner, whether through stimulation by hand of both people, or by sharing the excitement of a sexual fantasy, or oral sex.

The fear of HIV has increased rather than decreased the focus on erection; many men only became more nervous in the face of having to put on a condom without losing their erections or their sexual desire. Further new pressures have added more complications; not only are men asked to use a condom, they are expected to provide clitoral stimulation to orgasm in many cases, and to be emotionally sensitive to their partner, not (for example) turning over and falling asleep immediately after their own orgasm. While some men breeze through the art of providing clitoral stimulation by hand or mouth to orgasm, others prefer to think that a mythical "gspot" inside the vagina is the answer to the changes in sexuality that women have been talking about.

Masturbation is the one time when men express their sexuality without a focus on reproduction or coitus and when they do not worry about erection. As one man puts it, "I have more or less two sex lives, one with my wife and one with myself." Many women in my research were shocked to learn that a man who is their regular partner also regularly masturbates: "Why would he want to do that, when he can have sex with me almost any time he wants?" Men in my research say they enjoy masturbation or having sex alone because they can fantasize about whatever they want and there is no pressure on them to perform for another person. Also, laboratory studies show that self-stimulated orgasms (in men and women) are stronger (Masters & Johnson, 1966).

Men could enjoy their sexuality more if they focused less on penetration during sex and more on expressing themselves sexually in whatever form their emotions take, while making space for their partner to do the same. No man should ever fear lack of erection; perhaps he has only to reach down and touch himself.

### THE IMAGE OF MEN IN PORNOGRAPHY: THE UNCELEBRATED
### BEAUTY OF MEN'S SEXUALITY AS IT COULD BE

Clichés tacitly condone an underlying ideology: not only are women sexual servants, men are foolish beasts who "can't help themselves," and inside every man there is a lurking stranger, a beast who wants to rape and pillage. It's straight Dr. Jekyll and Mr. Hyde, appropriate for a culture that sees male sexuality as incompatible with the traditional family.

Of course this ideology is nonsense; pornography's depiction of male sexuality is nothing more than fantasy, not fact. In my view, the understanding of male sexuality in the clichés of pornography need revising. Male sexuality will be just as sexy and erotic when it takes a new direction.

Though many people think that the only position they can have is either "for" or "against" pornography, I would propose a more complex, in-depth critique of the underlying ideology, a more substantive debate.

The prevalent ideology is insidious because it is implicit; if text would state explicitly the premises (which we are beginning to delineate here), people would be more questioning. However most pornography consists of visuals, giving the impression that, well, everyone agrees, therefore the assumptions must be true.

A concurrent part of this belief system is that the end product of sexual feeling is violence, that if you let sex get out of hand or go too far, become bestial or instinctive, it will lead to violence. There is a belief that sex in its "uncontrolled, natural state" leads to violence, that the individual has to control sex or it could lead to something disastrous, like death. Of course, this is only true for those who have this wish in the first place; sexual feelings do not "naturally" lead to death or destruction— though they may be frenzied. Perhaps in the West the association of sex and savagery comes from the Bible. For centuries various "biblical scholars" or commentators argued that sexual women were "tools of the devil," "sexual temptresses" who could cause a man to go to his death if their "siren song" was heeded. Centuries of biblical commentators wrote interpretations of Old Testament scriptures "proving" that this was their meaning, just as today groups like the Taliban follow clerics who wrote texts exaggerating specific points of Islam, insisting that their interpretation is "the one true way." Of course, the assertion that sex leads to violence implies that sex has to be controlled by a series of moral imperatives —*especially* that women have to be controlled (a convenient conclusion for a society based on male inheritance and male dominance).

In addition to the clichés about men I have been describing, there are many silly clichés in pornography about women that have been analyzed by myself and others. One message is that women are there to be degraded, that in the end women like violence done to them. Pornography contains innumerable depictions of men being violent to women, such as depictions of women tied up, women bound and gagged. While such images can be exciting, nothing indicates that they represent "real human nature." Proving that women do not like to see themselves in these ways, sales of pornography to women have not increased (or have increased only in the most miniscule way) over the last three decades, though such an increase had been repeatedly predicted.

Pornography is unnecessarily stuck in old clichés. There should be many depictions of desire and physical interaction, not the same predictable script over and over played by the same characters, like Punch and Judy, eternally in opposition.

Pornography presents a highly distorted image of men. I don't believe that men are the monolithic beings depicted in most pornographic images, nor that they find "their authentic selves" in pornography. My research with thousands of men shows a different picture of "who men are sexually" whereas pornography represents the imposition of a rigid ideological view on male sexual feelings, expression, and behavior rather than a realistic depiction of male sexuality.

Ironically, while on the surface pornography seems friendly to men—more so than to women—its underlying message makes fun of men. Subliminally, *sotto voce*, it implies to men that their sexual expression is ridiculous, base, crude, or insensitive, even grotesque. Visually it frequently makes men look ugly and coarse, foolish and unappealing. Who hasn't seen these pornographic images? They're all around us, in sex magazines, email spam, on the internet, and even in "fine art." The makers and distributors of the images must believe that men like them, that they are generally making "what men like," because they market it "to men" and the industry is growing.

Do most men really like pornography? Do they identify with the images, or do they find them laughable, "not really me," or do they think to themselves, "I wish I could be like him, lucky guy"? Whether men like the way they are portrayed in pornography is difficult to know, since most men are brought up with the idea that if you find something revolting, you must not flinch but look it "straight in the eye" and say, "Wow! I like it! I'm bad!" Boys are not supposed to shy away from "vulgar things"; doing so makes you "girlish." Therefore, the more disgusting a pornographic visual is, the more a "real man" shouldn't show disgust. But privately, do most men really think they are "like that," or do they experience their sexuality as more subtle, more diverse, possibly more erotic and even spiritual?

Of course not all men look at pornography, so why is it generally considered "for men"? Is it because women supposedly don't need to "jerk off"? Or because the material puts "men on top" as "the winners," denigrating women as "the losers"? In porn, there is a subliminal "text" in addition to the actual visual depiction. Men are almost always presented as predators with erections—almost as rapists, really; one of the key unspoken clichés of pornography is that the man must show no feelings, no sentimentality, he must follow a strictly physical sexual scenario. Pornography portrays men as having pleasure focused on erection and ejaculation, especially inside a woman, rarely seeking eroticism for its own sake, or other purely sensual activity, but never "in love" or sexually active in a nonfocused way. They do not show men seeking full-length body contact or needing to hold another person and be held, or to be penetrated themselves in some way. Sexual exuberance, desire, elation, love-not-satisfied-by-orgasm, fantasy—these states are about something other than a biological drive to reproduce the species, the "male sex drive" that in pornography is central to "sex."

Today, "male sex drive" as a concept has taken on a sort of mystical ring. During the late twentieth century this term was used more and more often, so that it became "unquestionable truth," reality, and today this "drive" is assumed to be biological. But is it? Logically, if men supposedly have a biological drive to "thrust," then shouldn't women have a complementary reverse "drive" to "open"? Or, is the entire idea of a sex drive a fraudulent ideological category masquerading as scientific fact?

What about the other sexual states that men experience that are not seen in pornography? Are men as singularly mechanical and aggressive "by nature" as they are depicted? Society has tried to insist that a real man should "get hard" at will, whenever "appropriate," meaning in a private situation with a female of reproductive age, but it is impossible to will an erection into being. The penis is a delicate organ that responds with sensitivity to a man's emotional state, and most men report that it is desire they seek, not the mechanical means of orgasm or creating erection. Desire and arousal are the pleasures that spread through the body; orgasm, after all, can be attained alone during masturbation.

The beauty of male sexuality is not so much about erection as about all the gestures and subtle meaningful body movements, including the ups and downs of erection—tumescence and nontumescence, detumescence and retumescence—ways in which the body makes itself known or "speaks." These movements represent a man's beauty and personality and are very erotic. Pornography as we know it does not represent that variety and diversity of expression, it simply pretends to be "revolutionary" and "avant-garde" by being "shocking," passing itself off as "incredibly open" compared to the old value system of "prudery." But it is not revolutionary, such images do not address a more valuable and interesting view of "who men are sexually."

What is "male sexuality"? Why is it so closely identified with intercourse in a reproductive scenario? The answer involves an understanding of centuries of enforcement of the idea of "sex" as male reproductive desire or "instinct," to be socially controlled by putting it into a reproductive context within marriage. Yet this early ideology contained the seeds of its own destruction by furthering the idea that men are somehow in the harness of "reproduction within marriage," that their sexuality can only be "freely experienced" outside the family. In my research, it seems that the ideological split between "body" and "mind" or "soul"—as pornography depicts—is the crux of the problem men experience, not whether or not they are in a "reproductive relationship." The definition of sex created to go with our social order and family structure, originating about 3,000 years ago, has been focused on the reproductive act, to the detriment of other activities, because we have evolved from a culture that wanted to increase reproduction to one in which, now, most of us use birth control.

Men's "sexual nature" is very "polymorphous-perverse," as a *New York Times Book Review* characterized the picture of men that emerges from *The Hite Report on Men and Male Sexuality*. For example, during masturbation, my research shows, men stimulate themselves in many more places than they do when with a partner.

Consider this fact: Most urologists stimulate men to ejaculate during their examinations with a finger in the anus, since just inside the anus in men (but not in women) there is proximity to a gland that, when stimulated, causes orgasm. What does this fact imply?

Most men do not allow themselves to explore the various feelings they wish to express during sex with a partner, especially a female partner; instead they try to follow as "perfectly" as possible the reproductive scenario. Our sexual acts have been channeled into too limited a form of expression; sex could be more interesting if it was not always focused on one scenario: "foreplay" followed by "penetration," the high point being "fucking," coitus or "the act."

The appearance of Viagra and the fear of HIV have increased rather than decreased the focus on erection; for example, many men are nervous about having to put on a condom and consequently losing their erection or their sexual desire. Not only are men asked to use condoms, in many cases they are also expected to provide clitoral stimulation to orgasm. But many men cut short "foreplay" because they are afraid that they will lose the erection which, they have been taught, is necessary to the enjoyment of sex and which it would be "shameful" to lose. More men could reach much higher peaks of feeling and arousal if they did not feel anxious about how they "should" behave sexually.

Today many men seem to be withdrawing from "sex" and the erection/size scenario in various ways. This withdrawal can take the form of claiming "erectile dysfunction," "religious purity," deferring "commitment" or preferring nonstandard "kinky" sex. This may be a reaction to the clichés that surround society's view of men, seen increasingly through modern advertising as well as pornography. If men are told they are "cheap," their bodies mechanically obedient to "lurid" stimulus (akin to the response of Pavlov's dogs to a dinner bell), of course the more sensitive men will react by withdrawing. It would be better to change outdated stereotypes of "sex."

How do men feel about the way they are depicted as treating women in pornography and about the violence to women shown in most pornography? Most men feel perplexed and wonder why this picture can excite them. Although pornography frequently denigrates women—showing women beaten, black and blue, and so on, and liking it—it also denigrates men, cheapening and brutalizing their sensibilities, destroying their possibility of personal sexual discovery, implanting clichés such as "a real man is the one with the biggest, hardest erection," and so on, blocking their power to express themselves with others. In my interpretation, sex and violence are mixed during the Oedipal stage of boys' development, at a time when they are emotionally leaving "the mother" and simultaneously becoming increasingly sexual. But pornography's frequent implication that "men are beasts whose underlying unchangeable natures make them likely to be violent to women" is incorrect, misleading, and dangerous.

Pornography's messages bisect men psychologically, showing sexuality as separate from emotion and the soul. This view can affect men in a very negative way, though many remain unconscious of the origin of their discomfort; these nonverbal messages cause them to think that they are "two people"—the sexual "animal" and the thinking, spiritual individual. One thinks of the separation of women and men in Moslem mosques. For this reason, the vast majority of men find it confusing when they actually fall in love and mix "body" and "soul." The increasing male aversion to falling into these stereotypes of "male sexuality" can also be seen in a broader political sense: male Islamic extremists in Afghanistan proclaimed in many of their public statements that they wanted to "create a more pure society" that would be less sexual, a society in which women's bodies would be covered, hidden from sight (or were women being punished?). Both Western and Eastern traditions pose a problem for men in terms of integrating "mind," "body," and relationships with women.

Pornography is above all propaganda—an ideological construct used to direct men toward a certain style of reproductive sexual activity, to tell them the kind of attitude they should have toward sex and women. Women in pornography serve the basic purpose of legitimizing male sexual expression. Pretending to represent "nature," pornography touts an ideological view of how men should behave. It is a brainwashing device. In fact, the exportation of pornography is one of the areas of "globalization" that presents the most negative outdated versions of "who men are" to the rest of the world. Therefore, if we change our basic views of "what sex is," and if this change is reflected in pornography, we will be lessening, at least in this area of culture, the harmful effects of globalization.

### PORNOGRAPHY: MAN AS "RAGING BEAST"?

What does pornography really imply about men, what lessons does it give about men's supposed "sexual nature"?

Pornography—isn't it predictable? Even if it is, does it matter, since the point is having an orgasm with it, and it is the very clichés that help bring on the orgasm? For some, looking at pornography or having it around is a way of showing others that they're sexy.

For many, pornography feels out of date. It speaks to a passé value system, and it fails to understand (at all!) the new sexual woman. It makes as if to say, "Hey look at us! Aren't we being outrageous and bold?!" But tweaking the nose of traditional values (as pornography does, trying to shock) is not a revolutionary statement or ideological critique of the society. Such would be a shallow idea of politics.

I dislike the clichés most pornography presents about women (including pornography that shows women in the "new role" of dominatrix), as well as the clichéd way it portrays men. Pretending to represent "nature," pornography removes people's ability to relate naturally. In other words, it's a brainwashing device. It's an ideological tool masquerading as basic, raw human nature—which it is not.

Is pornography sexy? It's fun to be "just an animal" sometimes; no one would deny it. But it's also true that sex can carry an ecstatic spiritual emotion with it. Why do we allow one and not the other? Why is it OK to be animal, but not to be spiritual or joyous or in love in pornography? Basically pornography is aimed at men, or someone's idea of men. The female body is being marketed to paper-cut-out versions of "men," which, ironically, ridicule men and their sexuality.

While many remark on the negative image of women in most pornography, I am also interested in the distorted and negative image of men presented in pornography. I don't think that in pornography men are depicted as their authentic selves any more than women are.

Pornography is propaganda for an ideological construct that directs men toward a certain style of reproductive sexual activity, telling them the kind of attitude they should have toward sex, their bodies, and women. Women in pornography legitimize men; they do not act out of their own autonomy (not even when they are shown as dominatrixes, that is, figures that reverse the ideology). The underlying subtext of pornography revolves around the premise that inside every man lurks a raging beast, that this uncivilized, savage animal is the essence of his sexual being and part of his true nature. Thus, the implication is, any attempt by women or men to reshape their sexuality would be a false layer placed on top of a fixed, biological "reality." However, this is only the ideology itself declaring that it is taboo to make changes in it!

Many feminists believe that pornography should be banned as inciting hatred and violence against women. Pornography often does incite men against women, and it can lead to the murder of women and the abduction of girls. Currently in the United States there are 15,000 women missing, and in the United Kingdom, very young girls are regularly abducted, raped, and murdered, as the end of the fantasy; the number of girls and women sold into "sex trafficking" around the world is also very high, as is regularly reported. I would agree with those who want to ban pornography in that it incites hatred against women.

Pornography is teaching roles and behavior to those who look at it, both men and women. Pornography, via the Internet, is going global. It is a thriving business. Since none of us lives on Mars, you are likely to see it from time to time. What to do? While there is nothing wrong if you get excited looking at it, don't be naive; tell yourself: "If I look at it, I am exposed to messages that people want to fill me with, messages I am not aware of (and that they may not fully be aware of, either). No matter how smart I am, maybe some of these messages are going to penetrate and harm me." Try not to let yourself become brainwashed.

## PROBABLY MEN LIKE PORNOGRAPHY?

Not only does pornography denigrate women (it shows women tied up, beaten, and so on), it also denigrates men, destroying their "true sexuality" or possibility of personal sexual discovery and their power to initiate new sexual directions.

Pornography implants clichés, such as "a real man is the one with the biggest, hardest erection," and so on. In most pornography men are portrayed as being either stupid "jerks" who only want to stick their penis into something and "come," or as cynical manipulators with cruel dispositions. No joyousness is depicted.

However, men's sexual feelings are more complex and capable of interesting directions for the future. I studied seven thousand men for several years, asking them (anonymously) about their sexual and emotional feelings for *The Hite Report on Men and Male Sexuality*; that book presents intricate measurements of differences between men's feelings and their actual experiences. The books asks, How would men feel and behave without "performance pressures"? Are men focused on erection and coitus because they feel good, or because they are said to demonstrate manhood, virility, and potency? Why are men's orgasms measurably stronger during masturbation than during "the act"?

Men's bodies, like women's, are composed of a complex and amazingly rich number of systems, glands, hormones, and emotions. In the early embryo the "sex organs" of male and female are the same, it is only after three months that structures in boys develop outside the body, while the same structures in girls develop inside the body, as we see on page 180–181. (By the way, is there a parallel female "sex drive" to the hypothetical male "sex drive"? Logically, if men supposedly have a biological drive to "thrust," then—in this way of thinking—shouldn't women have a complementary or reverse "drive," for example to open?) Sexual exuberance, desire, elation, orgasm, fantasy—all are states that are about something other than a biological "drive."

A completely different kind of erotica is increasingly on view in women's fashion magazines—and sales of these to women, also increasing, show that women have a decided preference for this view of the body and its feelings over older clichés of pornography. (Please don't say that pornography is more naked than "fashion" layouts before taking a good look.)

Do men really like the way they are portrayed in pornography? It's difficult to know, since men are brought up with the idea that you must not flinch. If you find something revolting, you must embrace it, since you are not supposed to be afraid of vulgar things (and if you are, it makes you a girl). It follows that the more disgusting a pornographic image is, the more a "real man" should embrace it and say, "Yeah! That's me!" So it's hard to say if men really like it or not. At the same time, men are absorbing what I consider toxic pictures, often a view of themselves as rapists, really. And I can't think that this view could be good for a man's sexual development or sexual interaction with others. Pornography also reinforces the fear that, as he gets older, the man will lose IT, the big IT. Pornography is not making men sexually sophisticated.

Where does the all-too-frequent male tendency toward violence against women, combined with sexuality, come from? In my overall theory, it comes from a trauma that society forces on boys at puberty in order to disrupt their relationship with their mothers, a trauma Freud and other psychologists overlooked.[5] The depiction of men being violent to women in pornography may be a crime against humanity. Only recently has it been said that, generically, rape in war is a crime that should be punished. In the 1990s wars in Bosnia and parts of the former Yugoslavia, it was mostly Muslim women who were raped (at least this is what was reported), the idea being that the soldiers were trying to ruin the "purity" of that ethnic group. Widespread raping of women by soldiers in Rwanda was also reported in 1998.

Pornography is cashing in on our need to see depictions of some of what we feel and do, so that we don't feel so isolated and uncomfortable doing it; however, pornography is simultaneously feeding us antiquated stereotypes of who we are, loading us up with ideological baggage that equates male sexuality with brutality, and brainwashing us with an exaggerated focus on erection and intercourse. Pornography leaves out most of what men actually do feel and seems to deny the association of sex with positive emotions.

## DO MEN BELIEVE IN LOVE?

Men's descriptions of being in love often imply that intense feelings of being in love with a woman are unwanted, after early experiences that taught avoidance of intense emotion at all costs. "Real love" is seen as less passionately involving, family-oriented, a feeling divorced from "sex."

As one young man describes his feelings when he was in love:

> When she finally broke it off it was as if I had died. It was the only time in my life that I ever cried myself to sleep at night, and this I did frequently. I did not actually consciously think about suicide but I considered myself already dead. A greater emptiness and sense of loss I have not known. Since that time I have not been able to love a woman with such utter abandonment. I just haven't been able to do it. If I were to see her right now I know my heart would jump into my throat.
>
> There is the good kind of love, but then there is the kind that can't; the reasons don't make sense, nothing makes sense. It's like a form of mental illness, completely unexpected, even unwanted. Who in hell would want to feel jealous? Or possessive? But that's all part of it. I want this person so much it makes me feel guilty for wanting too much—guilty and bad. But this is what I live for and think about every day. I think that maybe today it will all work, even though I know that this is foolishness. And that makes me feel bad too. Makes me feel wrong, like I'm feeling something I'm not supposed to because it isn't shared, but I feel anyway.

Another mentions extreme distress:

*I have had thoughts of suicide, of my two arms opening up with the blood flowing out and, with it, my life and the pain. But I have never picked up the knife, there is always one little bit of brain left during these bouts with the Black Thoughts that says, "No." I'm a survivor. The Black Thoughts can come around during a crying jag, or in just silently thinking about "it" and what "it" is doing to me. I tell these things here because it is necessary for men to know that it happens, that a man can be that weak and that vulnerable and know that capacity for hurting. And that crazy, because that's just exactly what it is: crazy.*

## MOST MEN DON'T MARRY THE WOMAN THEY MOST PASSIONATELY LOVE

This is perhaps the central, most important finding of *The Hite Report on Men and Male Sexuality*; however, the real surprise is that most men not only do not marry the woman they most passionately love, but that they remain proud of this, proud of the fact that they "keep control." Why?

Traditionally men have been taught not to take love that seriously—not to "let a woman run your life." But as we have just seen, men do fall in love, and experience all the feelings of ecstasy and abandon, all the happiness that goes with it—for at least two weeks. At this point many men unfortunately become very confused and apprehensive. Being brought up not to let themselves be "out of control" or "overly emotional," men mistrust the excitement, the rush, thinking that feeling that much cannot be good, cannot be relied on, is not "rational"—and therefore not "masculine" and "strong."

Men's comments about these feelings are quite illuminating. "To be in love," as one man in his early twenties writes, "is to be uncomfortable because you are out of control, you do things you wouldn't normally do. Women are more willing to be dependent, or part of another person, than a man who wants to keep a separation, keep himself for himself, who fears losing his independence. Of course, one does sometimes start to fall in love, but you can always stop it before it's too late. It will be nice in the future if they invent a pill to neutralize you if you fell in love—to alleviate your dis-ease!"

Most men are so uncomfortable with feelings of love, desire/need, and vulnerability, that they do not marry the woman they are most "in love" with. Distrusting the feelings, they run from their own emotional openness and, furthermore, are proud that they "made the right decision," "didn't let their feelings carry them away" and "stayed in control"—made a "rational decision." They are proud and feel that they did the right thing, marrying "more sensibly."

And yet this decision, added to the fact that most men are brought up not to respect women—other than as mothers or mothering-type helping figures—puts most marriages in a very vulnerable, problematic position. An additional problem is most men's training not to talk about feelings or to solve emotional problems by discussing them, talking them out. Most men's reaction to a dispute would be to retain "manly" objectivity by going for a walk, and the like, expecting the air to have cleared on their return, and to feel proud of this solution, since they had not "lost control."

Many men in this study said that they were deeply frustrated, angry, or disappointed with their emotional relationships with women, at the same time that they treasured these relationships as providing the happiest and most intimate moments of their lives.

Most men had not married the women they most passionately loved. Most men did not feel comfortable being deeply in love.[6] Although they sounded very similar to women when they spoke of the first wonderful feelings of falling in love, very soon thereafter many began to feel uncomfortable, anxious, even trapped—and wanted to withdraw. Most men felt very out of control of their emotions when they were in love, not reasonable and "rational," and most men did not like this feeling; men have been taught that the worst thing possible is to be out of control, to be "overly emotional," as this behavior is "womanly" (uncool).

Thus, being in love, a man begins to feel out of control, "unmanly," and even worse, he begins to feel that he is controlled by the woman—that is, he would do anything to please her, he is afraid of her displeasure, and so he is "dominated" by her. This is an intolerable situation. Add to this the idea that most men still believe on some level that there are two kinds of women: "good," motherly women, and "bad," sexy women. The man, feeling very attracted when falling in love, is sure that he should not let himself go into his love, trust in it, and count on her. At this point he tends to pull back, to try to provoke a fight or find a problem in the relationship, in order to regain his former stance in life, his "control." He looks for, or believes he should look for, someone more "stable," someone who doesn't put him in a constant position of rethinking his life. Most men described this as a "rational" decision and took pride in having acted wisely, remaining cool and collected, and "using their heads"—even though they missed their lost love.

Most of the men in these marriages were not monogamous, as we shall see. Most marriages based on this "rational" idea tended to develop a pattern (at least in the man) of extramarital sex unknown to the woman—though, since there was such emotional distance in the marriage anyway, sometimes the wife did know but just did not care, since she herself had little interest in sex with her husband. These ("traditional") marriages, while not close in the romantic sense, could often be long-term. If reasons other than love were the basis of the marriage in the first place, it was not necessary to maintain a high level of communication, intimacy, or understanding to ensure continuation of the marriage. "Newer" marriages, in which emotional closeness and equality between the man and woman were goals, tended to be more monogamous and also to have quite different sexual patterns.

Are men getting the most they can out of life, preoccupied with being "on top," or are men being shortchanged?

## MEN'S GREAT SENSUALITY—AS YET UNTAPPED?

Why is male sexuality so closely identified with intercourse? Have men missed the boat because of the total focus on intercourse society teaches them, or because of the (also learned) dominating, goal-oriented definition of their sexuality?

Even if clitoral stimulation to orgasm is included before intercourse, as long as "sex" equals "foreplay," followed by "vaginal penetration" (why not call it "penile enfolding?"), and ends with male orgasm in the vagina, it means that sex will still be focused on intercourse and will retain its overly structured definition, making men worry about "performance pressures" and "what a man should do."

Defining sex as basically intercourse holds men back from getting to know and appreciate their own sensuality, forcing them into an unnecessary, anxious preoccupation with erection. The focus on coitus tends to cut off many men's erotic responses before they even get started. For example, many men cut short "foreplay" and physical affection because they are afraid they may lose their erection. But men could reach much higher peaks of feeling and arousal if they did not feel anxious about how they "should" behave sexually and if they did not focus so much on reaching orgasm.

Men's denial of their great sensuality is significant because it is part of the overall denial by men of their feelings and emotions. The traditional definition of masculinity tries to close men off from their full capacity to feel joy, sadness, love, the world, life. Men have everything to gain from leaving behind the mechanical view of "male sexuality" and at the same time developing a greater appreciation of their untapped sensuality, their own capacity for enjoyment and expression. Men's experience of their own bodies has been cut off, limited, falsified by the culture's insistence that "male sexuality" is a simple mechanistic drive for intercourse.

"Sex" could be redefined to become something with infinite variety, not always including intercourse or even orgasm (for either person). It can become part of an individual vocabulary of many ways to relate physically—including activities that express anger, tenderness, passion, and/or love, depending on the current feelings of the two people. Sex can be a way of expressing a thousand different feelings, saying a thousand different things.

Can men imagine a new conception of male sexuality and sensuality not necessarily focused on intercourse or orgasm? Would men like to diversify and expand, to eroticize their sexuality to become less constantly active, sometimes more passive, more receptive? Have most men ever experienced sex as less orgasm and more passion?

Why is intercourse so important to most men, or why is it portrayed in pornography as being the object of most men's lust? The usual assumption is that "men are made like that by their hormones, they can't help it." However, this belief is an assumption, not a fact, since no one can show how hormones create psychology. On the other hand, it is relatively easy to show—as this research does (no other research seems to have tried)—that there are many cultural messages to men coercing them to define themselves in this way.

Not only are men encouraged to want intercourse by a culture that claims this is how "real men" behave, but men are also left little other choice of ways to be truly close and intimate with other human beings. If men are cut off from each other—first from their fathers, by the "rules" of male behavior, and later, following that example, from their friends, at least in the sense of being able to talk intimately and show affec-tion—then men must turn to women for close companionship. But at the same time, they are "supposed" to dominate those women. For example, boys should not hang out with their sisters after a certain age. It is in this confused atmosphere that men and women experience "sex." Even more confusing, it is in the moments of sexual intimacy that most men feel most free to talk about their feelings, problems, hopes, and dreams. This, in combination with the need we all have for close, warm body contact, can make a sexual connection with a woman almost the most important need a man has. And the central focus of that sexual connection is intercourse. Only intercourse, per-haps, has the symbolic overtones to make this connection deep enough. But the sym-bolism has both a positive and negative aspect.

## ORIGINS OF THE DEFINITION OF SEX AS INTERCOURSE FOR MEN

In fact, the current definition of "sex"—basically, "foreplay" followed by intercourse and ending with male orgasm in the vagina as the "right" way to have sex—has not always been the definition of sex. Everything we think of as "male sexuality" is in very large part a reflection of the values and needs of the society we live in and the culture we have inherited. The definition of sex as we know it was begun approximately 2,500 years ago for the purpose of increasing reproduction. It was at this time that the Hebrew tribes returned from the Babylonian exile, a small, struggling group. These tribes passed a law, the first such law we know of, stating that henceforth, all sexual activ-ities other than heterosexual intercourse would be illegal. The Old Testament warned against other forms of sexuality, including "spilling one's seed" (masturbation), oral sex, and the sexual practices of the "heathens" (surrounding tribes), especially the Babylonians, who worshipped female and male goddesses and gods. This officially promoted focus on reproductive activities (and glorification of intercourse) was important for the small tribes, since only through increasing their populations could they become more powerful, consolidate their hold on their territory, cultivate and har-vest more crops, and maintain a large army to defend themselves.

This definition of sex also reflected a new male ascendancy in society at that time: henceforth, children (and women) were to belong to the fathers (or hus-bands), a situation that had not previously been the case. The Hebrew tribes (pos-sibly influenced by traditions of invading Indo-European or Aryan tribes) were organized along a patriarchal social structure. That is, the tribes were ruled by men; women and children were owned, legally, by an individual man (husband or father), who in turn owed his allegiance, legally, to a male king, who in turn owed his allegiance to a male priesthood and a male god. But the Babylonians, like many other societies of the time (for example the Canaanites), worshiped not one male god, but many deities, many of which were female; and indeed, it was women who were the priests. Queens in these societies were frequently more powerful than, or as powerful as, kings, harking back to earlier, nonpatriarchal civilizations.

The exact nature of the nonpatriarchal tradition is still a matter of debate,[7] but many scholars now agree that, based on archaeological evidence, early periods of history saw quite different forms of social organization from our own. Possibly women were held in higher esteem than today, and in general women were usually in charge of the temples and the distribution of food and goods. Whether women were also warriors is not known, although many goddesses were addressed as warrior-goddesses. And the "sex" (that is, physical relations between individuals) and family structures were in all probability quite different in these early forms of social organization from their forms in the later patriarchal structure.

The following are simplified versions of some hypotheses of the changes that seem to have taken place over a period of a thousand or more years, perhaps between 8000 to 5000 B.C.

The very earliest societies may have venerated women because women could bring forth new life. In fact, they could reproduce males as well as females like themselves. Some scholars believe that in early societies, much earlier than the Babylonians or the Egyptians, the relationship between intercourse and pregnancy was not known, and so the male's role in reproduction was unknown. Additionally, the earliest families we know of did not consist of the mother, father, and child as we know them today, but rather a group that included the mother, sisters, brothers, aunts, uncles, and children; children could be brought up by various members of the group, the biological mother having had the choice of whether to "stay at home" with the child or not. In other words, there has not always been the close tie between the biological mother and child (nor the father and child) we consider "natural" today; children of many mothers mixed together and were brought up by many members of the group. In fact, the concept of private property may not yet have existed or may have been very weak or unimportant to the society; certainly children were not "owned."

It has been theorized that when the male contribution to childbearing became known, possibly around 10,000 or more years ago (this knowledge coming at different times to different societies); there began a gradual shift to increased male involvement in religious functions, and gradually to the system of the patriarchal social order, in which men were almost entirely dominant. Scholars are only slowly piecing together fragments of records to understand what happened in these early times; much remains to be understood. However, some scholars see the Old Testament as, among other things, representing the story of the early patriarchal struggle against goddess worship and female-oriented societies, and the transition to a male-dominated, "one-god" society. The history of Greece, also, and the chronological changes in Greek mythology, have been seen as representing a changeover in thinking from goddess worship to God ascendancy.[8] A similar change from the ascendancy of queens to the ascendancy of kings can be seen in several centuries of early Egyptian history. The transition from Cretan culture to later Mycenaean/mainland Greek culture is another example. These interpretations, while steadily gaining adherents, are far from orthodox. However, scholars generally agree on a recent revision of the extent of our fully human ("civilized") history: according to the latest estimate, complex human societies existed as far back as 40,000 years ago—quite an increase over previous estimates.

What was the role of intercourse in prepatriarchal or "matriarchal" societies? Even in early patriarchal or transitional times, intercourse was not considered the greatest physical pleasure but basically was practiced for reproduction; this was true, for example, in most periods of Greek and Roman history. What must sex and physical relations have been like even earlier, then, 20,000 or 40,000 years ago, when it may have been believed (at least for some time) that women became pregnant simply by lying in the moonlight? When intercourse was not an especially noted symbol in the society?

Were sexual feelings tied to religious ("fertility") group activities, rather than to "romantic" personal activities? Or were sexual feelings and orgasm linked to "romantic" personal feelings, while fertility activities (whatever they may have been) were linked to group or religious activities? There is some evidence that the latter may have been the case, but we honestly do not know what people did.*

But to return to the present, it must now be clear how completely sex as we know it is tied to our own history and social organization. The definition of "sex" has come down to us from the early Judeo-Christian laws, which became the civil code of the entire West and which define our present civil code. In addition, old church laws are still enforced by many churches today. For example, the Catholic Church insists that women must not use birth control, since the purpose of sex is reproduction and since women should make their bodies available to their husbands for this purpose at all times and that the fathers will own the children.

It is also important to note that other societies, like those of Japan, China, India, and the Arab world, once they became patriarchal, also defined sex in much the same way—that is, regulated physical relations so that maximum reproduction, with the children being owned by the father. In other words, the reproductive definition of sexuality is an inherent part of a patriarchal society. In order for men to

---

* However, women then, as today, must have known about the importance of the clitoris, since, as discussed in *The Hite Report on Female Sexuality*, women in the twentieth century, without being given any information whatsoever on how, began to masturbate quite early in their lives; for the great majority of women this has meant manual clitoral stimulation. It is logical to assume that if women do this "instinctively" today, women must also have done this then, and known that the clitoris was a pleasurable area to have stimulated. Was this activity part of sexual institutions or customs at that time? Was masturbation considered private? What other activities were considered important?

control a society, it has been essential for men to control reproduction and to own the children.

Sexuality today is changing. Increasing population is not as necessary to the power of a society as it once was, since we now have very large populations and, even more importantly, machines (and computers) that can do much of the work large populations once performed, from farming to defending a country. As society feels it no longer needs to encourage reproduction to the extent that it once did, birth control is becoming more and more acceptable (legal) and male ownership of children (and marriage) less crucial, with "living together" arrangements more accepted.

However, this change has not yet deeply affected our idea of what sex is or could be. Even though we frequently use birth control, we still generally follow the traditional reproductive definition of physical relations, centered on intercourse. But, as seen in this book, some men are beginning to question the assumptions of our culture about "male sexuality" and our definition of sex: even though the issues are just beginning to surface, there is a gut feeling on the part of most men that something is wrong, that although there are beautiful elements to sex as we know it, somehow there are unnecessary problems, too.

DECONSTRUCTING INTERCOURSE: IS IT THE GREATEST MALE SEXUAL PLEASURE?

How much of men's desire for intercourse is due to our culture's insistence that all men "should" seek and want intercourse, that it is "natural" for men; and how much is due to an individual man's desire to have intercourse with a particular woman, for his own personal reasons? We can never know exactly. But it does seem clear that, without the accompanying cultural symbolism and pressures, intercourse would become a matter of choice during sexual activities, not the sine qua non of sexual encounter. This is not to say, of course, that men and women will not continue to enjoy intercourse with each other when they want, but simply that sex could be more enjoyable for both people if intercourse were not a "requirement"—if intercourse were a choice and not a given. Sex does not always have to include intercourse, and sex would become much freer if intercourse were not always its focus.

Intercourse is at once one of the most beautiful and at the same time most oppressive and exploitative acts of our society. It has been symbolic of men's ownership of women, as just described, for approximately the last 3,000 years. It is the central symbol of patriarchal society; without it, there could be no patriarchy. Intercourse culminating in male orgasm in the vagina is the sublime moment during which the male contribution to reproduction takes place. This is the reason for its glorification. And as such, men must love it; intercourse is a celebration of "male" patriarchal culture.

Surely the definition of sex as we know it (that is, intercourse) is guaranteed to make a man feel that his needs are serious, worthwhile, and important—at least his need for orgasm and his need for stimulation of the penis to reach that orgasm.

This fact is so obvious that it is usually overlooked or taken as a "given," a simple "bio-logical" imperative. However, our definition of sex is, to a large extent, culturally, and not biologically, created. Women's need for orgasm and for specific clitoral stimulation to reach that orgasm is not honored or respected in the traditional definition of sex. Certainly it is not enshrined within an institution, as is male orgasm. Although perhaps the institution we know as "sex" was created to lead to male orgasm in the vagina not because of male dominance but only because of the society's desire to increase reproduction, nevertheless the man himself, as eventual owner of the child (should pregnancy occur) and of the woman, must surely feel secure in the knowledge that this ritual honors him and enshrines and venerates his orgasm. Thus men feel that their orgasm during intercourse is good. However, men usually do not attribute creation of the institution to man-made society; they look, rather, to biological or religious sources—that is, "It's just the way things are," or as one man said, "Intercourse is a heavenly blessing which God created for man."

In addition, this cultural institution, this symbolic rite, is aided and attended to by another person, a woman. If male orgasm is the sacrament here, the woman functions as the priestess. This woman not only gives the man a sense of being accepted and desirable on an individual, personal level, but also gives him a further sense of acceptance by joining in and catering to the sequence of events that culminates in his orgasm. This woman, with perhaps varying degrees of enthusiasm, but almost never with withdrawal once "sex" (the ritual sequence of events), and especially intercourse, has begun, helps him along toward his orgasm and a sense of pleasure.

Both men and women feel that such is women's role. And yet most women still do not feel that they have a similar automatic right to clitoral stimulation to orgasm—and even less do they feel that they have the right to touch or stimulate themselves to orgasm, and still less do they feel they have the right to insist that men cater to their needs (especially if the woman is not also catering to the man's needs). Why does our society consider it perfectly acceptable to assume that "sex" can be defined as intercourse to male orgasm "every time," with clitoral stimulation to female orgasm included only "sometimes" or not at all, while considering it outrageous to define "sex" as clitoral stimulation to female orgasm "every time," with only rare penis stimulation/intercourse to male orgasm?

In addition, in traditional intercourse, the man was on top of the woman, adding to the symbolic impact of his culturally decreed superiority. Also, the fact that he almost always had an orgasm and she did not further encouraged him to think of himself as superior, more successful, healthier, and more sexual (more fully evolved, as some contemporary psychiatrists have recently asserted), as opposed to the "weaker" woman, who was not able to have a similar climax (despite the fact that she almost certainly was not getting the right stimulation).

In other words, during traditional intercourse the ancient patriarchal symbolism of the man on top comes to the fore: the man on top, "taking" his pleasure, the whole force of the social structure behind him, telling him that what he is doing is Good and Right and that he is a Strong Male, with the woman looking up into his eyes, not resisting and hopefully celebrating these feelings with him, saying Yes, you are great.

And there is yet another point: the symbolic acceptance of the sperm by the woman. As the woman accepts the semen, she accepts an intimate part of the man and, at least symbolically, she accepts the idea of carrying a child for him. Intercourse in patriarchy, as we remember, means power because a man can say, "I own this woman. I can make her pregnant." This process was equated with power in early patriarchy, because earlier societies had not known the connection between intercourse (sperm) and pregnancy; they thought women reproduced by themselves. After this connection was discovered, the erect penis gradually became the dominant symbol in society that it remains today. Before this, the female body, and especially the vulva and breasts (as seen in the thousands of fertility goddess statues that have been unearthed), was the primary symbol.

This is not to say, of course, that intercourse does not feel good to both women and men. It is just that superimposed on these basic feelings is an enormous cultural symbolism that has become so ingrained in all our minds, both male and female, that it is hard for us to be sure just why we do like intercourse.

Another facet of patriarchal ideology is that intercourse is both a rite of passage and a form of male bonding. Boys are told that they cannot have intercourse; only men can. Thus intercourse becomes a test of status and dominance through which males prove their membership in the male group—not only the first time they do it, but every time. One basic definition of a "man" is one who has intercourse with women. Why is this? Would this be a test of "masculinity" (whatever that may be) in a society that did not hold reproduction as a primary value? Historically speaking, the association of masculinity and intercourse (and the emphasis on "performance") grew out of a social system that wanted more soldiers and farmers. In fact, for quite a long time intercourse was not connected with love or romantic love, nor was it even considered necessarily the main thing a "man" would want to do: Greek men, for example, often seemed quite happy having sex among themselves—considering intercourse with their wives a duty necessary basically only for procreation. No doubt this was the way the wife viewed it as well, since her orgasm was not a consideration. (Was she having orgasms through masturbation? Or with her women acquaintances with whom she spent the day? No one knows.) And even earlier, Hebrew men had to be admonished in the Old Testament not to "spill their seed"—that is, masturbate—or practice sodomy, but instead to have vaginal intercourse. This implies that they may have found it more pleasurable or convenient to masturbate or to have other sex for orgasm, and that in fact such may have been their custom.

In patriarchal society, then, intercourse for a man has the whole force of a society's approval behind it: he is doing what the entire society says he should be praised for doing, and the woman's acceptance of him functions as a symbol of the acceptance of him by the entire social order—and especially by other men. However, intercourse does not bestow the same feeling of social acceptance upon women; the meaning of sex/intercourse for women is quite different. Although the woman, as an agent for the society (fulfilling her socially dictated role as nurturer, helper), is bestowing acceptance and approval (and the stimulation for male orgasm) on the man, she is frequently not getting any of the above in return. In addition, society does not praise her for having intercourse. Her orgasm is not enshrined, and she may be looked down on by the man for having "given herself." This is another issue, one that was covered in *The Hite Report on Female Sexuality*, but it is well to keep in mind how differently our culture has chosen to reward the two sexes for the same activity.

Still, women do enjoy intercourse, and women and men do often transcend these cultural meanings in their personal lives. Although intercourse has been a symbol of masculinity and male power, it need not continue to be. As women gain equality—economic, social, and legal—intercourse can lose these exploitative connotations to become once more a simple thing of beauty and freedom—and above all, a choice.

Finally, the point here is not that men are wrong for liking and wanting intercourse, but that they should be freed from feeling that they must have intercourse to have true sex—and to be "real" men. It would be senseless to "blame" anyone, either men or women, for traditional and stereotyped attitudes and behaviors that we all learn every day and endlessly hear repeated around us. The point now is to reexamine the part intercourse plays in our lives, to reassess our personal definitions of sex, and try to create more individual, and more equal, forms of physical relations.

In fact, it may be, on some level, just this cultural catering to men during intercourse that also makes men feel uncomfortable, uneasy, and ambivalent about it. Do they want to feel the object of so much unequal attention? Do men want to feel that the success or failure of the whole ritual rests on their performance? The ideal of masculinity glorifies men at the same time that it dehumanizes them.

## IS "MALE SEXUALITY" A SIMPLE HORMONAL DRIVE, A "BIOLOGICAL FACT OF LIFE," OR IS IT SOCIALLY CONSTRUCTED?

"Male" sexuality is central to the definition of masculinity, and masculinity is central to the entire culture—in a sense, it is the culture. Therefore what we are looking at here is far more than male sexuality, it is a way of life, the world itself, a culture in microcosm. To discuss sex is to discuss our most basic views of who we are, what we want life to be, and what kind of a society we believe in.

## IS MEN'S FOCUS ON COITUS "NATURAL"?*

Why do men want intercourse? Most men like and want intercourse. However, the reasons they give in response to the questions posed in my research are surprising.

---

* If coitus is really the basic expression of men's "sexual drive," why does society need so many laws and religious injunctions to insist that this is the only "right" way for them to have sex?

It is almost universally assumed that what men like/want from intercourse is orgasm. And yet men point out over and over that they can easily have an orgasm from their own stimulation (and often a stronger one than during coitus). In fact, what men want from intercourse is something else:

*I like intercourse more psychologically than physically. I get a lot of phys-ical pleasure from intercourse, but I can also get that from masturbating. The physical feeling of moving my penis back and forth inside my lover is pleasurable, but probably not as intense as a good hand job or fellatio combined with hands. Psychologically, though, there's much to want— the anticipation of putting my penis inside my lover, knowing I'm going to be surrounded by her, warmed by the inside of her. Then when I first slowly enter her, I want the instant to last and last. I like to stop moving, just lie there, and think and feel, "This is happening to me. This is so neat. I feel so good."*

Boys are brought up to equate intercourse with manhood:

*I felt (and still do, to a lesser extent) incredible pressure on me to prove my manhood by screwing women. This pressure made it harder on me to meet women and have sexual relations with them. I had to do it; if I didn't there was something wrong with me. Also, it was supposedly so great, look what I was missing. This pressure bred its own miserable rationales, e.g., "women always want it, even when they say 'no.'" Thus, I had no excuses. If I couldn't find a woman to fuck, it was my fault. I was a failure. I feel this pressure helped retard my sexual growth and expe-rience and placed undue importance on fucking.*

Some men did not answer whether they liked intercourse, or why, but simply stated that intercourse is what men do—the natural and inevitable expression of an "instinctive" male "sex drive."

*Sex identifies me to myself as a man; sex admits me to full citizenship in my species and my world. Without sex I would regard myself as somewhat less than a man and somewhat less than a person.*

*I feel that our Creator made men with a penis and women with a vagina for a reason, and that's for intercourse.*

*Being a healthy male, sex is very important to me. The purpose of sex is a normal function of the human mind and body.*

Many men's answers seem to suggest that they are not sure how often they would like to have intercourse, but that they are fairly sure that they should be having it more often than they are, or that other men are having it more than they are. There is also a vague sense of disquiet in some answers in which men say that it is not theirs to choose how often they will have intercourse, that at any moment the woman/women may "shut them out" and refuse to have intercourse with them.

In fact, the cultural pressure on men to have frequent intercourse is based on a purely mechanical definition of masculinity, in which the desire/"need" for intercourse is related solely to a man's supposed inner hormonal cycles, or some other mysterious innate sexual urges. Of course, how often a man has or wants to have an orgasm is a separate matter from how often he has or wants to have intercourse.

It is possible that our culture has pushed men to "want" intercourse more than they, without this pressure, might. Certainly it is possible to have sex without having intercourse. And certainly, men have the right to go without sex entirely or not to have sex with a partner (celibacy) if they want, as almost all men in fact do at some point in their lives. Men should not be made to feel that they "have to" have sex/intercourse to prove they are men or for any other reason.

The cultural emphasis on erection, which leads to an ever-present fear of lack of erection, forces most men to become focused on getting and maintaining an erection during sex. This in turn forces the activities to revolve around the erection, influencing the timing and sequence of events. Physical relations could develop a more spontaneous feeling if the importance of erection were greatly deemphasized. Older men, who may have trouble achieving or maintaining an erection (but not always), have been ridiculed and made to feel "less than men" by the society; in fact, often their diversification and rethinking of sexual pleasure has made them "better" lovers than younger men.

And some men did in fact feel repulsed by the vulgarization of their sexuality through cultural/advertising images of how "a real man is just naturally crazy for sex." Many men voiced a strong reaction against some of the ideas of the "sexual revolution," including the idea that men should want/have sex and intercourse at any time or place, not needing an emotional relationship or feelings:

> It's depressing. I don't usually have sex just for lust, it's more spiritual. I'm old-fashioned, romantic. I'm a dreamer, I guess.

> I hate the sexification of everything in which oppressive sex roles are just more visible and blatant, and everybody goes around acting terribly sexy and fucking each other's brains out, and sex is openly alluded to in aspirin commercials and toothpaste promos, etc. I think that's sometimes called the sexual revolution and I hate it.

The pressure on men to be "sexual" and to have frequent sex has been particularly strong during the last twenty years, especially since the 1940s and World War II, with the increasing equation of masculinity with aggressive characteristics. As mentioned elsewhere, in Victorian times men were often urged (by doctors and others) not to have sex and orgasm too often, lest they drain themselves of their "vital fluids" and become weak. Today just the opposite is urged. The idea of a male "biological need" for penetration and intercourse, an aggressive, animalistic "sex drive," was incorporated into the movement for sexual "freedom" known as the "sexual revolution."

## MALE "SEX DRIVE": REAL OR IMAGINED?

The term "male sex drive" is part of the larger reproductive ideology of our patriarchal society; there is no biological or physical proof of a male "sex drive" for intercourse. Although both men and women do have a need (or "drive") for orgasm from time to time, there is no evidence that men biologically "need" vaginas in which to orgasm or that there is anything hormonal or "instinctual" that drives men toward women or vaginas.

Many kinds of physical contact are enjoyed by other mammals just as frequently as, or more frequently than, coitus, which is practiced only when females are in estrus. (Humans do not have estrus in anything like the same way.) Most mammals spend more time on grooming and petting each other than they do on specifically sexual (genital) contact, as many primate researchers have described. Mammals and other animals also masturbate and quite commonly have homosexual relations. Among the animals for whom these activities have been recorded are the rat, chinchilla, rabbit, porcupine, squirrel, ferret, horse, cow, elephant, dog, baboon, monkey, chimpanzee, and many others.

Our culture seems to assume that since (theoretically) sexual feelings are provided by nature to ensure reproduction, intercourse is (or should be) "instinctive" behavior. Yet when one looks at other animals, it is obvious that other forms of touching and genital sexuality are just as "instinctive." Masturbation may even be a more natural behavior than intercourse, since chimpanzees brought up in isolation have no idea how to have intercourse but do masturbate almost from birth.

And finally, if (as is so frequently asserted) intercourse really is "instinctive" and all else is "unnatural," why do we need laws and social institutions that both glorify and require intercourse (especially in marriage), while setting up grave penalties and taboos against other forms of sexuality?

## BUILT-IN "INADEQUACY" FOR MEN IN THE CURRENT DEFINITION OF "SEX"

A constant source of anxiety among men is whether they continue intercourse long enough, remaining erect, or whether they reach orgasm "too soon." Most men, although they sometimes used the term "premature ejaculation," did not in fact refer to its standard clinical meaning—that is, orgasm before or just at the moment of penetration—but rather referred to widely varied amounts of time of intercourse.

In fact, most men who expressed this concern felt that this was probably the reason why a woman might not reach orgasm during intercourse with them; this thinking is inaccurate, however, as discussed in *The Hite Report on Female Sexuality*.

As many as 74 percent of the men who answered expressed concern over whether they continued intercourse long enough:

> *Sadly, so far, I have been climaxing too soon to suit me. I can't control it. And I feel as though I haven't really done much for my partner even though I do try to continue stimulation somehow. I consider it a failed test of virility.*

The popular media are constantly warning men against "coming too soon," insisting that this circumstance is the cause for most women failing to have orgasm from intercourse (coitus). Thus, most men feel it is their duty to the woman to have intercourse for as long as possible, so that the woman can have a chance to orgasm too. However, the results of *The Hite Report on Female Sexuality* suggest that this aim is a fallacy, since whether a woman has an orgasm is usually not related to length of intercourse. In fact, most women do not orgasm simply as a result of intercourse; and the minority of women who do, do so not so much from sustained thrusting as from specific clitoral stimulation during intercourse.

But the amount of pressure on men has been enormous. Men have been getting a double message: on the one hand they are told that it is very "virile" to become erect and excited and thrust home to orgasm; on the other hand, they are told not to orgasm "too soon." Since most men get rather good stimulation during thrusting, these suggestions provide a contradiction—leaving most men feeling slightly uneasy, guilty, and inadequate.

Although extending intercourse can be a pleasure in itself for both men and women, this guilt is unnecessary—as long as women's needs are acknowledged in a realistic manner at some time during sex, or any special needs of women desiring to orgasm during intercourse are fulfilled in a mutually agreeable fashion.

## PENIS SIZE: "DUDAS DE UN CHICO"

It seems that young men in their twenties today are still as worried about penis size as men have been for a long time. A young man (age eighteen) writes me with great sincerity, "I have a problem. My girlfriend reaches orgasm when I masturbate her or I practice oral sex on her, but not with penetration. I worry that the problem could be my penis size; I am in erection 20 cm tall and 12 cm around."

Although this cliché was overturned in the 1960s, it seems to have made a dramatic comeback. Discussions of the drug Viagra have added to the presumption on the part of the very young that "everybody knows" a man should have "a big hard one."

Many young men also have a prejudice against practicing c-spot stimulation with their female partners ("less manly than doing it to her with your dick"). As one puts it, "I understand that some women cannot reach orgasm with penetration, but I still want to try to make them happy." In what he thinks is an understanding statement, by his choice of words he has already put any female partner he might have on the defensive! First, he implies that only "some women" have this "lack of capacity," thus they are "incapable," "not like the others," and so on. In other words, they are "semifailures" and "not as good as" the others.

Rather than accept the reality of how most women reach orgasm, being happy about the variety and spontaneity offered, sharing that and changing the shape of "sex," some men worry about whether or not they have the "right" penis size, that is, "Whether or not I am big enough." The supposition is, "I'm sure that if I were big enough, she would have orgasm during penetration—just like in the porno movies!" Is it penis size such men are worried about, or do they feel a fear of learning the "ins-and-outs" of clitoral stimulation?

Maybe it is natural for people, when they find that life is different from what they have been told, to have doubts. Is it natural at this stage in our history that people would be filled with doubts? After all, for many centuries it has been said that "sex" should happen in one particular way. We are on the cutting edge of a new society, and it takes courage to live one's life authentically, believe in oneself and in one's partner.

An insistence on focusing on erection does a terrible disservice to both men and women. Any man who finds himself thinking something like this, should ask himself if he believes that he has been brainwashed by imposed beliefs about "having a hard penis"—or if he really is speaking about his own pleasure in feeling excited when he has an erection. Feeling the pleasure of one's own body is clearly the right of every human being; being brainwashed by slogans that are not good for you or your partner is another matter altogether.

### PRESSURE TO "MAKE HER COME"

Closely linked with the traditional pressure on men to maintain erection and thrusting during intercourse is the idea that it is a man's role to "give" the woman an orgasm during intercourse. Just as the man has traditionally been considered the "provider" economically—the man should "bring home the bacon" or buy the house—he has also been given the role of "providing" the woman with sexual satisfaction. A "real man" should "make her come."

This idea often puts the man in a no-win situation, since the information he has been given—that thrusting during intercourse should bring a woman to orgasm—is faulty. The result may be that he doubts his masculinity whenever female orgasm does not occur, or that the woman is pressured to fake orgasms. This needless pressure alienates men and women, as each blames the other when expectations are not met.

QUESTION:

Do you feel there is something wrong with your "performance," technique, or sensitivity if the woman does not orgasm from intercourse itself? That you're "not man enough"?

A few men insisted that women never fail to orgasm with them:

*Are you kidding? I never had a complaint.*

*I never have failed a woman yet to achieve orgasm.*

*Never had the problem.*

*Experience has shown that if a woman can't orgasm with me, she can't with anybody. I have brought out the first orgasm in several.*

But the overwhelming majority of men realized that women often did not orgasm during intercourse, and they found this a source of pressure. Many felt that the situation was their fault:

*If anything goes wrong, I'm blamed for it. Girls always seem to just lay there and say, "O.K., make it happen." I feel an immense pressure to perform and feel that it's all up to me.*

This pressure to orgasm from intercourse has been very oppressive to women, and has often led to faked orgasms. Although men say that they do not feel guilty, there is a tone of defensiveness. The unrealistic goal of women reaching orgasm simply from the rubbing of the penis in the vagina has placed undue pressure on both men and women.

### DOUBTS AND LACK OF INFORMATION ABOUT WOMEN'S ORGASMS

What is the cause of women's seeming lack of interest in sex? Of what many men call women's "passivity" during sex? Certainly it is not any innate biological difference from men in desire for orgasm[*] or desire for closeness and touching. Nor is it, for the most part, "Victorian upbringing," although this was the explanation to which many men turned. Nor is a woman's passivity related in older women to "menopause," since menopause does not in any way reduce or end women's sexual feelings.

One of the most obvious explanations: most women's need for specific (noncoital)

---

[*] Most women masturbate to orgasm very regularly, especially when they do not reach orgasm with a partner; just because women's desire for orgasm has often been hidden from society it is not any less than men's.

clitoral stimulation to orgasm is frequently not recognized, so many women never or rarely orgasm during sex with men. This habitual denial of women's sexual needs reflects the larger social system in which women have been given second-class status for hundreds of years.

Most men who participated in this research stated that they had experienced a great deal of insecurity and confusion over knowing when—or whether—a woman had had an orgasm. (The overwhelming majority were looking for this orgasm during intercourse.) In fact, most men had great doubts about whether, or how frequently, women had orgasms with them; 61 percent of the men who answered reported that they usually could not tell, or could not be sure, when a woman had an orgasm.

Most men still assume that women should orgasm from intercourse and lack information about the clitoris:

*I always assumed there was something wrong with them if they couldn't orgasm with each intercourse without clitoral stimulation. That prejudice dies hard. Although now I know what the truth is, doubts still remain just below rational consciousness.*

*One weekend my wife sent the kids off to their grandparents' house, and then she told me she had something to tell me. Well, what it was was that she didn't have orgasms the way I thought she did, that she didn't mean to hurt me, that she had really loved having sex with me all those years, but she just hadn't been honest. I was flabbergasted, I didn't know what to say. We started talking and she told me just how she did orgasm, and then I couldn't believe my eyes, she showed me how she did it. I have never been the same since, I mean for the better. I fell in love with her all over again, or anyway, I got a case of the hots for her that didn't quiet down for about six months. She was much more interested in sex than before. I learned how to make her come with my hand and we started specializing in weekend-long sex sessions. It was just too much. Bliss. Heaven. I was ready to die.*

*When I first read that women needed stimulation on their clitoris, and didn't usually orgasm with the penis, I thought, but what about all those women who had orgasms with me? Then I realized maybe they didn't really have orgasms, maybe they were just excited with me. I usually said something like "Was it good?" and they would say yeah—but maybe they didn't orgasm at all. That thought really shoots my ego down. Why don't they tell men? Why put men in such a stupid position? It made me feel like a fool, not knowing all those years, and acting like such a big jock. Were the women laughing at me behind my back? Or feeling sorry for me, or thinking I was stupid? Did other men treat them different? It's all just too hard to believe.*

The fact is that only approximately 30 percent of women do orgasm from intercourse itself* (usually from pubic-area contact, rather than thrusting per se); on the other hand, most women orgasm easily from more direct clitoral stimulation.

In spite of this, most men still assume women should orgasm from simple thrusting during intercourse, and would greatly prefer that they do.

QUESTION:
Would you prefer to have sex with a woman who has orgasm from intercourse (coitus), rather than clitoral stimulation?

Most men still assume that women should/would orgasm from simple intercourse (coitus):[†]

> *If she didn't come during intercourse I would wonder why she didn't.*

> *Some women will not orgasm from intercourse. Either they do not know how to make themselves orgasm or they do not want to. I feel a woman should orgasm during intercourse. She should try all different positions till she finds one that is best for her. If a woman can have fantasies when she is having intercourse and learn how to enjoy each movement, she will find that she will orgasm. I have taught this to many women with good results. Of course, the man has to know how to fuck.*

> *A lot of women have trouble reaching a climax. Some women should have surgery or go to a psychiatrist. I went with four women in a row that had to have manual stimulation to reach a climax. I was a little bit shaky, wondering if the entire sex had gone to pot.*

> *I believe that a woman's emotions play a large part in whether she has an orgasm. If I am tender and careful to be attentive to her during intercourse and still she doesn't have an orgasm, then the problem is in her head. She either doesn't love me enough or is preoccupied with something that's bothering her or something. If she wants to be orgasmic, I believe that a woman can be.*

---

* This figure reflects the answers of 3,019 women in *The Hite Report on Female Sexuality*.
† Answers seen here include men of all ages, points of view, and backgrounds; younger and older men alike were just as likely to expect women to orgasm from intercourse and to be unfamiliar with giving clitoral stimulation to orgasm.

And the overwhelming majority of men preferred the woman to orgasm from intercourse/coitus:

> *I prefer to have sex with a woman who orgasms from intercourse to a woman who only orgasms from clitoral stimulation.*

> *I like it if she gets off when I do; I feel like that is the most "natural" and free way for me.*

Others, in their answers to the question on preference, were unclear and confused:

> *I prefer intercourse because during intercourse you get the idea that you're both thoroughly involved at the same time.*

> *Coitus, because I want to feel her orgasm on my penis. Also, I think her orgasm would be more violent and all-encompassing.*

> *Coitus because otherwise it seems too one-sided.*

But most men in this study had not had the actual experience of giving a woman an orgasm from specific clitoral stimulation and thus were answering theoretically.

An almost equally large number answered "either" or "both." Often they included the phrases, "I don't care how she has orgasms—either way," or, "It doesn't matter to me how she does it," or, "Any way she wants to." These statements seemed to indicate less a willingness to try anything than a kind of lack of knowledge, or frustration with the "problem" of women's orgasms—or lack of interest. Perhaps it was easier for these men to say something like, "It doesn't matter to me as long as she gets pleasure" than to really distinguish what it is their partners specifically require:

> *It doesn't really matter—any way they want to get off is fine with me.*

> *It doesn't make much difference to me.*

> *It doesn't matter to me. They usually come during intercourse.*

> *I have only had intercourse with my wife. I don't care how she has orgasm, she can have it any way she wants to. If my wife wants to stimulate herself with a freight train she has my blessing. I will even be the conductor. But if my wife does not orgasm during intercourse I do not feel bad. In fact, I like it better when she does not orgasm because she will be warmer next time. She is best when she orgasms about once a week.*

*I enjoy the freedom of stimulation in any manner. I dislike any limitations.*

*I don't really prefer any certain way for the woman to get off. I don't think that much about whether she is getting off but I do what I can to make the experience the most exhilarating for the both of us.*

*It doesn't matter to me. I prefer to have sex with women that are sexually uninhibited, with open minds, and have clear thoughts about themselves and their sexuality. It doesn't really matter to me where she gets her orgasmic sensations.*

And several men said that they would prefer "both"—as long as her orgasm during intercourse was the grand finale:

*I prefer a woman who has both. The best times are when I can create at least a couple of clitoral orgasms before we begin to have intercourse and then be able to make her climax vaginally three or four times.*

*The woman who has orgasm first from clitoral, then again during intercourse with my orgasm is the best.*

However, some men who gave "both" as their answer indicated a more complete understanding of the alternatives:

*Sometimes I would prefer to have her orgasm from intercourse rather than from clitoral stimulation, but not always. It's a different sort of enjoyment. When she orgasms from intercourse, I have to exercise more self-discipline. However, it does cause contractions in her vagina which give me a good deal of pleasure, as well as her body movements just prior to orgasm. But if she orgasms from clitoral stimulation, I can then fuck at my own speed knowing that she is not depending on me to last a certain length of time. Also when she has her orgasm prior to my entry, it makes her very loose and slippery and sensual, which I like.*

*I don't feel it is very important whether the woman has orgasm from intercourse or clitoral stimulation. Most of the women I have known have had orgasms more readily, and apparently with as much pleasure, from clitoral stimulation. I get a big kick out of stimulating a woman to orgasm with my hand. Orgasm during actual intercourse is also nice. If I stimulate a woman with my hand during sex, it often is the case that the woman can experience more than one orgasm. If she only has orgasm during intercourse, it often excites me to the point of orgasm too, and the woman then has less chance of multiple orgasms, my potential for frequent orgasms being very small.*

Many men avoided answering this question directly, often discussing the importance of feelings while ignoring the issue of how the woman actually did orgasm:

*The partner's type of stimulation is not as important as that there be mutual physical satisfaction and love.*

*How she orgasms is not as important as if she feels love in the act.*

*This is a tricky question. Let's just say that I'll do whatever my partner needs to have done for an orgasm. I'm one of those fools who links sex and love as much as possible—in other words, I try just to make love to women I care a lot about—so giving a woman an orgasm is more important than the process of doing so. In summation of all this, I really don't have a preference.*

*I prefer to have sex with a woman who has knowledge of how to stimulate me and no hang-ups about any part of her own anatomy.*

*The question is whether she had pleasure from going to bed with me and not whether she had an orgasm.*

*I enjoy intercourse with a woman who also enjoys intercourse—however that is accomplished.*

Others expressed confusion over whether intercourse itself actually provides indirect clitoral stimulation for the woman:*

*Why separate orgasm from intercourse from orgasm from clitoral stimulation? Can't coitus also stimulate the clitoris? I do not really have a preference anyway—I want to give a woman what she wants, and as I observe orgasm, I can't tell any difference. Nearly all women can orgasm*

---

* For a discussion of the differences between *The Hite Report on Female Sexuality* and Masters and Johnson's research on this issue, see *The Hite Report on Female Sexuality*, Chapter 3. Basically, Masters and Johnson have said that women should get sufficient indirect clitoral stimulation from the penis's traction on the skin surrounding the vagina, which is indirectly connected to the skin covering the clitoris, to reach orgasm; however, *The Hite Report on Female Sexuality*, based on a much larger sample, found that, in practice, this was not effective for the large majority of women, who need more direct clitoral stimulation for orgasm.

*from finger/tongue stimulation directly to the clitoris. Some have a very hard time reaching orgasm from straight coitus.*

*I try to have my woman get off first during foreplay, then intercourse; both are clitoral stimulation just by different means—or am I mistaken? If they have an orgasm at all, I'm happy.*

*Aren't they the same? Isn't that question settled yet?*

Or they held the misconception that coitus always provides clitoral stimulation:

*I believe clitoral stimulation is the only way a woman can reach orgasm. What most people feel is coital stimulation is really a very gentle and indirect clitoral stimulation.*

A few men used the phrase, "She gets clitoral stimulation from my penis," without any explanation as to what the writer meant or how this might be true—implying a possible misunderstanding of female anatomy:

*During intercourse I never had a woman stimulate herself other than to rub her clitoris against my inserted penis.*

Women in *The Hite Report on Female Sexuality* who had orgasm during intercourse without the addition of manual clitoral stimulation usually got the needed clitoral stimulation from friction on their mons in contact with the man's pubic area, and not from simple thrusting inside the vagina, as these men explain:

*I believe that a woman who has coital orgasm can be easier stimulated to orgasm than one who has clitoral orgasm because of the location of the penis in the vaginal tract.*

*Standing up against a wall allows the woman to get more stimulation of her clitoris. As the penis goes into the vagina the outer lips are pulled down and in slightly. This allows the swollen clitoris to contact the top of the penis and thereby stimulate the woman. However, if the woman is shorter than the man, he must either bend slightly at the knees or she must stand in a little higher on some support.*

*All orgasms are from the clitoris. My penis comes in consistent contact with my wife's clitoris so she's really getting clitoral stimulation as part of our intercourse.*

One man commented:

*Some women like to rub the shaft of the penis against their clitoris as I move in and out, but that is agonizing because it bends the shaft where it isn't supposed to bend.*

However, the fact that these methods can work for some women in some situations does not imply that all women "should" be able to make them work. A great many women can orgasm only with their legs and thighs together.

Most men who had done clitoral stimulation clearly thought of the clitoris as something there to fall back on if nothing else worked; for a woman to have an orgasm from clitoral stimulation was second-best.

Surprisingly, many men whose partners did not orgasm from coitus said that they would still prefer the woman to orgasm in this way—even in cases where coital orgasm was impossible!

Other men, however, clearly expressed that—since it is the woman's anatomy!—it is the woman, not the man, who has the right to a preference:

*Whatever my wife wants is best. She's what I want.*

*I love whatever she loves. I love her, not a 'type' of woman who orgasms from one thing or another.*

*No preferences. You have to find what each woman prefers. I would simply adjust.*

*Her choice.*

A few men did say that not only is clitoral stimulation necessary but that they also enjoy it (!):[*]

*Clitoral stimulation is enjoyable because I can be one hundred percent aware of what is happening to her—preceding, during, and after her orgasm—without having my orgasm distract me from my attention to her.*

*I enjoy stimulating the clitoris and bringing on orgasm manually.*

---

[*] These statements are included here because, even though they seem unremarkable, they were very rare.

## BOTTOM LINE

There was a tendency in some of the answers to this question to hope or assume, if the respondent was aware of the statistics of *The Hite Report on Female Sexuality*, that his partner was among the 30 percent of women who do get clitoral stimulation during intercourse (adequate to orgasm)—and a further tendency to believe that the most "mature" and "best" women are naturally among the 30 percent.

Some men told how they had felt when they first realized that (contrary to cultural stereotypes) clitoral stimulation was more important for most women's orgasms than intercourse itself—that intercourse did not actually lead to orgasm for most women:

> *I used to think I understood feminine sexuality—you know, I was gentle, patient, understanding, etc.—if they "couldn't" orgasm, it was "O.K.," I let them get on top during intercourse and everything (a real sport, wasn't I?). Anyway, now I see that the sensitivity I had that I thought was about ninety percent was more like ten percent. [Age twenty-two]*

> *I guess I had personally observed in my own experience that the clitoris was the place of excitement in the female; I know that on many occasions I knocked myself out thrusting in the female with little effect. There was something wrong, but I must admit I was crestfallen when I finally became aware that what I had suspected was true—male thrusting of the penis in the female vagina is not what we males thought it was. [Age thirty-eight]*

> *I didn't feel good when I heard it. I didn't feel good for them, like a car with a defect that the dealer wouldn't fix. You're stuck with it and have to work around it. Or don't drive. [Age thirty]*

> *The other day a friend of mine told me that I was making a mistake expecting women to orgasm during intercourse with me, and that I should try to stimulate them some other way. This was radical news to me. It was odd, talking about it with another man like that. I have never really talked about sex with another man before, except the usual stories, etc. I wonder what he thought of my reaction, or if he thought I should have known or what. Anyway, I'm glad he told me. [Age thirty-one]*

> *Through almost eleven years of marriage, I believed that orgasm through intercourse was the rule rather than the exception. I "knew" that the clitoris was part of the female orgasm process—nothing more. In the last year*

*a lover entered my life (I am still married) and it is with her and through reading The Hite Report that I began to understand the function of the clitoris and the importance of manual stimulation. It has opened up a whole new side of sexuality, an addition. [Age forty]*

Certain men accepted the information with relief and a sense of pleasure, especially when it confirmed their own personal experience or when they thought that the "problem" had been their fault:

*My wife has never orgasmed from intercourse. I used to feel that something was wrong with my technique or with my wife's frame of mind (mental block). Now all that is gone and forgotten. She can always orgasm from clitoral stimulation, so we are not missing something. [Age forty-six]*

*I can't believe we have been deceived so long about the penis-vagina orgasm. I am sure my wife (and I) would have developed much more sensibly if we had known this fact thirty-five years ago. I often felt sad and puzzled that she did not orgasm from intercourse. I was relieved to find out that this is normal. [Age fifty-seven]*

One man had worried at first that the news that women needed more clitoral stimulation would mean even more work for him, and even more pressure to perform ("give the woman an orgasm"):

*At first I was worried because I thought this would mean more responsibility for me, that women needed more stimulation, not that it would make things easier in the long run. But that's how it worked out, really, because I don't have to strain so much during intercourse for a result that's impossible anyway—and besides, sometimes she helps me with her hand on top of mine stimulating her clitoris. I'm glad I learned. [Age forty-six]*

Some men expressed the difficulties of changing:

*I feel a great resistance in myself to the idea that a woman really needs direct clitoral or mons stimulation to orgasm. She should be able to orgasm during intercourse—that is what men have always said. And yet, if it isn't true, it isn't true. I know I should accept it, but it's really a revolutionary change in all my assumptions (and the way I've always behaved). I have to force myself to believe it. And yet, how egotistical can I be, with my very own love telling me it is so? Change is hard.*

> *It's a bit worrying to think of women not enjoying intercourse as we do—*
> *hope they're not going to lock us out of their vaginas forever. Still, the facts*
> *of female physiology can't be denied, even if they're not as men might*
> *wish. As Martin Luther declared: "There I stand. I can do no other."*

One man was grappling with the information and its implications—wondering how the woman felt about intercourse and how he himself should feel about it—and in the process rethinking his own definition of sex:

> *First of all my partner, my wife, has never orgasmed during intercourse,*
> *or in my presence, while nearly every time we have had intercourse, I*
> *have come to orgasm and ejaculation. Never! Here is the way I feel about*
> *it. Besides expecting to orgasm during sexual intercourse, I rejoice in the*
> *fact that I can orgasm during intercourse. I consider orgasm during mas-*
> *turbation and during intercourse as two different types of orgasm: mas-*
> *turbatory orgasm, for me, is a selfish orgasm, a self-love orgasm, all for*
> *myself. Orgasm during intercourse, to me, is a mutual orgasm, that is, I*
> *feel that I have not brought myself to "come," but also that my wife has*
> *helped me to "come." The fact I am enjoying the physical contact and*
> *closeness with her, the fact she has allowed me to penetrate her, make*
> *love to her, is an intricate/intimate articulation of the fact my orgasm is*
> *in part a gift from her. To me, emotionally and psychologically, this is*
> *ultimate, this kind of orgasm means so much more to me than my own*
> *masturbatory orgasm. This is how I feel I am.*
>
> *But I feel bothered I cannot bring her to orgasm during a mutual expe-*
> *rience of lovemaking and intercourse. I do not feel bothered because I*
> *feel responsible to bring her to "come," or that "it is my job." I have tran-*
> *scended this expectation. She is entitled to her orgasms as I am (mas-*
> *turbatorily). But, because I feel so much ecstasy when I have come while*
> *having coitus with her, I feel that I can be a part of an orgasm with her.*
> *I want to give or bring her to orgasm. Can you sympathize or empathize*
> *with me? When I come and she does not, I feel one-sided about the orgas-*
> *mic ecstasy: I feel I have reached a plateau she has not, which does make*
> *me feel alone in ecstasy, sometimes lonely. I desire my body, myself, and*
> *my lovemaking to be in part hers, for her, the gift of myself to her.*
>
> *As for helping my wife (if she wants it) to come before or after I come,*
> *I feel all game and willing to participate in this. But she feels a bit*
> *embarrassed to stimulate herself "in front of me." This is O.K. What I*
> *wish to make clear is that I am quite willing to help her come, in what-*
> *ever manner it takes.*

A popular response was to say that the woman's orgasm is her own responsibility:

*It's her business. She is responsible for her own orgasms.*

*I offer everything, if she doesn't accept, I'm clean.*

*The problem would be more hers than mine. She needs to know what turns her on.*

*It's not my problem. It's up to her.*

*I consider myself ultimately responsible for providing my own orgasms. To be hard-nosed about it, I frankly consider a woman ultimately responsible for hers too. None of my relationships has ever been so lacking in respect, tenderness, and diplomacy that we degenerated to fighting about orgasms, but if it didn't happen, and I was accused of "being not man enough," I would counter righteously that it takes two, and it is more than likely that she wasn't woman enough.*

These answers are certainly correct in one sense—that everyone does, finally, make his or her own orgasm. However, a woman's situation is different from that of a man. To imply that women are not taking their fair share of responsibility for what goes on overlooks the fact that most "sex" is still carried on according to the old rules—that is, the woman is supposed to orgasm from intercourse, intercourse is sex, it is assumed that intercourse will be included, and that the man has the right to the appropriate stimulation for his orgasm—that is, intercourse. The man has society behind him, encouraging him to have his orgasm, but the woman has society telling her that what she needs—that is, clitoral stimulation to orgasm, usually in the form of manual or oral stimulation—is not "normal," or that she has no right to assert herself. In other words, our pattern of sex does not put men in the position of having to ask for the stimulation they need; it is clear that "sex" should end with intercourse and male orgasm, whereas women must request "special" ("extra") stimulation, and/or stimulation not related to intercourse. As one man put it, "If the woman needs some special stimulation, she should let the guy know."

In summary, many men were very annoyed with women for not having orgasm more frequently or more easily during sex—feeling, "Why are women being so difficult? They could orgasm if they wanted to, if they would just try a little harder, or if they were not being overly emotionally complicated—why are they trying to make men feel bad?"—not realizing that it is the lack of adequate clitoral stimulation in traditional "sex" that makes orgasm difficult for most women, and not esoteric reasons.

## IS THE SOLUTION THAT "WOMEN SHOULD SPEAK UP"?

Other men felt that the situation was the woman's fault in the sense that the woman should tell the man what she needs, and should especially speak up about her need for clitoral stimulation outside of intercourse—although here again, many answers seemed still to imply that the woman would speak up about some particular preferences during intercourse. Men were frequently angry if they felt that women wouldn't tell them what they wanted: there was a great sense of annoyance, anger, and hostility in these answers—why are women so difficult, after all?

> There is something wrong with me only if a woman lets me know that she can orgasm if I do a certain thing, and I refuse to do it. Nothing works all the time for everyone, and I'm not going to stake my manhood on my ability to read minds.

> I would prefer she would tell me anything she wants rather than dead silence.

> It's her fault. I'm not a mind reader. She has to tell me what to do.

> I would help, if she would just tell me. It really pisses me off to think that a girl would tell me she had come when she hadn't and wanted to. Hell, that's what I'm there for!

> I wish I knew what they were scared of.

> It's the woman's fault for not telling!

> I assume that if she's not satisfied she'll tell me. But again, just try to find a woman this open—I think it's almost impossible. This is why I'm sick and tired of women's libbers telling everybody that men just like to "love 'em and leave 'em." This is bullshit. The truth is that women avoid being controlled by men by being secretive and unpredictable.

## MEN'S FEELINGS OF ALIENATION, BLAME, GUILT, AND ANGER

QUESTION:
How do you feel if the woman you are with does not have an orgasm at all in any way?

Doubts about how or if women were having orgasms frequently made men feel uncomfortable, guilty, inadequate, or defensive during sex—although some men said that they didn't care whether a woman had orgasms or not, since women's orgasms were not that important. But most men, still assuming that women should orgasm during intercourse, all too often wound up feeling alienated and either blaming themselves or blaming women for not achieving what really is very difficult or impossible to achieve:

*How do I feel? Like a doctor who loses a patient on the surgery table.*

*Inadequate, a poor lover, a failure.*

*Depressed, disappointed. Feelings of self-hatred.*

*She says it's O.K., but I worry.*

*There's no point in making love.*

*A selfish pig.*

*With my first wife, I became indifferent.*

*I feel parasitic or unexciting.*

*Disappointed because there was no mutuality.*

*Defeated. I would lose interest in her.*

Lack of women's orgasm, mainly a result of cultural imperatives that insist women should orgasm when men do, has been an unspoken source of alienation between men and women over the years. As one man put it, "I feel more respect for her and myself if I don't feel I am cheating her out of an orgasm—or I guess the word is 'using' her, since I have an orgasm and she doesn't. I feel relieved to be with an equal." And another man said, "I have been married for sixteen years. My wife reaches orgasm only with some difficulty. I have been trying all means of helping her gain confidence and relaxation during intercourse, but I believe that there is a shade of jealousy in her mind about my easy satisfaction."

All this could lead to feelings of guilt and negativity:

*I feel inadequate. Sometimes I wonder just how good a sex partner I am. But I guess we all have those doubts.*

*I feel I am at fault. It's something I have done wrong.*

*I have not done enough or the "right" thing.*

*I failed her.*

*I must be inadequate.*

## MEN AND THE CLITORIS

### MEN'S FEELINGS ABOUT GIVING A WOMAN CLITORAL STIMULATION TO ORGASM

What were men's general attitudes toward the clitoris? When men were asked, "How do you feel about the clitoris?" many answers included jokes or satirical remarks:

> *How do I feel about the clitoris? I feel in awe of the little bugger. It's got-*
> *ten so much publicity and become the focal point of so much rancor that*
> *I have the urge to salute it when I see it.*

> *A woman's clitoris is the greatest thing since the mop—other questions*
> *redundant.*

In many other answers, the importance of the clitoris was brought into question by the frequent use of diminutives:*

> *A woman's clitoris is a wonderful little thing.*

> *The clitoris is a mysterious little "love button."*

> *I think it is cute as it peeps out from its hiding place. Sometimes girls call*
> *it the "tickle button."*

> *Big surprises come in little packages.*

> *Cute little devil.*

But there were enthusiastic and positive remarks as well:

> *It is the primary erotic center of her body, tender and sensitive, and has*
> *to be treated with great care and emotion.*

---

* The exterior clitoris as we know it is only a part of a very large internal clitoral network, which is as large as the penis. See the drawing on pages 180–181.

*It's just as important to her as my penis is to me.*

*Beautiful, stimulating, the most sensual part of a woman's body.*

*The clitoris is the blasting cap on a stick of dynamite. It is the trigger mechanism which puts everything else into motion.*

*It's the most important part of the vulva. A man that has loved a woman and cares for her knows these things.*

*It amazes me. It's the center of my wife's entire sexual being. Every square micron must be packed with nerve endings because of her reaction when I touch it or even get near it.*

*Very beautiful and mysterious.*

A few men professed complete neutrality:

*What do I think about it? Nothing really.*

*I never really felt anything about it emotionally.*

*Nothing special.*

*. . . nothing to rave over. If that is the point she wants stimulated, I will stimulate it. But I don't have any special feeling about it any more than I have any special feeling about any other body part that isn't in plain sight. It's like asking me how I feel about her liver.*

Others had had no experience, or bad experiences:

*She won't let me touch it.*

*My wife says my finger hurts it.*

*The clitoris is a strange thing to me. It protrudes.*

*I could never find my wife's. She doesn't seem to have one. I'm not sure what the clitoris is.*

*I have no feelings about it. She shouldn't have one.*

When men were asked, "What does the clitoris look like?" there were a wide range of replies—many containing elements of discomfort and unfamiliarity, and even sometimes hostility, again often using diminutives:

*A small hooded pink bump which enlarges on arousal.*

*It looks like a tiny worm which needs sunlight . . . very pale.*

*It looks good and tasty.*

*When the hood is pulled back, it looks like a red pea coming out of its shell.*

*Like the tip of a male cat's penis. It looks like a funny little critter peeping out of its house.*

*A tiny titty jelly bean (I like the red ones).*

*Like a grapefruit seed in a translucent veil of tissue.*

*Small, round, pink, and sensitive. A pearly little head. I have not seen it as illustrated in books.*

*Like a dog's penis.*

*It looks like a woman's helmet or something similar at the tip.*

*Why, it looks like a clitoris, of course.*

But most men said that they had never actually seen the clitoris:

*Never seen one in real life.*

*Only seen them in books.*

*I've never seen one because the lights are off or my eyes are closed.*

*I've seen diagrams and photos but not my partner's clitoris—she admonished me not to "play doctor." Instead we have operated by verbal feedback, i.e., "further up . . . a little to the right." This seems to work O.K.*

*The clitoris swells and is easier to find as a woman becomes aroused. But*

*I have never turned on the lights, sat back, and examined one, so I am unclear about the exact description.*

*I was never told about the clitoris, nor about the shape of a woman's vulva (apart from there being a hole there). Nor did I hear where the urethra was. So I've had some difficulty in finding my way in on various occasions. I haven't seen it or examined it in detail, but believe I know where it is. Just inside the top of the main slit. Incredibly high up in fact, right out of the region that I used to consider as cunt.*

*I know where it's supposed to be according to the books but she's apparently fully hooded and it is never exposed. At the slightest pressure it rolls sideways and gets lost again.*

*I learned about the clitoris from pornographic books. [Age thirty]*

*I read about it recently in some anatomy literature. [Age seventy-four]*

*I first heard the word "clitoris" on the radio, and then looked it up in a few books. I was surprised to find that so important a part of human anatomy and sexuality was spoken of so little. [Age twenty-eight]*

*From texts I've tried to learn best how to stimulate it, especially with my tongue. [Age thirty-eight.]*

*I read in a book in college that the clitoris was anatomically synonymous with the glans penis. I got the impression that it was much more "like a penis" than it turned out to be. I thought it would be much bigger (longer) than it actually is. [Age thirty-three]*

When asked, "Where is the clitoris?," although most men knew basically where it is, many of the answers were rather vague. Although the most common answer was, "At the top of the vagina," it is unlikely that most men think that the clitoris is inside the vagina; therefore, are these men using the word "vagina" to mean "vulva"?

*High up on her vagina.*

*Just above the vagina.*

*Right at the top of the vagina.*

*It's between the lips above the vaginal opening.*

*Centered just above the vaginal opening.*

*Under the hood/sheath in front of/top of the vagina.*

*Very top edge of the vagina.*

*Top of the vaginal opening.*

Clearer descriptions included the following:

*It's near the top of the "crack."*

*It's higher up than one would think—and farther away from the vagina.*

*It's at the upper end of the outer lips, near the pelvic bone.*

*At the top (pubic bone) end of the vagina.*

*Right above the pee hole.*

*At the base of the mons, sandwiched between several folds of flesh.*

*Hiding under the covers above the vagina.*

Also notable is the emotional reaction this question created in some men:

*I could give an average location in centimeters from the top of the vagina, etc., but there are many more questions I could better spend the time on.*

*I would rather show than tell.*

*In the illustration on page six of "Sex for Third Graders."*

*Sure ain't in her nose.*

A few men admitted that they did not know for sure:

*I have never separated the clitoris from the whole genital area.*

*To tell the truth, I am not quite sure where a woman's clitoris is.*

*I was performing cunnilingus one time and all of a sudden I stopped and said to my girlfriend, "Where the heck is your clitoris anyway?"*

## SIMILARITIES BETWEEN CLITORAL AND PENILE ANATOMY: WHY IT IS HELPFUL TO UNDERSTAND THIS

There is a widespread misunderstanding of women's sexual anatomy. What we usually think of as the "clitoris" is simply the exterior part of a larger interior structure. The extent of this interior clitoral network is quite large—comparable to the size of the penis and testicles in men. Inside the penis there are two cavernous bulbs the length of the shaft that fill with blood and thus cause erection. These same two cavernous bulbs exist in the female; however, in the female they are separate, each extending on one side of the vulva, beginning at the pubic area (the exterior clitoris) and going back on either side of the vagina. During arousal these structures fill with blood and cause the entire area to swell: this is the reason a woman's vulva becomes swollen and puffy, pleasurably sensitive to the touch. When orgasm occurs, muscle contractions send the blood out of these structures in waves. In other words, the clitoral system is similar in size to the penis, but the clitoral system is interior, while the penis is exterior. Both systems are the same in the early embryo.

If men could understand the similarities of their structures to those of women, they could understand clitoral stimulation much more easily. For example, most men need stimulation at the top of their penis for orgasm, even though they feel the orgasm basically at the base of the penis and inside their bodies: stimulation at the sensitive tip and around the rim leads to sensations deeper inside the body. In the same way, stimulation of the exterior clitoral area causes sensations deeper in the body and vaginal area, culminating in orgasm.

Some men truly did not know where the clitoris is, sometimes stating that it is inside the vagina:

*It is inside the vagina.*

*It is deep down inside.*

*Between the lips up inside the vaginal opening.*

*An inch or so inside the vagina.*

*In the vagina just past the folds of skin.*

*Just inside her pussy.*

# SIMILARITIES BETWEEN CLITORIS

## Parts of the clitoris and penis

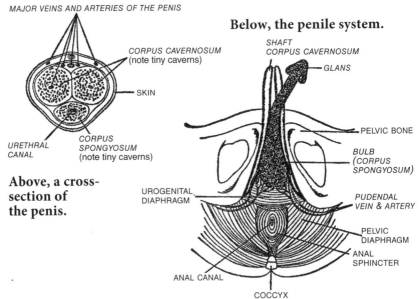

The clitoral system during arousal.

Below, the penile system.

Above, a cross-section of the penis.

# AND PENIS ANATOMY

**systems are underscored.**

## Side View

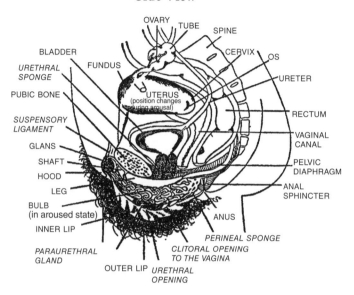

OVARY
TUBE
SPINE
BLADDER
CERVIX
OS
*URETHRAL SPONGE*
FUNDUS
URETER
PUBIC BONE
UTERUS
(position changes during arousal)
*SUSPENSORY LIGAMENT*
RECTUM
GLANS
VAGINAL CANAL
SHAFT
PELVIC DIAPHRAGM
HOOD
LEG
ANAL SPHINCTER
BULB
(in aroused state)
ANUS
INNER LIP
PERINEAL SPONGE
*PARAURETHRAL GLAND*
CLITORAL OPENING TO THE VAGINA
OUTER LIP  URETHRAL OPENING

## The Clitoral System During Arousal

There is a widespread misunderstanding of women's sexual anatomy. What we usually think of as the "clitoris" is simply the exterior part of a larger interior structure. The extent of this interior clitoral network is quite large—comparable to the size of the penis and testicles in men. Inside the penis there are two cavernous bulbs the length of the shaft that fill with blood and thus cause erection. These same two cavernous bulbs exist in the female; however, beginning at the pubic area (the exterior clitoris) and going back on either side of the vagina. During arousal they fill with blood and cause the entire area to swell: this is why a woman's vulva becomes swollen and puffy, pleasurably sensitive to touch. When orgasm occurs, the blood is sent out of these structures in waves by muscle contractions. In other words, the clitoral system is similar in size to the penis, but the clitoral system is *interior*, while the penis is exterior. Both systems are the same in the early embryo.

If men could understand the similarities of their structures to those of women, they could understand clitoral stimulation much more easily. For example, most men need stimulation at the top of their penis for orgasm, even though they feel the orgasm basically at the base of the penis and inside their bodies: stimulation at the sensitive tip and around the rim leads to sensations deeper inside the body. In the same way, stimulation of the exterior clitoral area causes sensations deeper in the body and vaginal area, culminating in orgasm.

*. . . feminine genitals are quite complicated, and it took me a long time, when I began to have sex, to find out exactly where everything was. It sounds silly, but it's true. I bet many men cannot really describe what a cunt is like. In college, I had a good school friend who insisted—joking, more or less—that in spite of having made love quite a few times, he had never found a clitoris, and suspected they didn't exist.*

## HOW DO MEN FEEL ABOUT STIMULATING A WOMAN TO ORGASM CLITORALLY BY HAND?

*I hate to admit it, but my wife's way of having orgasm used to really irritate me in the beginning. She always clenches her legs together, sometimes even twists them together while I am supposed to rub her clitoris. After all I had heard about a woman spreading her legs meaning she wants you, I felt that this was a rejection, and really, that there was something 'weird' about her. It took a couple of years before we could talk about this. In the beginning, I just did what I thought she wanted, but I really resented it, and gradually I began to do it less and less enthusiastically, I guess. Finally, we had a fight about it. She said she thought I resented her orgasms, and I said I thought she was being selfish when she had them. She didn't need me at all. I wasn't involved, I wasn't inside her, and I wasn't getting stimulated (although I have to admit that sometimes it was a pretty sexy situation, with her doing all that moaning and groaning, writhing and getting hot and sweaty, saying she loved me and grabbing me after—wow, very passionate kisses). Anyway, I still resented it. She was very hurt that I didn't enjoy her orgasms, and didn't want to have sex for a while. That got me started thinking, what was the point of sex anyway? It's taken me a long time to begin to accept that this is how she (women?) has orgasm, and that it doesn't mean that there is anything wrong with me because she doesn't do it during intercourse. I mean, I know rationally that this is it, clitoral stimulation, and I really dig it, but at the same time, the myth of how it should be is still there.*

Most men who had tried manual clitoral stimulation expressed doubts about their expertise at giving it. When asked, "Do you feel knowledgeable and comfortable stimulating a woman clitorally? How do you feel while giving clitoral stimulation with your hand?" most mentioned feelings of discomfort and replied that getting feedback from the woman was essential:

*I don't feel sublimely confident when dealing with a clitoris; the orgasm seems very picky about what it likes and what it doesn't like, and it's hard to know, until you get to know a girl pretty well, just what the right thing is.*

*Sometimes I can't find a woman's clitoris. I am either constantly getting lost—or the damn thing moves around a lot.*\*

*I feel knowledgeable about touching a clitoris up to a point (get it?), and then I want her to communicate to me what she likes. I'm no mind reader, and different women like different pressures and motions, although I find that they often are so glad to have their joy button get any attention at all that they go up the walls.*

*I don't think I'm doing it right. I've talked about it with the other guys, but all I hear are stories about "sticking-your-whole-god-damn-fist-up-there" while "she-was-getting-wet-to-her-ankles" crap.*

*It's exciting to stimulate a woman clitorally and see her sexual arousal. My girlfriend told me I was too rough sometimes. I was never too gentle, or then she didn't say anything.*

*Generally I feel knowledgeable about touching it, but some differ so radically in preferences that one can never be sure.*

*After ten years my wife finally conceded to letting me touch her, but was very embarrassed in those days but not today. I enjoy giving my wife stimulation, but I have to keep myself stimulated too with my other hand because she cannot hold my penis during her stimulation—it distracts her and she can't come.*

A few men replied that they felt they were doing something "abnormal" that they should not need to do. A few connected manual clitoral stimulation with "teenage" behavior, calling it a high-school activity, or adolescent behavior, something they had done only before intercourse was possible. Still, in 1981, according to my data, most men had never given a woman an orgasm with manual clitoral stimulation!

When asked, "Do you get sexually excited by stimulating your partner? Do you enjoy her orgasm physically? Emotionally?" many men were very enthusiastic and commented on how much they enjoyed stimulating their partner to orgasm in this way. Some reported that the activity was great, even stimulation to the woman's multiple orgasms:

---

\* Once again, these replies were much more likely to contain jokes than to give serious answers relating to intercourse or other topics.

*How do I feel? Proud!*

*It's an ego trip.*

*I feel flattered.*

But how do men feel about a woman stimulating herself? Can a woman also stimulate herself manually while she is with a man? In the same way that men said that women often don't give them the correct manual stimulation of their penis, isn't it difficult for one person (especially of the opposite sex) to know just how to stimulate another? Although learning to do just that with a specific partner can be very loving and exciting, it is also very important for men and women to feel that they can stimulate themselves during sex with a partner. This can be an extremely intimate activity, while at the same time removing many frustrations and pressures from both the woman and the man.

QUESTION:
How do you feel if a woman stimulates herself to orgasm with you? During intercourse?

Most men had never experienced a woman stimulating herself (manually) while close to them; for most men, having the woman give herself an orgasm was a new idea. As one man said, "No woman has ever shown me how or even admitted to masturbation."

In fact, many men were shocked by the idea that their partner could masturbate to orgasm at all, even when alone; most men did not know how (or if) she did it. When asked, "Does your partner masturbate to orgasm? How? If you don't know, would you like her to share this information with you?" many gave answers similar to the following:

*No. I don't think so.*

*I don't think she ever has.*

*Can't answer.*

*Don't know or care—probably on rare occasions.*

Many men did not like the idea of the woman stimulating herself while with them:

*It's O.K. if she has to, but I would feel let down that I can't please her.*

*I would feel inadequate if she did that.*

*There would be a tinge of personal failure.*

*I would resent it.*

*I hope it never happens. I would get up and leave.*

*I feel very uncomfortable when she masturbates while I watch. I feel left out, an audience, unimportant, merely an afterthought on her part.*

*It would be like I didn't satisfy her.*

*Why does she need me?*

And many had mixed feelings about their partner masturbating:

*It's not much fun being pushed out of the way, but I don't mind having expert guidance.*

*It wouldn't hurt my ego but it would disturb me if she climaxed that way only.*

*I feel strange—happy that she'll reach orgasm, but unhappy because I'm not doing it to her liking.*

*I don't feel too bad, as long as I'm the mental stimulation.*

*If I am feeling O.K. about myself, I feel O.K. when a woman reaches orgasm by stimulating herself on me. When I'm not feeling O.K., I tend to feel used.*

*. . . With a vibrator?*

*I'd rather she came without a vibrator.*

*A vibrator is cancerous, probably.*

*Anything to make her come.*

*I feel no good if she needs a vibrator to orgasm.*

*Clitoral stimulation is O.K. but it's carrying it too far when she uses a vibrator!*

*I am very happy she does not use one.*

*Something about vibrators bothers me, but I don't complain to the one person I know who likes to incorporate one into the act.*

*If a woman stimulates herself to orgasm with me, I feel cheated. I would like to bring her to orgasm, and if I'm not, why am I her lover? Vibrators are for shit as far as I'm concerned.*

But other men expressed an open attitude toward trying one:

*I intend to buy a vibrator to see if we can enhance our sex life. I hear they're great.*

*I never experienced it, but I would enjoy watching her use a vibrator.*

*I would not mind my partner using a vibrator if I also took part, e.g., manipulating or helping manipulate the vibrator while kissing and fondling her breasts, etc.*

And a few men enjoyed the use of the vibrator by a woman:

*I love to watch her body spasmodically orgasm while she uses her vibrator.*

*My lover does not orgasm from intercourse—but we do many things together besides intercourse. It is very exciting to masturbate together. She has orgasms when she wants to—she just grabs the vibrator.*

*I really loved using the vibrator we had on my lover, as I could give her intense orgasms that way.*

*I am thrilled, frankly, that she is so into sex. She apologizes, and I have to keep encouraging her. The nitwit. It's like me eating a whole meal, and her feeling she must nibble.*

## VIBRATORS AND MEN, VIBRATORS AND WOMEN (WHAT'S THE PROBLEM?)

Should men use vibrators with a woman? Should women use vibrators to reach orgasm when they are having sex with a man? Why not? After all, a man might enjoy doing this "to" a woman—and he wouldn't have to worry about his erection coming and going.

An increasing (and already large) number of women use a vibrator for orgasm when on their own, or during masturbation. (By the way, most women who use vibrators for orgasm during masturbation do not penetrate themselves with the vibrator, even if they have one that is shaped like a "dildo" or a penis—often they buy these only because they are the kind most commercially available.)

Even though an electric (battery-operated) massager is the easiest way for many women to reach orgasm, most women who normally masturbate using a vibrator do not try to use it during sex with a man. They fear his reaction; many of those who have tried to use one with a man say that most men resist incorporating a vibrator into sex, even if they accept the principle of clitoral stimulation to orgasm as necessary for women.

As one woman writes, "I am 33 years old, living happily with Pedro. He—the man I am living with for six years now—knows I use a vibrator when I masturbate (not the dildo kind you insert, just a small round neck-type massager that runs on a battery), but he never likes it when I try to use it in our lovemaking. I would love to use it because I think it's sexy and I can come very easily that way—I want to let myself go more with him, have orgasms while we are kissing and playing around, and not worry about it. But if I pull it out, it seems to stop him. Now, sometimes I come to orgasm with him, but not always. Whether I have an orgasm seems to be an unspoken question between us, and this makes me feel tense sometimes, even if I come. I feel guilty saying this (is there something wrong with me?), but to really really come to my heart's content (a lot), I have to have a serious session with my vibrator. Maybe he thinks I should 'give up my dependency on the vibrator'—but I've tried, I guess I'm just not as secure while he uses his hand, I worry he will stop (just when I'm starting to come), and won't give me the continuous smooth stimulation I need (will he be bored? feel oppressed?) So I can't really let go and fantasize or focus on feeling that increasing glorious sensation when he is doing it …."

There is no reason why a man and woman today cannot use a vibrator as a regular part of lovemaking.

Furthermore, a vibrator is a good way to break through the shyness and newness that can accompany the time when both people are getting to know what it is like for the woman to have an orgasm, often several orgasms in a row. In this way, a man can observe a woman's timing and habits, in the same way that women get to know the likes and dislikes of "their man" during sex, how he reaches orgasm.

Any man who fears that a vibrator is "unnatural" should ask himself if he listens to a radio or drives a car before criticizing women for using "gizmos" and "electronic devices." Men, after all, are receiving a time-honored form of adequate stimulation for their orgasm during coitus, therefore they do not need "mechanical help." This does not mean that they are biologically superior!

Some men see the vibrator as a pleasant enhancement of everything else that is going on. A vibrator of any size or shape can be held by the man and the woman together, or by either one of them. Most important: a man should not make a woman feel that she is alone while using it. For example, if a woman presses it to her mons/clitoral area or crotch, the man can put a finger in her vagina or caress her anus and kiss her, play with himself or "talk dirty" to her.

This is an activity for two, not one.

### MEN'S FEELINGS ABOUT CUNNILINGUS

Although most men in my research reported that they liked cunnilingus, and were more familiar with it than with manual stimulation, it was not a major way of giving women clitoral stimulation to orgasm. Only 32 percent of the men who answered said that they usually continued cunnilingus until the woman reached orgasm.

However, most men were extremely enthusiastic about cunnilingus. For just over half of the men who answered who enjoyed sex with women, cunnilingus was the second most popular sexual activity, after intercourse. But a large number of men felt squeamish about cunnilingus—including many of those who were enthusiastic about it. There were very few in-between opinions about cunnilingus, and the answers show a much greater emotional reaction than those to almost any other subject.

Although most men thought of cunnilingus as "foreplay," they felt more comfortable with this form of clitoral stimulation than with manual clitoral stimulation. In fact, when asked about "clitoral stimulation," most men began discussing oral sex, not mentioning manual stimulation unless it was specifically referred to by the question. Still, the form of cunnilingus practiced by most men did not include much specific clitoral stimulation but was more likely to concentrate on the general vulva and/or vaginal opening, rather than the clitoris. While this can be very pleasurable, both physically and emotionally, and even preferable in the view of many women, lack of precise clitoral stimulation for orgasm is a drawback if no other provision is made for the woman's orgasm during sex.

QUESTION:
Do you enjoy cunnilingus with a woman? What do you like and/or dislike about it?

Many men were extremely enthusiastic about cunnilingus:

> *More than anything else I enjoy oral sex. If my partner wants, I will eat her all day long. I feel very happy, content, secure, and loving doing so. I*

*adore the texture, feel, and taste, and also the lovely way a woman seems to respond while being eaten. The women I have had oral sex with seem to relax and very much enjoy being eaten. We both seem to have very good feelings about oral sex. There seems to be a very open feeling between us.*

*Oral sex with a woman is my favorite of all. I feel a great closeness, a deep intimacy burying my face in that dark secret place. I feel that she trusts me fully. I love to look up and see her eyes closed and her face contorted in exquisite agony. I love my face drenched in her secretions, and her clit dancing under my tongue and her rocking hard and arching her back. And especially her moaning, screaming, raising her arms above her head so I can see her armpits. I love the convulsive motions of her coming. I love it when it's over and I keep my face between her legs and it gets dry and sticky and our skin pulls when it peels apart.*

Others were ambivalent about the taste and smell:

*My wife repels me four out of five times. Sometimes her genitals smell like a chicken dinner.*

*First you sniff it, if you wouldn't lick it, don't lick it.*

*Some gals smell strong at first but if you just get going, it's like eating Limburger cheese. Smells rough but tastes great.*

*As the taste and smell are strong, I sometimes have to be slightly deliberate about first contact, but no more so than when eating, say, a particularly ripe cheese or unusual fruit, drink, spice, etc. —once you get a good sniff or taste, then whatever the initial apprehensions, it's enjoyable. And anyway, it's her.*

*Occasionally during a woman's cycle the smell is more of a turn-off than a turn-on initially. If I "kiss" her anyway the smell soon becomes a turn-on.*

Of course, yeast infections could disrupt the natural smell:

*Several minor vaginal infections, including trichomonas, produce an off odor. I'm confident that I can diagnose trichomonas by the odor-flavor.*

*Once in a while she's had some sort of vaginal infection that produces a strong and definitely unpleasant smell, an odor of old sweat and decaying fish. I don't like it. She understands . . . but I've never found a way to tell her that without making her feel hurt. I wish I could say, "Hey, you've got that symptom again," without making it sound like a moral accusation.*

Some men hadn't decided yet:

*Female genitals are fragrant. Taste wonderful and my only complaint is a really, really raunchy crotch that hasn't been washed. But it's not really a true complaint since I've never experienced one—I just think that if someone didn't wash for two weeks it would smell foul.*

*What I dislike is that some women have an offensive—well, not really offensive but strange—smell. I'm still trying to get used to it.*

But some men had none of these negative associations:

*Many men and women find a woman's sex to be unclean in some way. I enjoy showing the woman that not only do I find her sex not unclean, but in fact I find it extremely delightful.*

*Would you believe that some women are reluctant to engage in such an activity since a lot of them have hang-ups and prehistoric beliefs that they smell bad? Usually my partner showers before the activity and it smells clean and tastes great with all the woman juices.*

*Many women have a tendency to push your face away from their genitals as though they feel they've done something wrong or smell bad. It is hard to convince them that I enjoy the smell and taste—and I do.*

*My wife cleans too much.*

*For me, cunnilingus is beautiful but only when the woman enjoys it. Some get pretty freaked out about it. The smell and taste is something exquisite. It can get a bit raunchy at times, but on the other hand, a freshly scrubbed cunt can be pretty tasteless, and lose a lot of appeal.*

Some men emphasized that they liked the taste very much:

*Darndest thing: women taste so sweet down there. Without using anything added. Just reasonably clean. It's really nice.*

*Tastes and smells always excite me. Tastes vary—sometimes they are sweet and sometimes a little salty or tangy.*

*The taste is a very plain taste with just a slight distinctness which I like and which also arouses me.*

*Most are sweet and creamy.*

*I love the way my wife's genitals taste and smell, the way her pussy looks and feels, the heat and velvety wetness of it.*

*I like, in fact, just adore, the taste of women's genitals.*

Of men who mentioned "feminine hygiene sprays" or flavored creams, most indicated that they did not like them:

*Women taste great (if clean and if they're not using any of those hygiene sprays). Their odor is a definite sexual turn-on and the taste is superb.*

*All the women I've gone with have been clean and washed. I like the natural woman taste and smell and do not like the use of the "vaginal mouthwash" sometimes advertised.*

*I generally like the smell of women's genitals—I like the smell of sweat too. I don't believe in all this hype about anti-perspirants, etc. All that advertising serves to separate people from each other, makes them think they stink and are ugly, and uses sexuality for profit.*

And other men emphasized that they liked the smells:

*The taste is faintly salty; there's a delicate smell that's very distinctive, but I can't describe it. I like it. Sometimes I've gotten it on my fingers and long afterwards I can hold them to my nose and still get a trace of that lovely scent.*

*Smells (the healthy ones) have become increasingly attractive to me with age.*

*The taste is good but not as exciting as the smell.*

QUESTION:
Are women's genitals "clean"?

Although many men liked cunnilingus very much, almost half of those who answered were also preoccupied with whether the woman or her genitals were "clean":

> I'm learning more and more to enjoy cunnilingus. It's been hard to do— I have uncomfortable feelings about oozing: I was raised clean clean clean. I like to take a shower after sex.

> If you want to have oral sex with a gal, I am saying to her, "You are clean."

> I'm still kind of squeamish about cunnilingus, and still think of female genitalia as dirty. Most of my earliest sexual experiences were with women whose genitals were dirty and really did smell awful. I sometimes enjoy oral sex with women when I first establish that they're clean. I like the musky, sweet smell of a woman and get some pleasure from cunnilingus for myself, but mainly get into it to please the woman.

> My partner usually washes just before or at least a few hours before and is either tasteless or pleasantly scented. Stale, unwashed female genitals taste and smell bad to me.

> How does one ask a woman politely to wash?

> Female cunt is not good-looking but I love it, every inch of it, if it is clean.

> I like everything about oral sex with my lover-wife as long as she has secretly showered (I like my partners "clean")—taste, smell, texture, the pleasure it gives her, the turn-on to me.

> I think women usually consider their pubic area "unclean, smelly, dirty, slimy, etc." Pardon me, but I would rather make that distinction. If I find a distasteful (no pun intended) situation, I'll suggest an erotic, arousing shower together.

> I only like it after a bath. I don't like the taste of urine or stale secretions. Or the smell of feces. But a clean pussy tastes good, believe me!

One of men's most frequent "buts" about the vagina and vulva was related to whether the woman is clean or has washed recently. While the fact that all bodies need bathing rather regularly would seem to go without saying, no men mentioned the necessity for brushing teeth regularly to make kissing pleasant. The fact that so many men saw fit to stress this point with regard to women's vulvas seems to reflect the influence of the age-old patriarchal view of female sexuality (and women) as being "dirty," "nasty," or "not quite nice." Children still learn this in the story of Adam and Eve: it was Eve's sexuality and "desire for carnal knowledge" which ruined the Garden of Eden and for which men and women are still being punished—especially women, who are told that they must henceforth bring forth children in pain and suffering.

Unfortunately, for centuries in our society, women's sexuality has been considered "dirty": a sexual woman is a "tramp," "dirty," "filthy," and so on, whereas a sexual man is very masculine, admirable. The vulva, of which women are taught to be ashamed, has been hidden away for so long that few people really know what it looks like. The general impression many men have is of a dark wet place with an unfamiliar smell, a kind of unknown space into which the penis ventures courageously. One of the early triumphs of the women's movement was to reclaim the beauty, strength, and dignity of women's bodies for women, and to emphasize that it is women who own women's bodies, not men. For the first time women felt that they had the right to explore their own bodies and look inside them. With a mirror and a light and a plastic speculum a woman could see her interior, suddenly finding it to be a beautiful glossy pink, clean and dazzling—as opposed to the dark and unpleasant place she might have been led to believe she would find.

Perhaps men who still feel they are affected by these stereotypes about women's genitals can overcome the stereotypes by also looking inside a vagina once, with someone they care about. Some men have seen their wife's or partner's vagina during a joint physical examination, conducted by a gynecologist or sex therapist. This technique was originated by Drs. Leon and Shirley Zussman, and has had excellent results.

A few men commented on cunnilingus during menstruation:

*I like the warmth and moisture of my partner's genitals, and I enjoy the very pleasant odor of them. The only time I do not like cunnilingus is during her period, although I have done it and was surprised that I could not tell the difference in taste or odor.*

*I love the smell of my lover's vagina while she is menstruating. I want her to menstruate in my mouth and on my face—it tastes so sexy and smells so good.*

*The smell and taste of a menstruating vagina does not appeal to me, though I have never tasted one.*

*Some women have a psychological hang-up of feeling dirty during this time. Why should they? Aren't they proud to have such sophisticated bodies? Aren't they proud that they are women?*

*As I grew up I was led to believe that this was the time of the month when a woman discharged all the poison and disease germs from her womb. I know better now, but still am hung up about it.*

*Menstruation makes little difference to me. Oral sex with a tampon in place is just the same as when she is not menstruating. Without a tampon, I reserve the right to refuse but that is unlikely.*

*I feel more "afraid" of the vagina at that time. I'm less likely to play with it, to touch it or feel it. I rule out oral sex completely. She is hornier when menstruating. I will not hesitate to have intercourse.*

*I ate one girl who later said she was menstruating at the time, but I guess I was too wrapped up in it to care. Blood, blood, I had enough of it on me in Vietnam not to worry about it.*

QUESTION:
How do women's genitals look?

Many men had ambivalent feelings about the appearance of the vulva. On the other hand, some men liked it very much and offered beautiful descriptions. The range of answers covered every attitude imaginable:

*Better than men's.*

*Like "raw flesh"—a horrible mismatch.*

*I wish they were dry. Moisture bothers me. It looks like the skin of an old woman on a young one.*

*Gorgeous.*

*They look mysterious.*

*Inviting.*

*They look hairy, sensual, puffy, excited, red, and full.*

*A pretty furry pet animal.*

*Ugly but appealing and nice to touch.*

*Like a damp rose, petals blossoming.*

*Strange and compelling, inviting and ripe for explorations.*

Some men described why they liked how it looks:

*I love my wife's genitals. They look big, pink, wet, warm, ready for fun, ready to respond to me, mysterious, powerful, something to explore. Wow!*

*I think women's genitals are about as lovely as something on this earth can get. I love the way they taste and smell. There have been some genitals about which I held a near-religious feeling; this was because they were attached to women for whom I felt a deep love.*

*I think a woman's—my friends when I peeled off her pants—genitalia are so beautifully shaped and designed! What was very nice was that her pubic hair was very blond and the moon shone in the window as I put my head between her legs.*

## HOW DOES CLITORAL STIMULATION TO ORGASM AFFECT MEN'S SEXUALITY?

Is clitoral stimulation (whether by hand or mouth) something that men "should" learn to do because women need it, women "demand" it—or is clitoral stimulation an erotic and beautiful activity, as valuable and intense as intercourse? Is it pleasurable for men?

Most men sometimes doubt that women orgasm regularly during intercourse with them—and this makes them feel insecure, defensive or "inadequate." There was an undertone of anger and frustration in some answers: "When she doesn't have orgasm during intercourse, I feel like I've ripped her off. I wonder whether I should be sticking myself in her, or not. What's in it for her? Is this some sort of martyr shtick?"

And yet, as we have seen, even when men realize that women do not orgasm with them regularly during intercourse, most still also assume that women should orgasm from simple intercourse. Most men have very little expertise with clitoral stimulation to orgasm.

The stereotype in our society that says that women have a "problem" having orgasm is false: it is not women who have a "problem" having orgasm, but society that has a problem accepting how women do orgasm.

## WOMEN'S RESISTANCE TO TRADITIONAL SEX AND
## INTERCOURSE: NOT "NEUROTIC"

Many men are frustrated and dissatisfied with sex with women or have mixed feelings about the activity, even while they say that they want more. The situation is not intractable; though society has created inequality and separation between the sexes, which originally involved a struggle over the control of reproduction, these attitudes are slowly beginning to change.

Why aren't some women more frequently enthusiastic about sex with men? First, because women feel exploited sexually: they must help the man have his orgasm but must not take/make the stimulation they need to have their own. Given our definition of sex, the fact that men usually want sex more often than women should come as no surprise. Sex provides efficiently for male orgasm, and inefficiently and irregularly for female orgasm; sex is defined so that the woman expects to help the man orgasm every time, but the man is not realistically informed about how to help the woman orgasm,[*] and the woman is told that it is wrong to stimulate herself. Therefore, should we be surprised that men want sex more often than women do? Sex as we know it is a "male"-defined activity, and women, in not showing enthusiasm for many aspects of it, are displaying resistance to an institution that does not provide for them equally.

Where did the belief arise that women should orgasm from intercourse? The institution we know as "sex"—"foreplay" to intercourse ending with male orgasm—was first legislated into existence as the only acceptable form of sexual expression approximately 2,500 years ago, for purposes of increasing reproduction. But intercourse did not take on the connotations we give it today until much later; intercourse was not always considered a romantic activity during which women were supposed to orgasm. In the late nineteenth century, in fact, women were considered vulgar if they did orgasm. Then, in the early part of the twentieth century, with the increasing discussion of the rights of women, women's orgasm began to gain importance. Perhaps it seemed logical, in the beginning, to assume that women should orgasm from the same activity that led men to orgasm, especially since participation in this activity was glorified as being a form of "natural law." Of course men orgasm from other forms of stimulation too, but the "acceptable" time for men to orgasm was and is during intercourse.

Tragically, although most women have known how to stimulate themselves to orgasm easily during masturbation, they have not felt free to explain the stimulation they needed to men, or to stimulate themselves during sex with men. Being dependent on men, economically, socially, and politically has kept women silent: women have not felt that they had the right to challenge society's definition of sex or to assert their own needs and forms of sexual expression.

---

[*] Many women report that men, trying to find their clitoris, wind up touching their urethra.

But on another level, women have been resistant to intercourse because intercourse has not been a choice. The legal structure in which women were owned by either their fathers or their husbands included (and still includes in many countries today) the provision that a man has a right to intercourse with his wife on demand; there was (is) no such thing as "rape" in marriage. Further, many women have felt unable to protect themselves against pregnancy by using birth control, when it was (is) against the rules of the state or church. Thus, in a very real sense, women had no rights over their own bodies, as their husbands controlled them; and therefore many women, feeling that their husbands could do with them whatever they pleased and that any attempt at resistance or influence was futile, developed very passive and/or hostile attitudes about sexual relationships; they would participate in sex, but only when they had to, and would not be any more active during it than necessary.

Thus intercourse, far from being a simple pleasurable activity, has for centuries symbolized and celebrated male domination and ownership of women, children, and society. Conversely, it also symbolizes female subservience, or being owned. A woman, in having intercourse, especially in the traditional position with the woman on the bottom, helping the man have an orgasm but not having one herself, was reminded of her position vis-à-vis the man. It is obvious, in this context, why many men would feel much more drawn toward participating in this institution than would women.

Many women's resistance to "sex"—far from being simply negative "conditioning" about sex—can also be seen as a large-scale and healthy resistance to being dominated, and to their bodies being owned. Saying no to "sex" has become, for many women, a way of maintaining dignity and integrity, and some control over their own identity.

A basic cause of many women's resistance to sex/intercourse is emotional alienation. If women feel on some level that men think of them as second-class and value them only as "helpmates" and sexual partners, emotional alienation within the relationship is likely to result. This is another cause for women's passive resistance to having sex. One man embodied these attitudes quite clearly: "My wife is not perhaps the woman one might dream up, but she's steady, dependable, and consistent. She's the mother of my four kids, and in my own way I love her, even though she doesn't like sex too much. She doesn't initiate oral sex spontaneously, or intercourse either. She says the reason is because I don't show her enough kindness and affection throughout the day. She says if I did she'd be more active sexually. These things are not so bad that I can't live with them, but after twenty-seven years of marriage, they bug me if I don't watch out."

Another man commented on men's actions: "Most men are only attentive to women when they want sex, and women know it. From my experience as a minister listening to married women describe their sexual problems, men spend their time, energy, and interest elsewhere—then expect the women to want them when it's time for sex. This hurts the women considerably."

This emotional alienation can be directly traced to the inequality created by the society in giving men rights and privileges over women. This alienation is cemented by bringing up men and women with different psychological attitudes, and rewarding them for different types of behavior. Owning (or having the tradition of owning) women can lead men to have attitudes of condescension toward women while valuing other men more. If a woman is valued only sexually, sex (or not having sex) may be her only power. If a man expresses a real desire to spend time with a woman only when he wants her to have sex with him, is it any wonder that a woman often says no? In a society in which women are dependent on men, and in which men sometimes seem only to "need" women for sex, saying no is many women's only chance to gain recognition as an individual or to have some control in the relationship.*

How do men feel about all of this? Men often feel very angry with women who never initiate sex and too often don't want sex. But this anger has an undertone of alienation, guilt, and insecurity. Men feel instinctively that sex does not involve an equal sharing, especially when they are having an orgasm and the women are not—and this puts men on the defensive. As one man remarked, "I feel more respect for her and myself if I don't feel I am cheating her of an orgasm—or I guess the word is 'using' her, since I have an orgasm and she doesn't. I feel relieved to be with an equal." But many men covered this feeling over by bragging, accepting their "aggressiveness" as inherently "male," and insisting that they were only behaving as their "natures" compelled them to.

Although many men are very angry with women and suffer profound discomfort as the result of women's "passivity" regarding sex—possibly because of buried feelings of guilt and defensiveness, knowing that somehow women are being exploited—most men do not overtly connect this with the need for improving women's status. Most men prefer to think that the problem is simply a lingering vestige of "Victorian morality" and further to believe that somehow women can be sexually "free" even though they are not also economically and politically free.

Men are encouraged to accept this "difference" between men and women, and not to question it. Although many men instinctively feel uneasy on some level about what is going on, they are told by society that this is "just the way things are." Many men may feel that, by virtue of their having an orgasm and the woman failing to have one, they are exploiting the woman, that the situation is unfair, or that the woman is somehow in an inferior position, but they are nevertheless told that it is men's "nature" to continue wanting intercourse and having orgasm and that whether the woman does or not is "her own problem." Men's reaction to this is often to become

---

* As one man put it, "As a male, there is no question, we are always in control once she consents to lovemaking. We have the dick, that's all there is to it! We are the fucker and she is the fuckee. At the same time, in this society, the woman has the final choice as to sex or no sex. She can deny us (and herself) or she can engage in sex."

alienated from women, to feel "different," superior, uncomfortable, hostile, or insecure with them. But, they may still wonder, do women really accept their less privileged status, or are women angry?

Men are faced with the dilemma of either believing (1) that women are built differently from men and do not always need to orgasm to be satisfied; that women in fact do not mind simply watching/helping the man have an orgasm while they do not; or (2) that women can indeed orgasm (through masturbation, for example) but that they have been oppressed economically and socially into a position in which they have been forced to accede to men's wishes in sex and that women have a hidden residue of anger at men for this situation. In other words, either women are innately unequal or women have been forced to submit. These are not pleasant options. If a man believes (1), he must accept the idea that women are somehow fundamentally different from men in their basic humanity. This point of view was implied by Freud's famous question, "What does woman want?" which seemed to express the belief that what women want is so fundamentally different from what men want, that it is mysterious and unfathomable. If a man accepts this position, then his ability to be truly close to a woman is quite limited, as he feels himself so different from her.* On the other hand, if a man believes (2), he is in a much better position to achieve a close and fulfilling relationship with a woman, even though he may have to reexamine how sexuality is defined, and rethink the basis of male-female relationships. But this process can lead to much greater fulfillment and happiness for a man in his own sexuality and life.

Where do pressuring women into sex, rape (of various kinds), paying women for sex (either outright or, as many men stated, in marriage or on dates), and buying women in pornography fit into men's lives—if they do? Are these things only "abnormal" men are involved with, or did they in some way involve and affect all men's lives and relationships with women, because they somehow involve the basic underpinnings of the entire social structure?

If sex/intercourse has traditionally been the basic symbol of male domination and ownership of women (whether or not an individual man may feel this), rape and paying women for sex, or buying women though pornography, are basic extensions of this ideology—as opposed to biologic "urges" or part of a physical male "sex drive." Is it what "sex" means to men that makes them sometimes want to rape or buy women?

The general culture—in movies, books, jokes, and popular sayings—reinforces the idea that men "get" or "take" sex from women, men "have" women, men conquer and possess women, women say no but mean yes, women "give in" to men—and "penetration" is the symbol of this victory. Men, brought up to feel that a vital

---

* He may feel different not only sexually, but also in what he wants out of life; he may feel that he is more aggressive and demanding of life in general, in his career, and so on, than women—who are "naturally" content with home and security. This belief can make him feel alienated, emotionally unconnected, isolated, and angry.

part of being a male is to orgasm in a vagina, often resent women's "power" to withhold this "male need" from them; they fail to realize that this is in many ways the only "power" left to many women. It is in part this dynamic that sometimes leads men to claim that women are "more powerful" than men.

In fact, the model of sex as we know it has even been called the "rape model" of sex. If men have more power, money, and privilege than women, can the definition of "sex" change? Won't forcing women into sex (intercourse), either physically through rape or financially through paying a woman or buying pornography, continue its appeal? Arguably a real and profound change may occur. Right now, in many ways "fucking" and physical rape stand as an overwhelming metaphor for the rape—physical, emotional, and spiritual—of an entire gender by our culture.

## RAPE AND SEXUAL VIOLENCE:
## DO MEN "NATURALLY" WANT TO RAPE WOMEN?

*Sometimes I've found myself getting excited watching a show in which a man is planning a rape. It bothered me that I was being aroused by it. I'm not sure I understand why.*

*I have often wanted to rape a woman, and I fantasize about it a lot. But the idea disturbs me because it runs counter to my sense of mutual respect, humanism, feminism, etc. I'm really anxious to see what other men feel about rape.*

What does the physical rape of a woman mean to men? Is the desire sexual? A form of hostility and anger? Or a way to reassert an injured "masculine pride"?

Many men think of rape as a way of putting a woman "back in her place"—a man's right. Others believe that women are "asking for it," the implication being that women have no right to be sexual unless the attitude leads to intercourse with men and that men have the right to control women's sexuality:

*I've seen a lot of women who seem to be asking for it . . . just as a person with a fistful of money is asking for robbery by flaunting his money, especially in a gin mill or dark alley. I also feel sympathy for women. After all, when someone wants to protect one's money from being stolen, the money can be placed in a bank. But how does a woman protect her body from being raped? I wish I knew. A little more prudence, I guess. I'm glad I'm a man.*

*There is the provocation of "dry hustling." Dry hustling is making oneself available for sex and then withdrawing or withholding it. The brassiere-less woman in a public place is a dry hustler. The bra-less look is attractive. It is supposed to be. And it is a provocation.*

A few argue that rape is justified by the male "sex drive" and the "failure" of women to meet that "need." Underlying this point of view is the idea, strong in our culture and in all patriarchal cultures, that men own women's bodies. As one man noted, "She is mine. I have a right to orgasm through intercourse. God gave me the right when he made women for men." A man should not have to masturbate for orgasm when sexual desire is not mutual, according to this point of view; he should have his orgasm through a woman at all times (only an orgasm had through intercourse with a woman is legitimate), and it is a woman's duty at all times to help him do so.

Also implicit in many of the replies is the idea that a woman denying a man sex is somehow denying his manhood and that by raping a woman a man is reasserting his masculinity—not only with the woman, but in his own mind as well:

> *Once I was going with a woman (in high school) and she would not let me have sex. All my friends had done it with their girlfriends, and even did it with us when we went out on double dates and parked together after. I got to feel like a real reject. I could have lied to them about it, but then my girlfriend would have found out, and they probably wouldn't have believed me anyway, since I couldn't have described the feeling. This made me so angry I felt like raping her. Finally, without anybody knowing, I picked up a streetwalker and had intercourse. This did a lot for my feeling of confidence in my own masculinity. Soon after, I broke up with my girlfriend and started going with somebody else who would go all the way. Then I could tell the guys, and I felt like one of the group again.*

One man writes about his desire to rape being connected to the teachings of the culture:

> *It's pretty obvious that I have some hostility toward women that started way back—they have something I want, and I'm a "bad boy" for wanting it—they're excluding me—they have a secret—they have a sex organ, but dirty little boys don't get any, etc., etc., ad nauseam. I have become aware of these feelings and know when they are active; when I feel them, I back off whatever situation is causing them and find something else to do.*

Another man describes chillingly his generalized feeling of rejection—feeling left out of what "everyone else" is enjoying, what other men are having:

> *I have certainly wanted to. Usually this desire comes after I have been rejected by a very attractive woman, e.g., at the office. Then I fantasize following her, putting a gun to her head (I own a revolver), and asking*

*her something like "Now tell me who you want to go to bed with." In recent months, I have become more sympathetic toward rapists, because I see in myself the other side of the sexual revolution: it is all well and good for the Beautiful People to decide to bring their fantasies out of the closet and talk about the joys of sex in public—it is another to be tantalized day after day by the sight of beautiful women you desire but can't have. Apparently every one of them is experiencing the wildest sexual pleasures and fulfillment, because the media are everywhere saying so.*

The image of a rapist appeals to some men, who identify it with being strong and virile, passionate and powerful:

*I don't think I could. But I have been sort of impressed by people who pulled off what seemed to be an especially brilliant or daring rape.*

*I have fantasies of doing it, as a form of "proving" to the woman that I am really all "man," able to get and keep a hard-an and use it to force myself on her, whether she wants me or not.*

Some men even write that all "real" men have a desire to rape women because this is part of a male's innate makeup (a "natural" animal instinct):*

*Why do I want to rape women? Because I am basically, as a male, a predator and all women look to men like prey. I fantasize about the expression on a woman's face when I "capture" her and she realizes she cannot escape. It's like I won, I own her.*

*Rape behavior in males today probably exists because it has been selected for (this would take precedence over selection by females) in the Darwinian model of natural selection; as much as our contemporary society despises the rapist, we must admit that in man's history the rapist's genes were naturally selected because the behavior had survival value.*†

A few men wonder why they don't have these feelings, and whether they are "abnormal":

*I have never raped a woman, or wanted to. In this I guess I am somewhat*

---

\* This feeling is inaccurate, since animals are generally not known to rape. The implication in this answer is that rape is a "natural instinct," which only "civilization" can overcome. In fact, it is our "civilization" that has created the concept and encouraged it.

† Darwin's theory concerned selection between different species, not within species. This is a misunderstanding and misuse of the concept of "survival of the fittest."

*odd. Most of my friends talk about rape a lot and fantasize about it. The whole idea leaves me cold.*

In fact, despite the seeming secret admiration of some men for rapists as the ultimate "man," strong and powerful, the reality is usually just the opposite: it is the man with the lowest self-esteem who is most likely to rape women or pressure them for sex—the man who does not see himself as strong and powerful, the man who feels the most rejected, the most like a "loser."

The loner rapist who becomes violent is becoming more and more a common figure in our society, unfortunately:

> *I am single, never married, never lived with a woman, and I am so alone that I am slowly going crazy. I am fifty pounds overweight, work as a clerk in a welfare office and as a security guard at nights. I find going out to meet women very frustrating. Going to dances and no one wanting to dance with me gets me pissed. I get very depressed and antisocial. I have a perverse but vicarious thrill in other people (usually men) who go berserk in public places and kill innocent bystanders, such as David Berkowitz (Son of Sam). When I was in college, I wanted to shoot good-looking coeds on campus with a concealed automatic pistol. They never look at me or acknowledge my humanity, so maybe I'm not good enough for them. I think they're afraid I'm going to rape them. I would never rape a woman because I don't think I could convince them I'm serious, they'd probably scream and I would run. Berkowitz's strategy was more direct, hostile, vengeful, and up-front. I admire Berkowitz, Son of Sam, for what he did.*

### PORNOGRAPHY'S DEFINITION OF "MALE SEXUALITY": IS IT VIOLENT?

What is the reason for pornography's increasing visibility in our society? Sex is a larger business than the record and film industries combined, amounting to billions of dollars a year. Why do some men (and some women, of course, though many fewer) use and look at pornography? Is it for sexual stimulation or "male bonding"? What "turns men on" about pornography? Is it the viewing of female nudity or sexual activities? Or because of the fantasies of male power that accompany the viewing?

Certainly we all—men and women—have a right to see and read about intimate relationships between people, and in this way to make more sense of our own lives and feelings. But pornography as we know it does not for the most part serve this purpose. In fact, much of pornography shows a woman submitting to a stronger, threatening, perhaps hostile and violent male.[*] Even in "soft-core" pornography, in

---

[*] Pornography much more frequently shows women rather than men being dominated, tortured, and humiliated. Sadism against women is a cultural theme for the West that goes back to the "witch" burnings of the Middle Ages, during which several million women were killed.

which a woman is alone on the page or screen, perhaps making eye contact with the viewer but almost always in a "come and get me" pose, the woman is being dominated—not by a man in the picture, but directly by the viewer, who can use her in any way he pleases. Pornography as we know it—indeed, sex itself—is a reflection of the society, with women often being used for men's pleasure. Men dominating women in these pictures is such a commonplace that the implication is lost.

Pornography also reinforces in men the idea that all women can be bought; as one man said, "Pornography is a cheap way of buying a woman." Pornography does not glorify women. Most men have contempt for the women they see on the pages, no matter how beautiful. A common form of using pornography is for men to look at it together in a group and to make comments about the women. This is a form of male bonding and reinforces the idea of male ownership of women.[*] Pornography reminds one of slave markets and slave auctions: each man can appraise, select, and buy the body that suits him. The economic pressures on women, especially poor women, to sell their bodies in this way are great.

The continued spread of pornography will make relationships between men and women much slower to change, because pornography reinforces in men so many of the old and stereotypical attitudes toward women and toward themselves. This is just as true of pornography that shows the woman/women dominating men as it is of depictions of men dominating women, since the gender change is only a role reversal and still centers on the same definitions of sex involving all the issues we have discussed in this book so far. Pornography keeps men believing that women are the way they want women to be, or have been told women are (either submissive or dominant, "bitchy"), and fortifies men's belief in their own sex role. When reading and looking at pornography, men know that they are sharing in something other men see, and they therefore assume that this imagery is what all "real men" want, identify with, and enjoy.

## MEN, MARRIAGE, AND MONOGAMY[†]

Do most men have sex outside of marriage, and if so, why? In my research, according to men's descriptions of their feelings about their marriages and their wives, the majority of marriages were not based on the emotional intensity of being "in love." But most men said that they definitely loved their wives and had no intention

---

[*] Most men do not look at pornography with a woman, as most women do not like the way women are portrayed in pornography. Also, men looking at pornography together can find that this act is another way of proclaiming one's masculinity for other men to see and a way for men to have sexual feelings together while still focused on a "heterosexual" object.

[†] Many more single (never married) men were in favor of monogamy than were married men; in fact, the majority of single men planned to be monogamous in their marriages or were currently monogamous in their (nonliving together) relationships. Is this a reaction to the "sexual revolution," and the lives of their parents, or are younger men more idealistic—or both? Or had married men also intended to be monogamous before they married?

of leaving them, even though most of them also had sex outside of their marriages, unknown to their wives.

QUESTION:

Do you like extended periods of monogamy? Why, or why not? Have you had "extramarital" sexual experiences? If so, how many, and how long? Did/does your partner know about them? What was/is the effect on you as an individual and on your marriage?

The great majority of married men were not monogamous; 72 percent of men married two years or more had had sex outside of marriage; the overwhelming majority did not tell their wives, at least at the time.

*I have been married eighteen years. I like it, very much. We have a very good sexual relationship—I could not ask for a better sex life. I believe in monogamy. It is the moral and the religious thing to do. My outside sex has been unknown to my wife. It had no effect on my marriage. The only problem is it costs too much money to support a family and a girlfriend.*

*Married to the same woman thirty-nine years. Never more affection and pleasure than this morning. As far as extramarital, yes. Unknown to my wife. It has broadened my understanding of life.*

*Married seven years. I greatly enjoy being married. Marriage has given me a regular sex partner and opened more doors for us sexually. I love my wife very much. My love has gone from one of selfish, possessive love to a feeling of need, sharing, communication, protectiveness, and mutual enjoyment of our child and life. I do not believe in total monogamy. I feel that there are times in every person's life when they need outside input, even to the extent of intercourse, to renew their sexual feelings and stimulate their fantasies. I feel that it can improve the marriage relationship under the present circumstances. I have had ten "extramarital" experiences and they were of the one-time type. I do not now have one planned. I feel that these experiences greatly increased my sexual feelings for a while and added to my passion with my wife.*

*Eight years. I don't like being married. I'm still married because of our kid. I've had affairs and they were very satisfying to me. They were unknown to my wife. At first I was bitter, to be out in the street doing something which I thought I would be doing home with my wife. But I've resigned myself to her being as she is, and I try not to make comparisons between the women in my affairs and my wife. I just enjoy them. Even prostitutes.*

The most frequent reason men gave for having sex outside of marriage was sexual rejection by their wives and the boring nature of repeated sex with the same person in marriage. But since these two statements practically cancel each other out, are there other reasons? Why do men need to bolster their marriages on a continuing basis in this way? It would seem that there may be hidden tension or anger between men and women that focuses on sex.

Does sex automatically become boring in marriage or in a long relationship? Is the constant repetition of certain activities with one person inevitably less interesting as time passes? One way to answer this question is to ask whether it is less interesting to have dinner and a conversation with a friend you have known for twenty years than it is with a friend you have known for one? Obviously it depends on the friend, and on the status of the relationship at any particular time. But usually one can talk more deeply to an old and good friend than to a new one—although there is fun and excitement in discovering a new person.

Part of the reason for the "inevitable boringness" of sex in many of the marriages of men in this book is the fact that they have frequently shied away from marrying the women with whom they were most in love, the women who most excited them, the women toward whom they felt the most open and emotionally vulnerable. Men have tended to base their marriages more on practicalities, on a "rational" feeling of being "in control" over their lives and being able to foresee a stable and predictable future, than on a feeling of being overwhelmed by the sudden beauty (in manner and thought, in a total sense, not just physically) of another. But to be so totally in control is boring, eventually.

Another reason repeated sex with the same person may become "boring" has to do with the repetitive nature of the way we define sex—that is, as "foreplay," followed by "vaginal penetration," and ending with intercourse and male orgasm in the vagina. If the definition of sex is constantly static and filled with performance pressures, perhaps the only way to find variety is to change partners.

In some ways, also, the alienation that has been built into marriages, based on the inequality between men and women legislated by our society, can also lead to a feeling of "boredom"—as boredom often represents built-up and unexpressed anger, rage, or hopelessness. Men often feel this rage against their wives, and marriages often contain decades-long cold wars. Most men's reaction to this situation is to search secretly for an interim relationship outside of the marriage. But men seeking emotional intimacy and fulfillment through sex—first with one partner, then another, as a pattern throughout a marriage—were not, in this study, very happy in the end because of it. It was much more rewarding, as some men did, to seek out the causes of the "boredom" or lack of closeness, whether bottled up anger or something else. To deny that there are problems, to describe "male sexuality" as if it were a mechanical "drive," with a built-in need for "variety," as if men were "biologically programmed" to go from "blossom to blossom" spreading their "pollen," only increases loneliness and isolation.

## ARE MEN ANGRY AT WOMEN?

Are there other reasons for men's extramarital sex? Perhaps some men see it as their "right"—something they are privileged to do as men, when they feel like it; in fact, some men may even feel pressured to have extramarital sex by a culture that implies that all "real men" do it. Other reasons include maintaining a separate identity or individuality, getting affection or an ego boost when needed, or getting out of a marriage they want to end.

But the main reason for most extramarital sex, the reason most men give, was that it "makes the marriage workable"—that without these affairs, they would not be able to continue in the marriage. And in fact, some of the longest marriages did seem to have survived in just this way.

But why were these marriages "unworkable"? Is lack of sex, or "boring" sex, the reason, or is the trouble men so often describe as sexual merely a reflection of larger unresolved issues in the relationship? Are these unresolved or unacknowledged issues different in every relationship, or are there also more common, culturally created, problems between men and women? Of course there are always individual conflicts or problems unique to any two people that can lead to fighting or to alienated feelings; but there are also problems common to many couples, problems that therefore take on a larger meaning.

On one level many men find that they cannot reconcile in their own minds the idea of loving their wives as the mothers of their children (and the women who have the role of "mothering"—taking care of, feeding—the men themselves), and seeing her as a sexual being. Many men, raised to think of the mother as asexual or sexually taboo, find that they begin to have similar feelings about their wives, soon after marriage or after children arrive.

But another, perhaps more hidden or underlying, reason is unexpressed or unrecognized anger. In fact many men's extramarital affairs, kept secret from their wives, can be seen as an escape valve—a way of secretly or unconsciously expressing anger at their wives, "getting even," "showing her"—a kind of private revenge that does not, on the surface, disturb the relationship, but gives a feeling of relief, allowing one to return refreshed, feeling more loving than ever, now that the anger has been expressed.

What, underneath it all, are men angry about? Were there any underlying themes in the complaints men presented—any complaints that surfaced again and again, that could, on a larger scale, be a cause of much of the anger? Or was most of this anger hidden, even unrecognized? In fact in many, many replies, hidden anger, guilt, and ambivalence emerged as factors blocking relationships, especially long-term relationships.

All too often men learned from their fathers' attitudes toward their mothers to see women as weak and overly emotional, dependent, able to gain "power" only by relying on psychological domination and manipulation, using men for their own economic advantage. As one man put it, "My father taught me (by implication) that women are traps and burdens, but the best that's available for overcoming loneliness." It is remarkable, given these views—and, sadly, as a result of cultural and economic pressures on women, these stereotypes have, at times, been true—that relationships between men and women ever manage to succeed.

## MEN'S PERCEPTION OF WOMEN AS WEAK

But how does men's view of women basically as "sex partners" or mothers, as generally weak and inferior, lead to men's anger with women? The first reason is that men feel guilty and conflicted in their loyalties, and angry with women for making them feel guilty:

> Since she loves me so much, I feel guilty that maybe I don't love her as much. She really looks up to me. Sometimes I feel like she worships me. This makes me feel funny. I know that as a man it is my duty to help her, but sometimes I feel annoyed with her. Why can't she stand on her own two feet?

> I can't help looking down on women. You can get anything you want from them by telling them they are "special." They love to be told they are "special."

> I guess what makes me maddest about women is when they lack pride, underestimate themselves, and are over-careful. When I see a woman with intelligence and abilities take a passive role in life because she lacks self-confidence, it upsets me and I tend to become critical.

A great deal of the alienation of men from women is caused by men's knowledge, on some level, of their superior, privileged class status over women—or at least of a difference in status. This issue, too emotionally charged to discuss in most cases, is taken for granted by most men and women, but with unrecognized consequences for the entire relationship. Although men felt somewhat free to voice these feelings about their mothers, and to recognize their mothers' subordinate position vis-à-vis their fathers—often calling their mothers "weak"—many men did not feel free to express, or perhaps even to recognize, such feelings about their own wives and lovers.

A further problem is economic. Since the society has kept women economically, socially, and even emotionally dependent on men, it is no wonder that men sometimes feel "trapped" in marriage. And yet most men do not explicitly connect problems with the social and legal role assigned women (for their own role as "caretaker") and their own feeling of lack of satisfaction in marriage, or suffocation. Most seem to feel that their marital problems related to their wife is assertiveness, that she was being unreasonable and making too many demands, or that she was not responding with a sufficient amount of affection (gratitude?) by participating in sex more frequently. Or she was not being "giving" enough. Thus, men felt perfectly justified in going outside the marriage for sex and pleasure, since they felt that they were being cheated inside the marriage.

However—even though most men did not connect society's assigning women a second-class or dependent role with their own feelings of dissatisfaction, accompanied by their endless search for a gratifying "sexual" relationship with a woman— a majority of men did recognize the potential drain on the spirit from being supported by, or dependent on another. When asked, "Do you envy women the choice of having someone support them, the seeming lack of pressure on them to make money?" almost no men said they envied women, and most stated strongly that they would not like to be supported by someone else.

The traditional marriage, in which the man controlled the money while the woman's domain was the house, was the type of marriage most likely to include a pattern of extramarital sex for the man.* Newer marriages, struggling to create more equal relationships, were more likely to be monogamous—with the partners also more likely to end the marriage if the closeness dissolved, rather than patching up the marriage with outside sex. But "newer" marriages were not necessarily between younger men and women, by any means. A more equal marriage could be something a couple of any age might strive for.

The happiest men in this study were those with the closest, most functioning relationships with women—that is, a minority of (in most cases, married) men. Trying to live by the male code, being totally self-sufficient, emotionally and economically, always providing shelter and food (or sex and orgasms), never receiving or needing anything, never needing a woman's love more than she needs the man's— all this hurts and stunts men.

Some men were beginning to see that their own welfare is tied up with women's fight to restructure their lives and relationships for the better, to redefine themselves above and beyond the traditional confines of "femininity." "Masculinity" can be just as much of a pressure on men as an enforced "femininity" can be on women.

But one of the deepest problems still prevalent in many men's minds is the connection they made between money and sex with women. Most men believed that women were somehow for sale. When asked, "How do you feel about paying a woman for sex?" meaning prostitution, many answered, "You always pay anyway"—meaning that whether it is in marriage, where the man provides support in return for (what he considers should be) domestic and sexual services, or on a date, in which the man pays for dinner expecting sex in return, he is always paying. Many men replied that it was more honest, and more of a bargain, to pay a

---

* Studies have implied that women engage in extramarital sex somewhat less frequently; many men have outside sex with unmarried women. Actually women's traditional patterns of extramarital sex are largely unknown.

woman outright. In fact the number one reason given by men for their anger with women was the financial burden. Men mentioned frequently that you can't trust women, that women often "use" men to get financial support. Many men feel that they can never be sure that a woman loves them just for themselves: "Maybe she is just staying with me as a meal ticket."

The unfortunate part in this respect is that most men do not accept the women's movement, which could change the situation. If women had equal rights with men, equal access to jobs and education, and equal pay (in the United States, women earn only 59 percent of what men are paid for the same work), then men would not have to fear that women loved them only for their money or for financial support. Most men gave lip service to women's rights, admitting that women should be "equal," but disapproved of most of the ways that this change could be brought about. Men were afraid that women's liberation would mean less love: if women got equal rights, and especially if they were financially independent, they would not love men anymore. Most men did not seem to feel secure that they were worthy of love on a deeper level. And most men did not want to give up their so-called masculine privileges, even though these "privileges" had not made them particularly happy. Perhaps the less happy some men are, the more they cling, paradoxically, to the very ideas and beliefs that have left them so unfulfilled.

## DO MEN NOW WANT TO REDEFINE THEIR RELATIONSHIPS WITH WOMEN?

The inequalities pervading men's and women's traditional roles have placed a tremendous burden on relationships between men and women, often creating an adversarial, distrusting situation. If individuals were free to choose their role in a relationship, to create new types of relationships with each other, more equal relationships, there would be less need for distrust, and more mutual respect and communication would be possible.

Since our society has kept women in a secondary position, economically and socially, most women remain somehow dependent on men.[*] Traditionally a woman with children had to depend on the good will of her husband for her and her children's support. This situation may have created a subtle pressure on her to fear her husband and to cater to his wishes, no matter what her own feelings—preventing a free and spontaneous relationship between equals.

Many men in my study did not see the relevance to them of the women's movement; they did not see the connection between their own feelings of being trapped and alienated—in their role in marriage, in their jobs, in their lifestyle, in their lack of closeness—and the critique of society and relationships that the women's movement poses, the suggestions the women's movement has made for improving things.

---

[*] According to the U.S. Bureau of Labor statistics, women in 1980 still earned only 59 percent of what men earn for the same work.

Many men tended to see the women's movement more as "women complaining, raising a ruckus" than understanding how both men and women, working to change and restructure their relationships (and the family), could make increased happiness for both. In fact, many men were angry that now women might be "getting ahead," because their own lives had often left them feeling unappreciated, unsatisfied, angry, and stifled.

## WHAT DO MEN THINK OF WOMEN'S LIBERATION?

*I think women's liberation is great. It has not affected any of my relationships.*

*A man and woman can't live and love each other as husband and wife unless the man is the head of the house and the wife considers her husband as the master over her in everything.*

*I can't respect women, because why did they let themselves be subjugated, owned and ruled?*

*I think it's important to mention the guilt I sometimes feel very acutely when I realize the privileges I enjoy as opposed to what the majority of women enjoy. I think of all the hidden ways that this privilege is handed to me by the culture in which I live, and the ways women are short-changed of those same privileges. It makes me uncomfortable to be given extra points for being a white, middle-class male with an education, but the ingredient that provides the most credence in this society is gender.*

Many of the answers to the question "What do you think about women's liberation?" brought out a huge amount of anger at women, or anger with men's own situation, their own role in society and tremendous lack of fulfillment. Many men felt that now, with the women's movement and the emphasis on women achieving more independence and equality, they were being falsely maligned and misunderstood:

*All I ever hear about these days is how brutal men are, how women are always getting fucked over by men, and how the sisterhood is gonna go it alone. Well, men get the same kind of shit, and I do not like being put in a category. I'm no better or worse than anyone else, regardless of gender. Just like a woman, I want to be loved and give love in return.*

*There seems to be a growing stereotype of what bastards men are. Although I suppose some do live up to this stereotype, I know many men who don't (including, I believe, myself). I don't like this trend and find it similar to the black backlash against all whites once they achieved greater control over their lives ... alienating even those whites who had fought alongside them for equal opportunities, etc. Some men are stronger feminists than many women. Why condemn all of us? Society has dictated not only to women the roles they should play but also to men. Men have been stereotyped and enslaved into following traditional approaches to life just as much as women, and the more moderate feminists are willing to accept this and seem to be turning towards a cooperation with men in changing society.*

Many answers seemed to imply that the women's movement is merely something having to do with women's "self-esteem," rather than being a fundamental critique of the society and both men's and women's roles in it, and therefore something to which men must address themselves directly, as it involves a basic readjustment in "their" world:*

*The "movement" has not affected my relationships because the women I like do things as individuals, not as part of movements. However, if some subtle change in the general atmosphere has helped them to reach a more open state, that's good. Most, though, still want the man to take the initiative in the early stages of dating and sex. So it has not changed my relationships.*

*I feel that it has helped my wife.*

*Women's liberation provides a medium of support for women who can't otherwise feel good about their womanhood. As such it has its benefits to our society.*

A minority of men, still misunderstanding the movement, replied that they were totally against women's liberation:

*It stinks. Women should be feminine, but with equal rights. American women should make men feel like men, not competitors.*

*I believe men and women are not equal. They each have their own jobs in life. Let me explain. First of all, a woman can have a child, a man cannot. He doesn't even have to be there for conception. A sperm bank can do that. A woman's skeleton matures faster than a man's. Women have faster reaction times in general. The list is endless in comparing men and*

---

* But they have—it's fundamentalism!

*women. They were each put on this earth with all their differences. However, if men and women stopped competing with each other it would be a better world.*

*It made women feel like they can do it all, as if they don't need men to keep up a house. I think being pregnant should be the woman's natural desire.*

*I think it's the worst thing that ever happened to women and their relations with men.*

*I don't like it. The vital role women play as mothers who mold the future generation has been deemphasized. We are on a self-destruction course. If you think we have a lot of crazies now—you ain't seen nothing. Day care centers are sadly run by people who raise children as a business. The children are second-class children, they are entitled to more. Up with Mother Power. It's all marketing and media hype. If some women want to work in this cold, often boring life outside the home, fine. But never degrade the role of the mother. Also, some women are getting socially aggressive. I'm flattered and respond—but if they didn't make advances to me I probably wouldn't go after them, therefore after the initial thrill is over I dump them, and I got a depressed liberated broad to deal with.*

*Women just need to sound off. The greatest people alive have been men, including Jesus Christ Himself. No woman has yet lived and been great enough to be the Daughter of God! Print it!*

*A farcical gyration of dykes. It has afforded me many laughs.*

The largest number of men claimed to be "in favor of women's liberation, BUT":

*It's O.K. but I wouldn't want a woman for a boss.*

*It is righting some wrongs, but also causing disruptions in established patterns which have been beneficial to society.*

*Women's liberation is a just cause when it pursues equality of opportunity in life, and the desire to be judged as a person first, not on a prejudicial basis. But the women's movement is unjust when it chooses anti-male attitudes instead of the pursuit of justice. Anti-male is no better than anti-female.*

*I'm in favor of it when it comes to getting rid of discrimination, but it's overblown. Women have always been able to get what they want.*

*I am all for women being equal, but nothing they or I can do will change biological differences. It is wrong when women "want to be men," and I feel sorry for those who do. The world would be a miserable place if most men and women were not happy to be what they are. But basically I am open-minded and want to be fair, so I can't say I'm against women's liberation, but women's liberation turns me off when it becomes hatred of things masculine.*

## A TIME OF CHANGE?

Today many men—men of every age, not just younger men—are privately anguished over how to define their own masculinity, what it means to be a man. The majority feel an enormous amount of pressure and frustration, too often focusing on women as the cause, rather than taking on the social values that need to be confronted. Many men feel that they cannot talk to other men about their frustrations with "masculinity"—because to do so might make them look less "masculine" to other men, as if they couldn't "make it" as a man.

Men want to be close to women to express their emotional lives. This is especially true since, as we have seen, men learned from their fathers that closeness, personal talks, and affection were not an appropriate part of a relationship with another man; men feel that they can only express this part of themselves with a woman—and even then, all too many men have mixed feelings, believing that these urges, these needs, represent weakness, are needs they should not have.

Most men are cautious about falling in love. Men's first feelings on falling in love are as joyous and ecstatic as women's—in fact, men's take on love is one of the only parts of this section that could have been written by women—but after their initial feelings of happiness (and erotic attraction), most men backed off or distrusted their feelings—ironically, the very feelings that had given them such pleasure. In fact, most men distrusted these feelings so much that the majority of marriages were not based on this kind of emotional intensity, at least as men in this study described their feelings about their marriages and their wives. Most men did not marry the women they had been most "in love" with, although they emphasize that they love their wives and do not want to leave them, even when they are having regular sex with someone they care about outside the marriage.

The men in this study who most accepted traditional stereotypes of masculinity were those who were most unhappy with their lives. There has been a built-in contradiction between the so-called male lifestyle and human closeness. Lack of emotionality and closeness make men feel isolated, angry, and cynical. Men today are faced with the rather formidable choice of either continuing to live their lives as in the past, feeling torn apart by constantly having to suppress and deny their own needs (and suffering with their early death rate and illnesses)—or creating something new.

## WHO ARE MEN TODAY? WHO IS THE MODERN MAN?

The last twenty-five years are thought of as an era of change for women, but men have been changing as well. How much have men "undefined" their ideas of masculinity, of who a real man is—and how much are men carrying on with an old point of view dressed up in a new style?

Many men have a perpetual sense that "the party is going on somewhere else," that they are missing out, that they might die without ever having really lived. (Clearly, being "masculine" is not the most satisfying way of life.) Though most men believe in equality for women, they simultaneously worry that the Brave New World "run by women" won't have a place for them. They feel subliminally anxious and guilty because they may possibly benefit from a system of male-privilege— though this guilt may be hidden, unacknowledged. Amidst such pressures, many are inclined to revolt and cry out, "Hell with it, I can't do anything right, I'm going to act like the mean macho maverick I really am deep down!"

This may be one of the first generations of men to be preoccupied with sexually pleasing their mates/women both physically and emotionally—an adjustment that requires a sea change in a man's conception of his own sexual identity.

Yet current popular clichés with a "biological determinist" slant imply that a man's nature can't really change. Men are destined biologically, this thinking goes, to be competitive and aggressive, to bond with other groups of men and not include women, who are also "destined by biology" to be "different"—that is, less adventurous, preferring home. This "unchangeable human nature in their genes" makes them lust to be warriors and hunters, to fight battles.

But images of mythic masculinity are not the great gift to men they may appear to be, as men sometimes realize. Most don't really identify with warrior images, and they worry that they won't live up to them. Questions men ask themselves include: Is a "real man" monogamous or not? Is he a "good husband and father" or not? Is he married or single, lover or husband? While most men somehow believe in marriage, ironically, most also believe that they should be free, less "tied down," and many fault themselves for not being sure what they really want.

This inner turmoil may mean that many men today are quietly staging a revolution within themselves, questioning the beliefs they were brought up with, redesigning their inner value system, rethinking the importance of work and private life, asking how much time should be spent at work/at home, what love is about.

Based on my research, I would like to propose a new theory of "male nature," one based on social pressures rather than on biology or hormones, one that takes into account how, during their formative years, boys are pressured to completely change their identity.

My research, conducted over many years with thousands of men, brought out the fact that most boys are subjected to taunts or bullying (even being beaten up) by bigger boys or older male members of the family ("Don't be a sissy, grow up and be a man!"). This situation causes boys to undergo a powerful process of self-questioning, ending in a basic identity change.

Though most boys are close to their mothers when they are young, at a certain stage the pressures placed on them to "act like a man" become overwhelming.

Many boys in this situation turn to their mothers for protection or resort to staying at home; they are surprised when she too says, "You can't come home to mother anymore, now you have to go out and tell off the boys who are bothering you, or beat them up!" Then boys, according to my data, are filled with doubt and spend on average a year or more questioning themselves about how they should adapt to the new situation. The problem is not only that they are supposed to "act tough," but also that they must cut off their relationship with their mother or other women or girls; a boy is seen as a "sissy" if his best friend is a girl or if he "hangs out with girls all the time."

Though many boys like being with girls who are their friends, they soon learn that they have to make peace with the men around them, find a way to get along, and learn to exclude women, "leave the women at home." Joining the "world of the fathers" is a frightening experience for many boys; most describe feeling alone and insecure in a new, colder and more competitive world, a world, men state, over and over, their fathers did not explain to them. Later men can come to feel that conquering this new world is the biggest adventure they undertake in life.

What happens in private life? If a man falls in love with a woman, this event usually forces him to reexamine his relationship with men and his own idea of himself. This is more difficult if a man feels "real men don't fall deeply in love!" Most men included in my research do not marry the women they most passionately love, often adding that they are proud of this decision. Why?

Men feel that they can better follow "the rules" if they stay in control of their feelings. Other boys do not fall in love at all; their reaction to "male" puberty pressures is to decide that they are not "joiners" (they feel that they do not legitimately belong to the group of men, and are "faking" fitting in) and decide to be "loners," "independent," close to neither men nor women.

Men's relationships with other men are generally deeply unsatisfying: like the Michaelangelo fresco of Adam reaching for God's hand in *The Creation*, in which their fingers never quite touch, men often feel a tantalizing sense of "almost, almost." Most boys grow up with only a distant relationship with their fathers, which carries over into relationships with other men. Men are left with a feeling that "he" is unattainable, and that this is how it must be.

Many men cope by living with split personalities, one for work and another for "private life" and "love." During the last two decades books on "personal growth" ("self-help" for women and "business secrets" for men) have helped individuals think through issues of identity change. Most men no longer want the "traditional manhood" of the 1950s and 1980s but a new way of life, which they are inventing now, engaged in a momentous interior transformation that has as yet to go public.

## DO MEN LIKE MARRIAGE?

Joke after joke tells us that men try to "escape the trap of matrimony" and "remain free," that it is women who are "desperate to get married."

Yet statistics tells us that the majority of divorces all over the world (even those of previous centuries) are usually brought by women, not men. We have no statistics on who asks whom to get married: could it be that it is also women who are "popping the question"? Tradition has it that the proposal is a man's privilege and honor, that it is for the man to "choose" the woman and ask for "her hand," yet hearsay reveals that women have to ask men.

However, most married men like marriage, though they often hide this fact. For example, most men in my research stated that their wife is their best friend, as well as lover, and that they like this close companionship. Men like long-term stable relationships with women (why shouldn't they?), though "male images" normally portray men as liking to be together with other men, as the "norm."

When I asked men in my research why they like marriage, they usually mention such elements as love for their wife, sleeping together in the same bed, sharing a family and a history, and future plans. If men have complaints about marriage, they generally voice them only as complaints about a particular behavior of their wife's, not the whole idea. Significantly, very few men indeed say that their marriage makes them feel "tied down;" contrary to the stereotype, the sense of being trapped does not seem to be an issue. (Men often find that they have plenty of time and freedom to "have sex elsewhere" if they so desire to, or to go out on their own, go to work, and the like.)

Why do men hide the fact that they like marriage? Most male movie heroes and rock stars are single; in fact, it is hard to think of any male film heroes who portray married heroes (they may be married in real life, but not in films). Though it is simplistically said that this phenomenon is because "female fans like men single," in fact it is mostly a male audience that dictates the choices of what films to attend. Men especially like single male heroes who are "free" and have adventures, men who are admired for their gutsiness. Rock stars guard their images as nonmarried, "free," and single, adventurous males. Male trendy phrases refer to the terror of being "tied down to a woman," wanting to "avoid marriage like the plague," and "needing my freedom, my space," and so on.

Does this imply that men are married against their will?? That men are basically against the idea of "family?" How do men grow to connect the idea of being "free," being a "real male," with not being married—or even "too much in love"?

Usually women are blamed for the changes going on in the family, for attacking the family and demanding that it change. In fact, the rebellion against marriage and family was largely begun by men. Even in the "golden family age" of the 1950s, jokes were commonly made by men (echoed by male comedians on television) about "the old lady," "my nagging wife" or "that gold digger, my wife." A 1953 film, *Shane*, created a new male heroic image, marking a turning point: it featured a cowboy "loner" who drifts into a small town and helps the wife and son of a passive father-of-the-family, portrayed as a wimp and quasi-coward, as they survive Indian attacks. By the end of the film, as Shane is leaving (his destiny is "to roam"), both the mother and her small son seem under his spell, calling his name plaintively, looking after him as he rides off into the sunset on his palomino horse. This film firmly established the new male "loner"-hero (seen later worldwide on Marlboro cigarette ads), a tough, lone man who "keeps his independence and is proud of it," who "doesn't need anyone." Other famous films, such as *Midnight Cowboy* and current detective thrillers, continue this worship of the single male.

Men's revolt against marriage grew after World War II. Was this because of the "sexual revolution" and the fact that men had more access to sex outside marriage after the advent of the birth-control pill? Or were the pill and change in attitudes ("sexual revolution") the result of men's new drive to be "free" rather than its cause?

In fact men's drive to "shake off the shackles of marriage" came before the "sexual revolution." Contributing to men's revolt against marriage were wartime propaganda images of men, which were created by governments to get more men to enlist in the armed forces. The myths governments needed to create during World War II to convince men that they wanted to enlist and go to war (rather than stay home with their wives and loved ones) changed ideas of male psychology. During the war years, the United States government poured enormous sums of money into the Hollywood film industry, as is documented. No longer were men portrayed as being happy "getting their girl" at home; now "real men" were those who sought adventure far from home, relishing the thrill of battle with other men at their side—or, sometimes, heroically on their own.

These images of masculinity—"man as fighting animal"—left the impression that a "real man" is a killer, not a family man. This cliché continues in films today. Is this image wrong? Why, even now, sixty or more years after that war, does the stereotype of "real man as single loner" seem almost to intensify rather than fade? Though research shows that men like marriage—the vast majority of men do marry, most do not want to divorce, and men even live longer when they sleep (sleep, whether or not they have sex) together regularly with a woman(!)—and though all the indications are that men like and need marriage or long-term positive relationships with women (living together), still the idea of the need for "freedom" and "space" has the greatest cachet. Why?

Possibly it is the tightness of the "traditional family" institution that men don't like, the way marriage has been defined, rather than long-term relationships with women.

### ARE MEN MONOGAMOUS?

How often have you heard jokes about, "What can you expect from a man? Men can't help having a roving eye—it's their nature!"

Women's eyes are not expected to "rove," women are (or have been, at least) expected to love one man only, no matter what. People remind women today that "not long ago" it was the custom for men to have "more than one wife" and that therefore women should realize their good fortune and not push their luck, not "ask for too much"!

Fortunately women today are beginning to have enough economic autonomy to declare to a man that either they will both be monogamous or neither will be—depending on how a woman feels about her relationship. In some countries in the Middle East, with extremist Islamic governments, a woman can be "legitimately" killed for being "unfaithful"—a man, however, cannot.

Though men sometimes celebrate a monogamous love for "one woman only," often they hide such feelings in shame. Some men are embarrassed and think that they will look "wimpy," not like a "superstud," if they proclaim how happy they are in being monogamous. In some cultures men are encouraged to "display" their masculinity by showing how many women they can have; in others, "fidelity to marriage and family" is considered a virtue for a man.

One young man in my research describes doubting his focus on one woman: "I feel this unbelievable sexual, physical, and personal attraction to her, and have ever since the minute I met her. She is irresistibly sexy, I can't control myself when I'm around her or I just think of her. When I see other women at work, even if they are attractive, neat bodies, etc., it's like they're not even there for me. I only want her. I never tell this to the other guys at work."

But what if the other guys are largely putting on an act too? What if most of them really like being married but are afraid to say so? One older man, married for thirty years, puts it this way: "I never wanted to leave my wife, even at times when we were not so happy. Yes, there were other women along the way who attracted me, but before everything else comes my relationship with her. We are in the business of life together, I mean we have raised three children, we have seen each other at our best and worst, she is still beautiful to me and interesting. But no one believes it when I say this, they think it can't be true. So I don't talk about it much."

So much fun has been made of men who are married ("He's henpecked, his wife nags him all the time"), rather than giving them respect and admiration for forming a good relationship with a woman, that many men feel embarrassed at their monogamous tendencies. They fight them like crazy. Even when men fall truly in love, they sometimes try—no matter how happy they are—to extricate themselves from being "in too deeply" or "totally committed," since they don't want to be called a "sissy" by other men! (Or by their own inner policeman.)

The old idea that decrees that "being a man" means making lots of sexual conquests with many women, penetrating them once or twice but not thereafter being "tied down" or "committed" in any way, comes from an ancient preoccupation with increasing reproduction. Some early societies trained men to feel that they should "spread as much seed as possible to prove that they are men" in order to increase the population. If a man does feel deeply involved with and attracted to one woman, but tries not to have such feelings, this is unfortunate.

When they first fall in love, many men try, according to my research, to "lower the temperature," cool down the relationship, "get it under control"—though they usually succeed only in confusing the other person and causing rifts. A chance for extraordinary happiness is lost. Men kill part of themselves in killing these "wilder" feelings.

In a culture in which men are trained to graft their emotions primarily to the system, men often try to reject the passionate love they feel, going through three stages. First, they feel "swept away"; second, they struggle against the passion within them to "regain control"; third, they fight with the loved one, seeing her as the "enemy" or "guilty" of "provoking too many feelings," and (most ironic of all) "creating a lack of stability"! This stage often leads to a breakup.

A man who does not allow himself to love fully—or forces himself to cut off his passionate feelings—can feel empty, leading to a quest for multiple partners in an attempt to satisfy an appetite that can never be satisfied without truly loving. Monogamous men are generally much happier than other men, by the way—not because they are monogamous, but because they want to be monogamous, because they live with someone they do love and with whom they have a real relationship.

Of course not every life—male or female—contains a "happy ending," not all of us wind up living with the person of our dreams so that being monogamous comes naturally.

Monogamy is not always right for every part of everyone's life, but monogamy for men is at least as rewarding and satisfying as it is (or is not) for women. And it allows love to grow, based on stability and time spent together for the growth of real closeness.

## COMBAT BETWEEN FATHERS AND SONS FOR POWER/TURMOIL IN THE KINGDOM OF FATHERS AND SONS: MALE CONFORMITY AT WORK

For several decades corporations did not challenge men's identity. The corporate landscape was predominantly male, so nothing was out of sync with the traditional social order. Male competition could follow the old models of sons with or against fathers, brother with or against brother, and so on.

Corporations have traditionally been kingdoms in which "sons" and "fathers" by turn compete with each other or work together. Young and old men jousted or fought together for power, glory, and money. Thus corporations did not pose a challenge to the traditional social order but seemed to affirm it: men were "hunters," whether in a natural jungle or in a corporate jungle.

The arrival of large numbers of women in the workplace, however, means the office no longer resembles the traditional social order based on the family and its prototype relationships. This means the office as we know it could be like a blank page on which we can design a new social order if we were to shake off our embedded gender identities. However, most people unconsciously project old stereotypes of family relationships or love relationships (even sexual relationships) onto situations at work.[9]

Today men question their place in the sun: if work is not exclusively theirs, what is? Does it matter? How much time should be devoted to work, how much to private life? Is time at work real life? One way of understanding relationships between men at work is the Freudian view: men are in combat (competition), and the son fights his father for power. Some would claim that this is "basic male nature."

But while Freud might claim that it is natural for sons to try to overtake and dominate their fathers, one does not find this scenario in such classics as Shakespeare's *Romeo and Juliet* (the son of Capulet does not try to wrest power from his father), nor does Arthur Miller portray the son of Willie Loman in *Death of a Salesman* as trying to dominate his father. On the other hand, many men in corporations do feel that part of the fun lies in competing with the other guys.

The "human nature is unchangeable" view implies that men can't change, that sons will always challenge fathers. But is this true? My research has turned up two different reasons for males' attitudes to each other inside corporations, whether they are fighting or bonding. Both imply that flexibility is a large part of human nature and that change is not only possible but probable. The conclusion that emerges is that what we call "human nature" is very much shaped and created by society.

First, men's loyalty to other men (and desire to be accepted by them, to work with them) is rooted in the lack of closeness with their fathers most boys felt as they were growing up, according to my research.

Boys form their understanding of relationships with men from this early encounter, no matter how distant it may have been. Boys in my research for the *Hite Report on Male Sexuality* and *The Hite Report on the Family*, repeatedly stated that they did not know their fathers very well, and that their fathers rarely talked to them about their feelings, personal thoughts, or relationships. In fact, most boys said that they had never had a real conversation with their fathers about a personal topic. Most expressed a longing to have had some deeper communication. Boys often become fascinated by the power of this emotionally silent and mysterious monolith, the "older man." One noted, "I didn't know my father, really, I didn't know what went on in his head. He went to work, he came home, he got angry at odd moments and everybody seemed to have to help rearrange things so his anger would go away and he, the god, would be pacified. I used to ask my mother what was I supposed to be like—him?" Another reported, "My one-year-old son said to his mother (when they thought I wasn't around) 'Why doesn't Daddy say anything?' I had managed to look just like my dad looked to me."

A spiral is created in which the younger man, or a woman, is unable to get through to the grown-up, perfectly closed-off man, who in turn feels less and less loved. My research shows that what we call male nature is in good part socially created at puberty. Harsh puberty initiation rites teach boys to bond with and/or fear men in groups; boys learn to try to conform (at least by appearance) to the behavior of the men around them. These pressures of boyhood, not noticed (or taken seriously) by Freud and others, came out strikingly in my research, showing that boys at puberty learn a bitter lesson: they speak repeatedly of their extended pain and emotional turmoil at ages ten to twelve.

What most of them describe is that early in life they felt very close to their mothers, but then, especially from the ages of ten to twelve, pressure was put on them, usually by older boys at school, to "shape up," "be a man." Failure to heed these messages meant loss of status within the group or worse.

Most boys were emotionally distressed during this period: they didn't want to betray their mother by taking on new, disdainful attitudes, but eventually they came to realize that they had no choice but to join the male group.

Many men apply the same logic at work, concluding that they must conform to the group of men in an office or a corporation (or on a construction site) or they will not fit in and will certainly not get ahead. Many men thus feel nervous with the new presence of career women and about breaking the rules of conformity to male groups.

Many younger men now want to find a new way forward, a new way to relate to women as well as to other men, but they find it difficult to behave in new ways at work. As they learned as boys, the approval of other men is very hard to come by; once you've got it, you'd better not lose it. These boyhood lessons are internalized and forgotten, so that men in corporations behave the same as ever without knowing why.

Corporate executives today could feel unconsciously uncomfortable being "disloyal" to the men's group at work (working closely with women on an equal level or promoting women above men would mean being a "sissy"). If men can break the spell of this fear, which they learned early in life, a fear that to many has become unrecognizable, then the meritocracy that was promised in the "capitalist dream" could become a reality. Once people realize that corporate boardrooms resemble the boys' bully system at school, and that they don't have to carry on this tradition, things can change quickly.

Today many men at work have ambivalent feelings: they want to "let women be equal," an idea with justice on its side but one that involves a trade-off. Should men work easily with women, blend in, make new choices; or should they try to please older male authority figures (controlling their jobs and their promotions), who may prefer signals of an old male-bonding variety?

## WILL THE "NEW MAN" CHANGE CORPORATE CULTURE?

Originally corporations did not pose a challenge to the traditional social order (the social order for the last millennium has been based on the family and its prototypical relationships) because men were "hunters," whether in a natural jungle or a corporate jungle. However, with the arrival of large numbers of women in the workplace, offices no longer reflect the traditional social order.

For several decades corporations did not challenge men's traditional identity. Except for secretaries, it was mostly men who inhabited the corporate landscape, so nothing was out of sync with the traditional social order: male competition could follow the biblical model of Cain and Abel, brother against brother, son against father, or brother working with brother. Traditionally corporations have been kingdoms in which sons and fathers by turns competed with each other or worked together. Younger and older men jousted or fought together for power, glory, and money.

## ARE MEN QUESTIONING THE CLICHÉS? CHANGING THE SYSTEM AND THEMSELVES?

Various factors have come together to set men thinking, embarking on a momentous interior transformation that has as yet to go public. Most no longer want the extreme "revolution" of the 1960s, nor the "return to traditional manhood" of the 1980s; they want a new, third way, something they are inventing.

This change in perspective has been in the making for some time. Related to history rather than to hormones, an entire century of social experimentation underlies many men's deep desire for change. They may have lived through twenty-five years of rethinking or some were raised by mothers and fathers who had also done major rethinking. Though twentieth century media spoke more often of the changes women have made, men have changed dramatically too. During the second half of the century men revolted en masse against the family; as shown in the playboy revolution (reflected by James Bond films, showing the ever-single, glamorously nonmonogamous Agent 007), the 1960s flower power, civil rights, and black pride, as well as the birth-control pill and "sexual revolution" movement. With all these, men stressed the fact that they wanted more individual self-determination and less conformity (in some cases they wrongly targeted women as the cause of feeling "tied down"). Through the feminist movement of the 1970s, men's self-concept was challenged in a new way. All of these changes made a heady mix, and by the 1980s and 1990s many men were ready to call a halt and "go back to traditional values." But could they go back? The divorce rate passed 50 percent, and the number of people living "single" neared half. The late 1990s saw an increasing media focus on extreme versions of sex—sadomasochism, internet pornography, and sexual violence—as fun ("You're not a real man unless you like it and participate . . ."). Of course earlier tendencies throughout the century had also been noted with novels such as *The Story of O* and advertising work such as that done by Helmut Newton. What made the 1990s more extreme would be hard to say in any case. Perhaps what had been written about in the nineteenth century by more elite writers such as Marcel Proust now became a more general trend.

Out of all this twentieth century turmoil, what emerged? While media images of men stressed the importance of being "different," there was simultaneously great pressure on men at work to conform and "be traditional"—to give off an image of respectable, traditional stability if one wanted to get ahead.

Though we now have one of the greatest opportunities in centuries or even millennia (after all, how often do we get the chance to design a new society?), will we be able to take advantage of it? Will men be able to overcome their unremembered fear of other men, their irrational bonding with a system that claims to help them, to prefer them to "the other half" of the population (women) as if they could not create another, new, and better system? Will women be able to think in a new way, "insist on their rights," act as if empowered?

## THE JANUS-HEADS OF MALE PSYCHOLOGY: HEROIC ACTIONS AND FEAR

Glorious, heroic images of masculinity abound in history—mythic figures who sail out to find their destiny, rescue their countries, create great science and art. These heroic efforts do not seem to imply any negative attitudes toward women—except, of course, that women were not allowed on any of these expeditions. The heroic quest has been a male preserve .

There are but few noble images of women in standard history books, Catherine of Russia, Empress Maria Theresa of the Holy Roman Empire, and Queen Elizabeth I of England are the best known. But generally the role of hero has been reserved for men. When Jeanne d'Arc, for example, lived a heroic life on her own initiative, and in male terms, she was eventually subjected to an inquisition and killed. Today's parliaments and scientific expeditions still include a small number of women compared to a large number of men. How does this situation affect men?

To be "male" and admired by other men seems to have two traditions: masculinity as being courageous, brave, and noble—and masculinity as being macho with women, aggressive, and competitive, "conquering nature," all attitudes that are justified as "natural behavior." Which is the "real" masculinity?

How can such a tradition as the noble male—going into space, building mathematical systems, discovering the laws of the universe—exist side by side with the lowly tradition of oppressing women—keeping women out of educational institutions, excluding women from power in governments, and generally treating women as second class, even less than fully human? How is one to reconcile in one's mind that a great tradition could also contain the least noble of traditions?

Has there always been this split in the culture's possibilities offered to men? Or is the "macho" side of being male more with us today? Gore Vidal, the famous writer, once quipped, when I asked him what he thought about "masculinity": "Oh, masculinity—I hear they had a bad outbreak of it down near Tampa, but I think now they're getting it under control."

Historically the classical Greek state, so admired for its balanced ideas of government and philosophy, was, we remember, not balanced: it was a male upper-class democracy—excluding women and slaves from free speech and government, already using the stereotypes of the "talkative" woman (Socrates' wife was said to "nag" him), the only philosophical women or women of letters being categorized as "mistresses." Does this mean that they had lovers? That they were not married? That famous men were attracted to them, and they allowed these men to make love with them? Men who have lovers are not categorized by history as "lovers," and yet women are frequently presented by the history books as no more than "mistresses," "harlots," or "courtesans."

At puberty boys are faced with pressure to prove that they are "one of the guys," not "at home hanging out with their mother, hanging onto her apron strings—a sissy." This role involves showing disrespect to or domination over her in public. Most boys find this change very upsetting, according to my research. Although they eventually must accept it and demonstrate their status over their mothers, lest they risk nonacceptance by other boys and men, they then ingest a double-values system that can create a bisected, Janus-headed mentality—one that believes that magnificent, heroic behavior should be displayed with other men, but different behavior with women. They learn to respect male heroic or aggressive traditions while they learn to look down on "things female." This situation sets up a psychological dichotomy, plus an inner moral compromise, that many men have difficulty overcoming later in life: how can a man think of himself as "noble and heroic" while at the same time "keeping a woman in her place"?

Of course this psychology is not something a man is automatically part of just because he is anatomically male; it is an imposed way of life and way of thinking. Some men confront the issues here discussed, others do not.

Most men look to women for love; 90 percent get married during their late twenties. Rarely are men the ones to initiate divorce. Men want a home, warmth, and children, just as women do. But they also have deeply ambiguous feelings: real closeness is a threatening state of emotionality that most can't afford, since a "real man" never completely lets his guard down or loses control of a situation; a man must continually assert his "independence" (or "dominance"). Real closeness is forbidden to a man because it makes him vulnerable.

So exactly what is heroic in men? If many men experience their minds as being in conflict over how they should behave in "matters of the heart," how does this sense affect their decisions? In fact this "two minds" situation often plays havoc with men's logic, tricking them into believing that only by "following the tried and true path" are they being "rational"—no matter what their experience may tell them.

The basic ideological structure of "male psychology" is only beginning to be understood; for many centuries it was thought to emanate automatically from "human nature" rather than being part of a social system, not the "essential nature" of human beings—one that can be analyzed.*

What is heroism in this setting?

NOTES

1  See Appendix for the *Hite Report on Male Sexuality* questionnaire.

2  Parts of this essay appeared in different form in the *Washington Post* Outlook Section. See also the Preface.

3  Some of this material appeared originally in different form in the *Guardian*, 1996.

4  This heading originally appeared in the *Sydney Morning Herald*'s excerpt series of *The Hite Report on the Family* in 1994.

5  See "Oedipus Revisited," above.

6  The complete data relating to this overview can be found in *The Hite Report on Men and Male Sexuality* (Knopf, 1981; Ballantine, 1982; still in print with Ballantine).

7  Books related to this subject include W. Boscawen, *Egypt and Chaldea* (London: Harper, 1894); Roland deVaux, *Ancient Israel* (New York: McGraw Hill, 1965); Walter Hinz, *The Lost World of Elam* (New York: New York University Press, 1973); Margaret Murray, *The Splendor That Was Egypt* (London: Sidgwick & Jackson, 1949); Merlin Stone, *When God Was a Woman* (New York: Dial Press, 1976); and Jacquetta Hawkes and Sir Leonard Woolley, *Prehistory and the Beginning of Civilization* (New York: Harper & Row, 1963). Also helpful is the extensive bibliography contained in *When God Was a Woman*; there are an increasing number of books in this area.

8  See Jane Harrison, *Prologomena to the Study of Greek Religion* (New York: Meridian, 1955), and E. A. Butterworth, *Some Traces of the Pre-Olympian World* (Berlin and New York: De Gruyter, 1966).

9  See Shere Hite, *Sex & Business: Ethics at Work* (London: Financial Times Prentice Hall, 2000).

---

* By 2004 this analysis has moved forward, specifically in the context of the public debates over the military invasions of Iraq and Afghanistan and the debates about the 2004 United States presidential candidates' military records.

# Part 3

# Women's View of Love
## (1987)

*Perhaps the most complex, least generally understood, and most controversial of the Hite Reports,* Women and Love: A Cultural Revolution in Progress *was first published in 1987. Based on eight years of research involving over 3,500 women,[1] it originated such concepts as "emotional harassment," "emotional inequality," and the emotional contract and was the first extensive documentation of a system of gender discrimination and harassment in private relationships under the name of "love." It challenged a system of psychological gender discrimination in private relationships, including such reigning ideas as the accusation that "women love too much." The categories in which Hite presents the results of her vast enquiry are themselves groundbreaking: the first new categories for analyzing women's emotions and psychology in personal relationships ever presented in scholarly form. Yet an intense media attack followed the publication of* Women and Love, *despite the best attempts of a committee formed in Hite's defense to counteract it, which issued a statement defending Hite's work and placing the attack in the context of the beginning backlash against feminism.[2] The ongoing personal attack on Hite and her work's "methodology" and validity largely obscured the true meaning of Hite's work on women's definition and redefinition of love relationships to such an extent that its theories remain unclear and unanalyzed until this day.*

# Redesigning and Renaming Female Psychology

### 4,500 Women Describe their Emotions, Falling in Love, in Relationships and Marriage

If traditionally women were assigned the role of providing love and comfort to their families and others, now that women have developed new work roles for themselves and changed in other ways, have women also changed how they see "love" or their basic role as "love-givers"?

## WHAT IS LOVE?

*I like being in love with him, it gives me a great feeling to know that we want each other, that even though we are both working very hard every day, when night time comes, we will be close, in each other's arms, sleep together and eat together and share little daily things, like taking a shower one after the other, being naked together, having breakfast together—and, I don't know, just sharing life. If I weren't in love with him, if I didn't love him, this wouldn't mean anything to me, being with him would just be a pain.*

*I have gone through many stages of love, sometimes I thought it wasn't worth it, but now at sixty I'm glad we're still together, the kind of love we are sharing now is based on companionship and this lies underneath everything I do, it gives me a quiet happy feeling.*

*I really like being with my boyfriend, I've known him two months and I never felt anything like this—when we first had sex—I mean, the first time he kissed me (I was really surprised), the earth shook (in my mind and my body), it was like an earthquake happened inside me, I began to desire him so strongly, my passion really overcame me and so far it has kept on growing and growing, I crave his body and what he can make me feel in my body. I really am passionately in love with him—sometimes I fantasize that I want to have his baby, but so far I'm afraid to tell him this,*

*I'm afraid he would be scared and run off! I don't know if this love will last, or where it is going. . . .*

*I'm in love with him, but I wish I weren't. He is making my life a turmoil in which I seem to be always there to love him, but he frequently changes his mind about whether he is serious about our relationship—sometimes yes, sometimes no. This is driving me crazy. My friends never treated me like this. I am asking myself if I really need this crazy feeling of love, the only thing is that if we broke up, I would miss the deep embraces we give each other in bed at night. Why can't I just enjoy the embraces, and not care so much? On the other hand, if I didn't care, the embraces would not feel so good—so what's the answer?*

*I felt like I was facing a great mystery, the strength of the feelings surprised me and gave me a sense of wonder. . . .*

Although many women are enjoying love relationships with men (and other women), how they see these relationships is changing. Women are in the midst of a cultural revolution, a profound shift in their idea of what love is and what place it should have in their lives. Some women have decided to "give up on love," to make love only a part of life, less important than work, career, and other matters. But many women refuse to give up their view of life and still choose to have love at its center.

Women in my research express mixed feelings about their love relationships with men, often stating that they do not feel able to "be themselves" in them, and that the men they love are not sustaining the emotions of trust, closeness, and pleasure they need to "make it all worthwhile."

Such mixed feelings are not unique to this research, of course. Undoubtedly the large number of bestselling "self-help books for women" are finding a market because mixed feelings plague so many women; women want to improve their relationships or change their own thinking about them. The "high divorce rate" also indicates that there is "a problem."*

What is that problem? This research is focused on asking women to describe their relationships, so that a social-science analysis can be made, based on this first-person, large-scale data—something never before attempted (a scientific study of emotions), yet necessary today in order to move forward and create more harmony.

---

* Women, not men, as discovered here and later confirmed by United States and United Kingdom government statistics, initiate most divorces.

## "THE EMOTIONAL CONTRACT": HIDDEN GENDER DISCRIMINATION IN PSYCHOLOGICAL PATTERNS

What is going on in love relationships "in private" as women describe them—in marriage, "living together," or falling in love in a short-term relationship?*

*Although I find that I'm funny, sarcastic, and energetic when in mixed groups, "the life of the party"—when my boyfriend's there . . . boom. I'm very quiet. Almost like I don't want to steal his "spotlight." Am I alone in this?*

*Initially, being in love is fun but something happens and it becomes frustrating, painful, and disappointing. What is the thing that happens? With my husband (whom I love very much, we have been together for years and have a wonderful family), I try to open him up. I want to talk about our relationship, feelings and problems, and develop solutions or compromises, but he goes quiet, so I have to initiate talking and drag it out of him. I usually work the hardest to resolve the problem. Sometimes, when he finds it hard to express himself, he withdraws. Without communicating, how can you solve anything?*

*I am fighting with him all the time to preserve our relationship. He is happier when I never bring anything up. But if I don't, I feel unhappy, because emotional issues are never discussed—and I feel isolated, at a distance, alone. If we can't really be together, I'd rather leave the relationship. He probably doesn't realize this, because when I try to discuss things, he acts very put-upon, martyred, or bitchy—certainly he shows no serious attempt to listen (although I am always there for him). He just seems to want to get any discussion over as quickly as possible, saying as little as possible. But later, when he's ready to cuddle in bed and have sex, he doesn't expect me to be distant because of his previous attitude. He doesn't realize it's all connected for me—wanting to have sex is, for me, connected to our warmth and closeness. And I do love these things too, so lots of times I just put out and enjoy.*

*When I was three or four, my mother was already teaching me to see dust and other people's feelings. ("Don't bother your father, he's tired.") Men don't learn the same sensitivity. My father was somewhat affectionate, as much as he knew how to be—you know, that masculine way, by being*

---

* Thousands more of these testimonies, of all viewpoints, appear in the original work *Women and Love* (1987).

*insulting. Generally men have a tendency to bottle up their thoughts and emotions so that you have to use all your energy trying to get them to speak out and share their inner selves. I like sex with them.*

*I don't know if my short relationships with men are at all typical. The main thing that struck me was that there was virtually no discussion of anyone's feelings. Things that I kept finding myself doing/feeling around men: Feeling like they were the important ones. Feeling too big, in all ways. Too tall, too large, said too much, felt too much, occupied more space than I had a right to. Wanting to please them. Wanting to appear femininely pretty. I like it when they give me a lot of attention, it's very romantic.*

*He often tells me he loves me, and I believe he does—I love to hear him say this—but I'm not always convinced. To me, being involved with another person means asking them about things they have expressed concern over, giving them a chance to talk about things they are wondering about, being with them emotionally, to toss around whatever's on their mind that day, if they're worried or if they're excited about something. My friends and I do this all the time, but my husband never seems to do this with me. When I ask him, finally, to ask me how I'm feeling about something I've told him about, it is like pulling teeth to get him to do it even a little bit. Then he doesn't bring up the things later, he forgets about them. It's so frustrating. I love him, but why isn't he more interested in what's on my mind?*

## NAMING THE PROBLEM

It is useful to invent new vocabulary creating terms such as "the emotional contract." The emotional contract is the spiritual core of a relationship—the roles each plays, the implicit understanding between two people about how each should behave, the assumptions in words and behavior, how each expects the other to express emotions, how each interprets the emotional outcries and silences of the other. These tender and often brief moments are the lifeblood of the emotional closeness between the two people.

This normal flow of relationships and the emotional interaction is troubled by an unclear, demeaning, and gender-oriented set of subliminal attitudes that reflect outdated beliefs and assumptions.

The emotional contract we inherit contains psychological stereotypes that put women at a disadvantage and give men superior psychological clout via assumptions that have not been examined (but will be here); indeed, these assumptions were and are often declared to be "human nature." This pseudorealistic mind-set is a fundamental cause of many problems between women and men in love relationships.

## "REAL LOVE": WILL IT COME LATER?

Strangely, hauntingly, most women in this study—whether married, single, or divorced, of all ages—stated that they had not yet found the love they were looking for, that they hoped their greatest love was yet to come:

*My family, it is O.K. But I think I will never find what I truly want in love.*

*My greatest love was too unstable, too much hurt. I am still looking for the love I need to share in my life and I hope I have time for it to come later.*

*I have not found what I need in love and family. This gives me a desperate feeling in the pit of my stomach. I am losing faith and hope of realizing it in my lifetime.*

*I have not as yet been able to give the love I would like to give, neither have I received it. I would like to have a love that is openly expressed without fear of rejection.*

## THE COVERT EMOTIONAL CONTRACT

There is an unwritten emotional contract that even today puts men in the "driver's seat" and women in the "emotionally irrational" role, people who may be ridiculed and made fun of "in the normal course of things."

Based on this research, it seems clear that women are explaining that they are trying to live and love in a system that, without admitting it is doing so, discriminates heavily against them, penalizing them for in fact trying to create emotionally equal relationships. (The result of this struggle is "the battle of the sexes.") This uncoded emotional system (reflected in choices of vocabulary, such as "she was left") reflects the larger social system, with women today still having second-class status compared to men. (How many female presidents and prime ministers are there?)

The words used to describe what goes on in relationships have been highly influenced by social-status categories: men are expected to be emotionally "strong" and "in charge" of relationships. There is as yet little understanding of what equal emotional interaction might be, although, of course, there are some beautiful examples of exceptional relationships. The way that the emotions inside relationships between men and women are viewed, even by some "helping professions," generally puts women in the passive or receiving (weak) position, on the defensive; this happens generally via words used to characterize relationships, frequently tinged with prejudice against women. Examples follow that illustrate the problem.

Most women in this study, no matter how frustrating their relationship, or how clearly they saw the difficulty of coming to a real, mutual recognition with a man they love, still hoped and longed for a way to make love work. As one woman stated, love keeps resurfacing, perhaps as some kind of key: "In some way which I cannot find the words for yet, romantic love contains the key toward my identity—toward discovering myself, my inner being." Many women feel this way; perhaps they are right to come back, to try again and again to make love work.

### HOW DO WOMEN FEEL ABOUT THEIR LOVE RELATIONSHIPS?

Is injustice built into an unwritten "emotional contract" that exists in love affairs and relationships/marriages? Does love hide a subtle system of discrimination?

Listen to what women reported about what goes on in their relationships.* Since most of what they describe takes place in private, this may be the first time that the dynamics of such personal emotions have been looked at from a sociological point of view.

Despite the rhetoric of the "sexual revolution" that insists women and men are now equal, women report that subtle but extremely painful (and powerful) forms of discrimination are still built into the very structure of relationships, lodged into small wedges of daily interaction.

What women describe is an entrenched, largely unrecognized system of emotional discrimination, a system whose roots are entwined so deeply in the psyche of the culture as to underlie our entire social structure. As many women point out, the incidents that upset them can be small—and yet these incidents are troubling because they reflect an overall attitude, part of a fabric of denial of women as complete human beings.

How does one begin to name and demonstrate a pattern that has had no name for so long, these subtle interactions and subliminal messages that are much more deadly to love than arguing over money or children?

### WHAT IS "EMOTIONAL EQUALITY"?[†]

One woman describes what it isn't:

> *Like today, R. just turned his back on me while I was talking to him, thinking that would be the end of it. Was he surprised when I grabbed him by the arm and jerked him around! I could tell he wanted to really hit me, but he didn't. Then he said something like, "You can't make me*

---

* Please see the original volume, *Women and Love*, for the majority of testimonies, which have been omitted here in the interest of space.

† This term, like "the emotional contract," was first used in the third Hite Report, *Women and Love*.

*do anything you want. I don't take orders from you." I suppose that*
*refers to the chores I asked him to do. He could help me a little—like*
*maybe screw in a light bulb without being asked. If I ask him, he says,*
*"Oh, I didn't notice it." I can't believe it. Incredibly juvenile. Men can*
*get away with it, because they run things. Or they think they can. But*
*if women would stick together and not put up with this stuff, we could*
*change it. If England could run the whole world for a time, and David*
*could beat Goliath, we as women can get ourselves out of this hole and*
*end the stupidity of the whole male thing.*

Signs of an unequal emotional "contract" are thrown at women every day in a thousand ways. Indeed, the patterns are so subtle and accepted, coloring everything, that they make discussion of the "problem" almost impossible. As one woman puts it, "There are no words, to begin with, and when you do use words, they are viewed by men through a reversing telescope (when they are heard at all)—taking what I said for something totally NOT what I meant."

Lack of emotional equality is the fundamental stumbling block to harmony in relationships. It is embedded in many words currently used to describe love relationships—and these words greatly influence our way of seeing and experiencing ourselves. The underlying inequalities are built into the culture, so that women can become angry without knowing exactly why. As one states, "I wonder if our relationship could get better, because I resent him and don't know why. I feel on the defensive a lot."

The purpose here is to unravel these "invisible" dynamics in relationships (the "emotional contract") and build a better framework.

The assumption in the traditional emotional contract is that women's role is to be tranquil, loving and "mothering." Less frequently noted is the role the ideology assigns to men: being dynamic, "dominant," "starring" in relationships.

However, looking at women's testimony in my research, it appears that if a woman wants to love a man—give and receive or exchange feelings with a man she loves—but the man has little practice in emotional equality with a woman (but has learned he should not be "pussy-whipped"), then this puts a woman in an awkward position. The advice that is often offered to her now as to how to end the "frustration" (and "stop complaining") is to stop loving "too much."

## DO WOMEN "LOVE TOO MUCH"?

Women are often been criticized for being "too loving," too giving, too nurturing, obsessed with "romance." The theory has been that women rely too much on love for their fulfillment in life, that women "cling" because they are brought up to be psychologically "dependent," even that women are "crippled" psychologically(!). If women would only give up these behaviors and stop loving "too much," be more "like men," they would find that they would be happier, they wouldn't have so many problems with love—so the idea goes.

In fact, women are considering anew how they want to live their lives, engaged in redefining love for themselves. Most women agree that too much giving without receiving, nonreciprocal giving, can eventually threaten one's personality and self-confidence, even identity. On the other hand, to "love less" is not a solution for most women.

Feeling themselves faced with these alternatives, many women are struggling to maintain love in their relationships, while not letting themselves be intimidated by those who ridicule them for being more giving, not wanting to fight.

## IDENTIFYING GENDER DISCRIMINATION IN LOVE: GOOD-BYE TO FREUD AND ASSORTED OTHERS

It is sometimes said that if women feel "needy" and "insecure," looking for reassurance that men love them, this feeling is a sign of women's "biology": women (the assumption goes) have an innate fear of "being left," resulting from the fact that they may get pregnant and "must" have a man to take care of them. That is, since women become pregnant and need men to take care of them, they are somehow hormonally and psychologically disposed to being "dependent" on men. I find this explanation false. In some prehistoric societies, groups of women cared for newborn children. In fact one could argue that if society were constructed differently (as it has been in other times and places), maternal clans, mothers, uncles, and brothers, female lovers and friends, could protect pregnant women and, later, the baby. Thus biology cannot be the reason for women's psychology or feeling of being "insecure."

If a woman complains of bad treatment from a man (and it is usually part-time bad treatment, not full-time), she is apt to be told she is a "masochist," and she must "like it"—that is, "If you don't like it, why do you stay and take it?" But this attitude is "blaming the victim": for within a social structure in which women have been brought up and are still brought up to make love the wellspring of their identity, to put down women for being "too focused on love," "obsessed with love," is astonishing. Women are being blamed for doing what the social system asks of them.

And women do what the system asks in the confusing context of having to love individually those of a "superior" group socially: men. In other words, women are told to focus love on a group—men—whose status is "above" their own. Being told that they should love people of a "superior" group automatically proposes that women be second-status, that they must give to those who do not see them as fully equal.

This makes the labeling of women as "masochistic" particularly ironic and even sadistic: women are told to love men, who (as a group) are "above" them, then told to endure men's condescending or superior behavior (because men "don't mean it" and "really love you")—and when women do so and still keep on loving, they can be rewarded by being called "masochistic"! And so women are told that it is their own fault if their status in society doesn't change: "Why don't you change it if you don't like it?" they are taunted, aggressively.

According to women's testimony, men are often psychologically aggressive and provocative with them but are rarely called to account for this; instead, society criticizes women as the culprits for being "too emotional," too easily upset, too needful of reassurances of love, too obsessed with "romance." People rarely think to criticize the man involved, to try to get him to change, because our mind-set is focused on women as "the problem child," the "problem gender." And so many women live with the frustration of this unfair, unidentified, and unacknowledged system of discrimination, finding that they can really talk only to one another about it.

Instead of being called "masochists," why aren't women admired for their loyalty? Women in unhappy love relationships are often courageous in trying to see a bad relationship through, trying to help the one they love, remaining loyal even when the other person is difficult, but this behavior is almost never seen as heroic. Instead women are often put down or called "clinging," "needy," or "despicable females who only want something" for staying. Should they at times be admired? Would men be admired for the same behavior? Aren't men often seen as great romantic heroes when love is unrequited or doesn't work out?

Women in some of these relationships are making a positive statement in that they are not reacting to what the man does but expressing their own view of the potential of the relationship, their own feelings. They are defining the situation.

A love affair that is unstable is not necessarily a failure if it gives poetry and beauty: this may be what a woman wants. It may not be that a woman is "picking the wrong men," but in poor relationships she is usually made to feel bad by society. ("It didn't work out! She can't get her life in order!") Society has penalized women severely when they do not form permanent alliances with men.

Many women in this study do make themselves leave men they love, even while still loving them—if they need to. But sometimes there is a real reason for staying. What if a woman pledges her soul and then is "betrayed," or hurt? This situation does not mean that she should not have pledged her soul, should not have loved. It is good to have the capacity to believe in the reality of one's own feelings and to live one's own experience; society should not ridicule anyone for this.

## WOMEN'S REBELLION AGAINST POTENTIAL SLURS ON FEMALE IDENTITY: CULTURE CREATES PSYCHOLOGY

The standard understanding of women's psychology is inaccurate—or lacking in subtlety, to say the least.

Women who want love are all too often forced into compromise after compromise, seen as emotionally inferior or "needy." Ironically they are also required not to notice that their thoughts and points of view are disregarded—or how they are perceived by men as less important than work, friends, football on TV, and so on. For their patience they are frequently labeled as "weak" or "nonassertive," "pushovers" and so on.

A woman faced with a daily lack of communication and lack of respect is placed in a position of having to choose either leaving the relationship or staying and living with this pattern of subtle belittling and condescension (and possibly creating some balance by "nagging"). The outward symptoms of her inner struggle to maintain dignity and self respect are usually bickering and small daily hostilities, silences, or feeling emotionally "insecure." But although bickering can be "normal" in human relationships, in our world it is more frequent and bitter than need be because female-male relationships are "political"—that is, the socially condoned way of seeing women as "emotionally unstable" or "irrational," the emotional contract's lopsided view, places women on the defensive. Does this situation make men feel guilty and distant?

Phyllis Chesler has made this point forcefully in her classic, *Women and Madness*, a reference for all discussions of this topic. Professor Naomi Weisstein, of the State University of New York, almost simultaneously wrote "Psychology Creates the Female," a landmark theoretical treatise on this subject. However, women's behavior in love relationships has long been interpreted by "studies" done from a "male" (status quo) ideological perspective. As Simone de Beauvoir explained in 1984, "Although I admire Freud . . . I find that in the case of women, as he said himself, there's a dark continent; he understood nothing of what women want. Anyone who wants to work on women has to break completely with Freud." (Interview by Helene Wenzel, published in the *Women's Review of Books*, July 1985.) The views of the vast majority of "psychologists" are lacking in scientific objectivity: by the terms of "social science," if the majority of people display certain feelings, this preponderance makes those feelings "normal in that group." The conclusion to be drawn if women stay with men who treat them badly is not that this means women are "by nature" "masochists" who love men who hurt them.*

If one takes a historical and philosophical perspective, one can see both female and male behaviors in quite another way—that is, as logical responses to the specific cultural setup. Indeed, if we are to lift ourselves out of the forest, to see our alternatives, envision another mind-set, and make plans, we must take this broader perspective, see the current situation between women and men as only the creation of the larger overall ideology or set of beliefs.

Women must no longer be "defined" and "judged" through the lens of a culture that for centuries has seen them as "second-class" psychologically, as less than the standard of "normality." Data must be looked at from a new standpoint. The myriad findings and statements in my research present the field of psychology with a wealth of basic

---

* My research shows that men do not hurt women in the beginning of the vast majority of relationships; though they may begin to do so later, by then women have developed complex emotions that combine with their upbringing and socialization as women to "try to understand."

new information. Psychology currently has little vocabulary that can encompass the real form of women's thinking and possible psychologies, and needs to reinvent itself.

## "WOMEN LACK SELF-ESTEEM"—OR DO THEY?

Contrary to popular belief, it may be that men's double messages to women, not women's "lack of self-esteem," make women feel "insecure."

If men withhold equal companionship with women, distance themselves emotionally (the one who is less vulnerable has more power) and trivialize women in relationships, and then turn to those same women looking for love, affection, and understanding, believing that the women should "be there" for them (as well as provide domestic services such as cooking and housekeeping)—what effect must this process have?

How should a woman react to being with someone who, on the one hand, frequently acts emotionally distant and inaccessible—and then, on the other, periodically expects love and affection, telling her that he loves her? If a woman loves a man, and he says that he loves her (even though he exhibits the two-sided behavior just described), she may feel off-balance and disoriented, though she will probably want to stay and "make it work." But which is the "real" other person? she may wonder. The one who loves her, or the one who is distant and ridiculing? How can she break through that distance, when it occurs, to the "good parts"? So she tries to "bring up the issues," and keeps on trying, but often goes through an agony of frustration at the cruelty and emotional coldness she encounters along the way. She is accused of "nagging."

Though it is often heard that women have "low self-esteem," is this accusation an instance of "blaming the victim"?

In fact women are doing quite well, considering all the propaganda coming their way to the effect that they aren't worth as much as men. But there is great social pressure on women to prove they have "self-esteem" by becoming as aggressive and aloof as many men. One woman's statement portrays the equation of aggressiveness with having a sense of self: "It seems to me that many women—myself included—don't have the sense of self that men are trained to have. Men are supposed to beat up other people, in a way—even their mothers probably told them, 'Go back to school and beat him up, whoever gives you a hard time'; men are always pushed to win competitions. This makes for the difference in women's rules and men's rules."

Do women really undervalue themselves as much as is popularly believed? Thinking about relationships is causing women to question the whole system.

## EVERYDAY LANGUAGE AS IDEOLOGY: EMOTIONAL AGGRESSION AGAINST WOMEN

Do many of our everyday terms—those used typically for or about women—carry implicit messages of emotional aggression?

Names—what things are called, which feelings are given "reality" by having words that refer to them (and which are not)—are among the most powerful tools of a society for carrying on and reinforcing its ideology. In the case of gender, words embedded in the language act as hidden, subliminal value judgments, leading to specific (often irrational) interpretations of behavior.

The language that exists dictates what "reality" will consist of. For this reason we need to find new terms for women's experiences which may have been misnamed. For example, terming women "emotionally needy" or "overly emotional"—with "male" "detached" and "objective" behavior considered to be the norm—is not objective. To reverse the point of view, one might call "male" behavior "emotionally repressed," and "female" behavior "gloriously expressive." But in our society, non-communicative "male" behavior is more generally seen as something like "heroically in control."

The frequent use of words and phrases with built-in gender insults for women (words that have special meaning when used for/about women) creates an atmosphere of emotional intimidation, which weighs just as heavily on women as economic intimidation has. Through using this vocabulary, subtly, often unconsciously, and in a socially acceptable way, many men bully women emotionally, and thus control relationships. The implied threat often is that if the woman "complains" too much, or wants a better relationship (is "demanding" or "nagging")—she will be unlovable and therefore a man will leave her.

Also relevant here is the phrase, "Treat her like a lady"—which implies that, at any moment, if the woman doesn't behave correctly, "like a lady," she can be turned against, treated without respect, called the opposite, "a bitch." One woman reports poignantly, "I remember my father calling my mother a whore because she wasn't tidy enough in the kitchen."

Or consider the common use of diminutives when referring to women, the tendency to see women's achievements as "good" rather than "great" (women are "brilliant," but almost never "geniuses"). Women can be counselors or advice givers, but not philosophers. People belittle women also by using their first names, though they have just been introduced, or worse, by calling them "dear" and "honey," even when they are complete strangers. In a similar situation a man would probably be addressed as "Mr. Smith"; he would not be called "dear."

## A. CLICHÉS ABOUT WOMEN

Further gender-biased remarks made to women include, "I think you've got a complex," as a retort to a "complaint" a woman might have about a man's treatment of her. Or consider the remark, "You're too sensitive." In the midst of "trying to talk," a woman can find herself being put down by a "caring" or "solicitous" (condescending) response; the word "sensitive," with its two meanings, illustrates the sexism of words as they are applied to women's behavior: to be "sensitive" to the world and others is good, but to be a "sensitive" woman (that is, a woman who is always having her feelings hurt) is bad.

"I'm sorry you feel that way" is another frequent retort referred to over and over by women in this study, occurring when a woman has just described her injured feelings in a relationship to a man. This remark, rather than opening up the topic for discussion and serious consideration, places the burden for the "feelings" on the person experiencing the pain and no responsibility on the person making the comment. In other words, the man has no emotional responsibility. Do men who make this kind of retort realize that they are being emotionally destructive? Or do they simply believe that they are right, that women are too "emotionally demanding" and "difficult," and that it is the proper role of men to make sure women don't "go too far" and "dominate" a relationship? Some men use this and similar statements to end a conversation rather than examine in more depth what a woman is trying to express. It is a form of emotional violence—the cutting off of communication—and is very harmful to relationships.

Many women, of course, have interiorized second-class attitudes about themselves and each other, such as in the put-down of herself contained in one woman's response to being asked if she can talk easily to her husband: "If I want to whine, moan and groan and be dramatic, I'd best talk to a woman friend. My husband comes from a place of analyzing and being rational. I need a little drama."*

The gender-biased choice of words is one we might all make (since such words are used all around us and seem to be the only words available sometimes) without intending the implications.

## B. TEASING AND OTHER PUT-DOWNS

One of the most frustrating aspects of the stereotyped put-downs women live with is that the words frequently crop up in conversation "in passing." They are so enmeshed in the larger conversation that it would seem disruptive and "out of proportion" to stop the discussion to point them out (or be accused of lacking a sense of humor). Women often find such built-in, loaded words and jokes offensive, but not to such an extent that they want to risk being called "obnoxious" or "aggressive" by making an issue out of them. On the other hand, this situation leaves the woman to swallow the words said and, even worse, to seem to be condoning both it and the assumptions it embodies.

These comments can be subtle and almost "unretortable," according to most women:

> I hate it when men say something to the effect of "Isn't that just like a woman," or "All women are like that." I feel we deserve to be judged on

---

* Making this very analysis, one could characterize what women are saying about their relationships as "Women often complain that . . ." rather than "Women often report that . . ."

> *a one-to-one basis, not as part of a vague mob. It is the main thing I am*
> *trying to correct in my attitude toward men. Whenever I catch myself say-*
> *ing, "You men are all alike," I stop and try to see the man as himself, not*
> *as a group. Also I hate it when a man I like calls me his "old lady,"*
> *"broad," or "the little woman."*

Even more subtle may be the put-downs contained in what is not said, for example, the way the language celebrates masculinity—with the traditional cry of delight
on the birth of a male child, "It's a boy!" There is no equivalent cry of delight when
it is a girl, although many people are thrilled to have girls. However, the fact that one
phrase is standard, and no equivalent other phrase is, carries a significant message
to women and men every time they hear it, whether they recognize it or not: boys
are more valuable than girls.

### C. SEXIST VOCABULARY: "BEING LEFT"

Many, perhaps most, people display a subtle gender bias in their choice of the adjectives they apply to the end of a relationship, depending on whether it is a man or a
woman's behavior they are describing: people may watch a man do exactly the same
thing they watch a woman do—argue with a taxi driver over the fare, for example—and characterize what they have seen in a totally different way. The man may
be seen as "righteous," as not a fool, not letting himself be taken; the woman may
be seen as argumentative, loud, "bitchy," aggressive, and so on.

Many particularly ideologically laden words and phrases relate to the supposedly
"dependent" nature of women in relationships. "Being left" almost always refers to
a woman "being left"—with the implication that now the woman is sad and alone,
rejected. When marriages break up, it is usually assumed that it was the man who
wanted to leave, although, according to this study and other studies, it is usually
women who decide to do so. "Deserted" and "abandoned" are other words with similar connotations applied almost exclusively to women. It does not fit in with beliefs
about men's superior status to think that women could be the less "needy" ones.

Another related stereotype is the idea that women have difficulty accepting men's
departure because they fear "being left"; as noted, this is said to be a woman's "syndrome," part of women's "psychology," its origin existing in women's "nature"; that
is, women are biologically dependent on men because of becoming pregnant and
needing men to stay and protect them and their babies. (But in other societies
women bond together, or the clan takes care of mother and child.) In fact needing
men's support is not something that grows out of women's "innate" or "biological"
psychology. Rather, in our society, it is more likely that women have sometimes felt
uncomfortable about men's departures because of economic dependence—and
because of men's noncommunicative attitudes, which leave women feeling emotionally uneasy, unclear about what will happen next.

## D."EMOTIONAL HARASSMENT"*

Emotional harassment or a put-down can be a pattern in a relationship, but even more importantly, it is a pattern in society, a pattern that is socially acceptable. Therefore it can happen at any moment, when a woman is least expecting it—a kind of emotional terrorism. (Unfortunately, "teasing" is also one of the few ways women are allowed to express anger at men, so that a common pattern on TV sitcoms is bantering to see who can ridicule the other's remark first.) Men have more social credibility when "teasing" women, legitimized by society's seeing women as "foolish"; a notorious example of this "accepted" teasing or poking fun at women was White House chief of staff Donald Regan's statement in 1986 that women would not really be interested in the problems of South Africa, for they are "more interested in diamond bracelets."

## EMOTIONAL VIOLENCE†

There are extreme cases of emotional harassment that amount to emotional violence (for which the perpetrator need never answer, will never be called to justice):

*My ex-husband destroyed my confidence in myself. I remember once he wanted me to make a soup like his mother, so I spent all afternoon shopping and preparing it from scratch. Then he came home, and when he tasted it, he said that I put too much paprika in it and flushed the whole thing down the toilet and then slapped me. You can't just start living again after many experiences like that.*

*In my sixth month of my first pregnancy I was spotting and the doctor put me to bed. That night my husband insisted on having intercourse. The next day I went to the hospital and gave birth to my first child prematurely, who weighed only one pound fourteen ounces, but who survived. I'm sure I would have given birth (prematurely) anyway, but I felt very hurt by that for a long time.*

*We had been going together for six months, and told each other how much we loved each other. Then I realized I was pregnant, and bought one of those home tests. I was nervous about taking it, and before doing it, I told him. I said, "You won't believe this, darling, but I think I'm pregnant." After a while he said, "How can I be sure it's mine?"*

---

* This term was first used in the third Hite Report, *Women and Love*.
† This term was also first used in *Women and Love*.

*Years ago, when I was pregnant with my second baby, we had gone to a dance. I was sick, exhausted, and a number of other things, and had gone only because I didn't want to be a party pooper and spoil his fun. I made the best of a totally miserable evening, but by 1:30 a.m. I had had it and told him that I wasn't feeling well, had not been all evening (he didn't even notice), and could we please leave now. He agreed and I got my coat and stood by the door while he table-hopped and said goodbye for another forty-five minutes. I finally left without him, in tears. This leads to the worst thing that I ever did to him . . . I took the car out of the parking lot, and by this time I was furious. He was leaving the building as I drove down the street, so I swerved the car to run him over, just missing him. I drove like a maniac for three blocks, then parked the car and got hold of myself. I almost left him that night when I got home. I started to pack and we had a terrible argument. I didn't leave him, and now I'm glad I didn't. It was uncharacteristic of him to be so thoughtless, and uncharacteristic of me to react the way I did.*

*I was very hurt that he just left without a word. I thought we should have been able to talk about it. I thought he knew me well enough to know I would not create a scene. He was my first real love and everything was so good. It had taken me a long time to put myself back together, and to accept the fact that I will never see him again.*

Emotional harassment and put-downs of women (those many small layers of habit, verbal and nonverbal cues—not one of which one would want to start a fight about, or if one did, one might be called "hysterical") are more or less a pattern in society and in many women's personal love relationships, so that a cutting remark can be made at any moment, when a woman is least expecting it. This situation amounts to a kind of emotional terrorism.

Gender-biased attitudes are particularly harmful in a deep, intimate personal relationship. If the butcher or a salesperson makes a demeaning remark (which, as every woman knows, can happen), it is one thing: something unpleasant but something one can overlook as coming from a prejudiced person. But if the person one loves, is closest to, and depends on for one's most intimate contact with humanity makes such a remark—that is another matter. And this seems to be, in case after case, exactly what is happening. It is possible that many men have no idea what they are doing. Most do seem to be quite unaware of the residual stereotypes they hold. They think, "Oh, this is just Mary, she is like that. She had a childhood that . . ." Or, "She is a specialist with children, who cannot understand all that I, having been in the world so long, can know . . .," and so on.

If these attitudes were blatantly expressed, they would be easier to fight. But the subtle distancing and harassment that have been accepted for millennia not as "put-downs" but as just describing "how women are," are very difficult to deal with, their effects insidious.

What is the answer then, what will women do? Keep putting time in relationships to explain that their ideas *do* matter (and also to rebuild their own damaged self-esteem)? Or stop investing so much energy in "love," begin placing love second after work or career?

Women could easily decide to take this second route as the path of least resistance, unless emotional equality becomes the hallmark of gender relationships—so that women do not wind up feeling burned out and lonely inside relationships.

## ANGER AND ALIENATION—INEVITABLE REACTIONS?

Another woman describes the increasing alienation many women talk about:

> *I suppose trying to be honest is the worst thing I ever did to him, yelling at him. (He loves it too, though, because then he looks like the knight in white armor and I look like the whore/screamer.) I finally explode and say all the wrong things in front of anybody, mostly the children. I talk and he does nothing. He doesn't listen. I would have shared all of myself if only I were loved, but I've tried and been rejected for it. It is hard to share with a person who just doesn't talk to you.*

Many women believe that they are not getting equal emotional support, esteem, or respect in their relationships, but they find this lack difficult or impossible to explain. It can be difficult to describe definitively to a man just how he is projecting diminishing attitudes, since some of the ways this happens are so subtle that pointing to the thing said or done would look petty, like overreacting. But taken all together, it is no surprise when even one of these incidents can set off a major fight—or, more typically, another round of alienation, which never gets resolved. These little incidents cut away at the relationship, making women angry and finally causing love to dwindle down to a mere modest toleration.

Here we are focusing on the imbalance of power built into male-female dynamics, hoping that by analyzing them, making them visible, the paradigm can be shifted, and more harmony will come into being.

## DOES FIGHTING, "BRINGING UP THE ISSUES," WORK?

Many women wind up screaming or shouting at men from time to time because they so often feel that they that can't be heard, that men don't hear them. Since women generally have low credibility in the culture, men often do not hear them.

The statistics on the number of women taking tranquilizers and consulting psychologists further attests to the fact that women are having a rough time constructing satisfying personal relationships with men.

### HOW DOES CHANGE COME ABOUT?

Negotiating for respect in a relationship is important, something that should be accomplished with grace and good humor. But women say that they often find a need to overwork, just to get a balance. What should a woman do when there are frequent subtle hints of condescension toward her because of her gender and when mentioning these to her partner does not change his attitude?

The issues women are bringing up may appear on the surface to be "petty," but the pattern of condescension that is provoking women is so widespread that it is noticeable in this research. Women are forced to fight back, yet individual fighting back doesn't always work because men don't always understand what it is women are trying to point out to them. Perhaps it will be necessary for women to change the status of women as a whole before gaining enough respect and dignity to make it possible for their love relationships to thrive.

On the other hand, expressing anger can be a first step. One woman makes an excellent point about where women should direct their anger, and why they usually don't:

> Depression is, for me, taking out my anger on myself because it's too scary to face up to the real person who is making me angry. If you have been taught by your parents that you are worthless, it is then easier to consider self-destructive acts and behavior than to fight back against the people who you think are better than you. You don't know that you have any rights.

Anger unexpressed can become a fog that pervades everything, leading to a perpetual low-level anxiety. Indeed, women's frustration and/or anger is responsible in large part for much of the psychological counseling, tranquilizers, and so on women use.* And yet it is considered almost treasonous for a woman to express her anger with men or with "male" culture—either for personal reasons or for larger social reasons (that is, because men still do not share their social and political power equally with women).

In fact anger against men is the most verboten feeling a woman can have. A woman who states that she is angry at men or, even more, at "male" culture or the

---

* Statistically, in the United States twice as many women as men go to psychiatrists, psychologists, and counselors; this figure has not changed since the 1950s, despite monumental feminist works, including "Psychology Constructs the Female" by Naomi Weisstein, works by Shulamith Firestone, and *Women and Madness* by Phyllis Chesler. Today women are by far the largest consumers of tranquilizers, so that it could be said that a large percentage of the female population is chemically pacified.

system is frequently labeled a "manhater" or "hysterical." To be made outcasts or pariahs is the unspoken threat to which so many women react by noting that they fear their fate will be to become a "bag lady." This fear is frequently expressed in magazine articles and the like; when women worry that they cannot keep up with all that is expected of them—that is, maintain their looks, make men desire them, and now, earn money too. Even though we joke about this, it is significant; we wonder if there is really a place in society for us, especially as older women. We cannot afford psychologically to be angry with men because we fear that we may wind up as outcasts. This feeling is changing, but very slowly.

The initial impulse might be to say, well, why don't women get even with men in their lives, revolt? But the matter is more complicated. Women don't take violent revenge on individual men (or society) because to do so is not in accord with their most basic values.

Most women in my research do not believe in fighting, especially not "male" style, considering it beneath them. Instead most prefer nonviolent resistance, even if they are then sometimes seen as "wimps," as too "stupid" to fight, "peaceful" only because they are afraid or have been "brainwashed" not to fight back. In fact women often fight back by leaving unsatisfying relationships: 90 percent of the high number of divorces in the United States, the United Kingdom, and Germany are initiated and carried through by women.

## MEN SHOULD WELCOME WOMEN'S ANGER, NOT FEAR IT

For men simply to ignore the problem of the status of women in society and/or problems in relationships, or to think of them as "women's issues" and turn their attention to other matters, rather than making an effort to do something about the situation, makes the problem worse. Women often state that they "bring up issues," then men fall silent, hoping the "problem" will go away—which only makes women angrier and the problem worse. Women's so-called passive nature could be mainly a form of depression, a screen for women's fury, channeled in the wrong direction; if this energy were directed correctly, it could become a positive force for society.

## DOES THERAPY HELP—OR IS IT HARMFUL TO WOMEN?

*There came a time when I realized that the pain of my romances was essentially the same pain and conflict I experienced in dealing with my mother and that I was using romance as a way of dealing with my mother, of trying to be separate—individual.*

The situations described here in terms of the emotional contract results from large social issues; they are not something one person can or should have to fight alone. Although it is productive to understand one's own history and personality, to come away from "therapy" without it having been acknowledged that the culture also has a strong hand in creating these situations is wrong. After all, women will have to continue dealing with society's messages about women's status and "characteristics"; what tools would a therapy, which usually does not acknowledge the existence of this gender bias in the culture, give to a woman to help her go on with her life?

Even worse, some schools of therapy seem to blame women by labeling their socially created problems with such epithets as "masochistic," "dependent," and so on—completely ignoring the concrete phenomenon of women's economic fragility or outright dependency during most of the twentieth century and the effects this situation has had on women's (and men's) "psychologies."

A new psychocultural therapy should be developed.

Some forms of counseling are more progressive. One woman describes a very good experience she had with an unusual therapist, who did not deny the reality of gender bias against women in society, and took her anger against "male" society into realistic account:

> *Therapy can be wonderful—with the right therapist. At the point when I was in despair after the breakup of my affair after my marriage, I needed a therapist—and after trying two I didn't like, I found one who proved just right. I knew he would be right when he suggested at the initial session that if I really would prefer a woman therapist, he'd help me find one.*
>
> *We worked together for nearly three years—I say "worked together" very much on purpose, for I felt very much an equal in the relationship—perhaps the only relationship with any man in which I've really felt an equal. My initial "love relationship problem" faded, and most of the therapy delved into the causes for my tendency toward depressions—which basically has to do with my frequent feeling of helplessness to be equal to men in the world as it exists. This starting from the birth of my brother and being reinforced at every point in my life. I could never be outstanding enough in anything I did to be taken as seriously as men were—it is a fight I will fight all the rest of my life.*
>
> *Therapy helped me understand that this is the structure of our social milieu, and that I do not lack something essential. Thanks to the therapy, and to my own strengths, I understand now that I don't have to be perfect and invulnerable. I see some of my hang-ups and realize that I'll never get over some of them. I know that, as a woman playwright in a world where men pull the puppet and purse strings, I will have to work twice as hard as men and there will be a lot of unfairness and enormous frustrations. I won't like it one bit, but mostly I won't think my failures are because there is something inherently wrong with me. Therapy went a long way beyond curing a "broken heart."*

## CLICHÉS ABOUT PRIVATE LIFE THAT NEED TO CHANGE

Women's complaints about relationships should be taken seriously—not trivialized and "psychologized" away.

This study shows that most women are not in love relationships they consider to be anywhere near what they would like: 95 percent of the married women in this study want to make basic changes in their marriages, and 84 percent of single women reply that love relationships with men are more often than not filled with anxiety, fear of being "uncool" (by wanting commitment), and so on.

Woman after woman notes that she is putting enormous amounts of energy into trying to make her relationship work—but that the man doesn't seem to be putting in the same effort. This situation makes women alienated, frustrated, and often angry.

Many women lie in bed at night knowing that matters could be so much better, wondering how to reach the man sleeping next to them, or wondering why a man they love doesn't call—or how to get out of a relationship although they can't really explain just why they don't like it. So many women lie there thinking, "It's too bad that things are like this. . . ."

Women have been "complaining" about love relationships for some time, at least since Freud, but these complaints have rarely been taken seriously. What women express has rarely been given credibility, instead being discounted as "women bitching and moaning." Society blames women's feelings of frustration with men on women's "psychology"—not on the fact that many men may be practicing discrimination, or that most women have a legitimate complaint, that is, that they live with discrimination.

It is usually implied that if a woman is having problems, the problem is with the woman—with her outdated values, "demanding" behavior, "neediness," upbringing, "dependency," and so forth. Women daily hear themselves referred to as "messed up," "masochistic," or "neurotic" if they step the least bit out of line, and some part of them wonders if the accusations could be true. They wonder, "Do I send out vibrations that attract the wrong men," or they fault themselves for not recognizing or disengaging quickly enough from "destructive" relationships. Alternately, women worry that they may not be patient enough, understanding enough, expect too much, are too "idealistic." But are women really doing something wrong? Will the clichés change to create more understanding and love?

## BEING SINGLE: WOMEN AND AUTONOMY

### HOW THE EMOTIONAL CONTRACT APPLIES TO THE DATING SCENARIO

The dynamics of an unwritten "emotional contract," with its psychological roles, are quite pronounced in "singles dating." Bluntly, single women are defined by the system as needing men more than men need women. This puts women in a vulnerable position psychologically with men—women must "catch" men, not seem too "needy" of a relationship, not "complain" about men's lack of emotional support or condescension, bad manners, and so on. Yet when they don't, they are further defined as "easy" and "not very important"!

There is an undercurrent in most dating relationships of this unstated imbalance of power status between women and men—that is, the so-called desirability of females versus the desirability of males. The suspense in a relationship for a woman hovers around the question, "Is it love, or is he just using you?" Women have a realistic fear of being tricked—then being left to end up feeling taken, yet emotionally open and still loving.

Single women are having relationships with men who have grown up with images of the Marlboro man (the idealized "loner") and single male movie heroes, men who don't want to commit themselves and who believe in "freedom"—at least freedom from relationships with women, according to women in my research. Thus, when most men are in relationships, they act ambivalently. This puts women emotionally on the defensive.* The rules are: "Don't cling," "Don't ask for monogamy, there is something wrong with you if you feel insecure," and so on.

Indeed, some women want to get married just to escape the endless "trying out," the doubts and upsets of single life.

One woman offers her thoughts about what is going on in the whole singles area:

> In a desperation to get the supposed security of having a man, single women may hurt their own self-esteem. They cater to what they feel the man wants, while completely ignoring their own needs, which are reasonable and correct. For example, they are having sex with men after just a date, hoping the man will love and be close to them, marry them, and it doesn't ever work. The tragedy is how much women are hurt along the way. Women are answering to men's needs, believing that men's ideology about marriage and love is correct, not being true to themselves. They're afraid to be rejected if they state their real hopes and dreams—and try to be "loose" the way the "male" culture is. But they should have more belief in themselves. Their ideas have dignity and depth and profundity. Women should set the standards, and not listen to "male" standards.

Many women are torn over whether they are making the right choices, whether they have the "right" feelings about love, whether they are assessing clearly what is happening in their lives: "Sometimes I'm depressed or sad for a short while after leaving a lover. The first few times, I thought I might die, but I guess I'm getting used

---

* Also, of course, there is great pressure on women—a feeling (after the age of twenty-eight or so) that marriage is the only basic way to fit into society; most women feel that there will be no place for them in society after their twenties if they don't "find someone" and get married.

to it. It seems the older I get, the easier the break-ups become. I'm not sure how great that is, and it depresses me, all this long string of love affairs—even if some of them are 'good friends' later. What does it mean?"

Many women's relationships seem degrading (though no one wants to say so), since many men treat women condescendingly, according to women in my study (for example, they may drop a woman at any time, talk of love but never feel obliged to discuss the pros and cons of plans for the future). There is very little idea of team sharing; the "lone hero" version of the "male" ideology does not stop to consider women as having equal rights. Hence, women's pride can be whittled away during the course of a relationship with a man.

Women frequently feel that they are being "fucked over" emotionally by men who reflect the values of a culture that is trivializing women's lives, bodies and beliefs.

Many women take this treatment, even though they know what is going on, because they truly love someone, or they like other parts of what they get in the relationship (for example, physical intimacy and companionship). They may also feel that they have little choice, since every woman "has" to get married eventually.

All of this can lead to what one woman described as "relationship burnout."

## PATTERNS IN SINGLE RELATIONSHIPS

*You want to forget the feeling of being so hurt and just go on—like in a break-up—but is life serious? Does one event imply thinking about it, and changing your view of life? Or can you just forget and cover everything over?*

The whole scenario—a woman feeling, when meeting someone or starting a relationship, that if she doesn't sleep with him relatively quickly, he may never call her again; but if she does sleep with him, he may not take her seriously or treat her respectfully and may never call again anyway—puts women in an awkward position. Even worse, it never allows a woman to be the "judge" of a relationship: women hardly have a chance to think about what they actually feel, because they are so busy having to deal with the man's prejudices, stereotypes, and possibly condescending remarks. She has to judge situations in an atmosphere that makes the man a possible adversary.

During recent years, some men's "male" pattern of no-holds-barred competition and aggression has become much harsher in the "singles world," and the pressure on single women to try to appease men and fit in with their system has become stronger. Women in the "singles scene" often rightly feel anxiety about whether men will drop or dump them—the man first acting loving, then unfriendly, then later returning to act loving again (meanwhile wondering why she is "so unstable" and demanding to know if he loves her). What is going on in this atmosphere?

Many men's casual treatment of women in single relationships seems remarkably hostile and confrontational; the wild impoliteness of some men in the "dating scene" documented here (in *Women and Love*) seems to represent an enormous increase over previous years. Almost a flagrant show of power and contempt, the message is: since a woman is so "powerless," it cannot hurt a man to be rude or treat her callously.

In the world of noncommitted, fluctuating relationships, men's leaving immediately after sex, not calling, calling at random times, keeping unpredictable schedules but still expecting the woman to be available—all these have become standard behaviors, so that a woman often correctly finds it hard to enjoy the "date" or "relationship," or even to know if she is in a relationship. The attitude of "I deserve a woman to love me and be nice to me, but I don't have to be nice back" is widespread. As one woman asks, "Are they afraid and nervous, or did someone tell them it's macho to be mean?" Many men seem to have leaped mentally from the 1950s attitude that women who are not playing the role of mothers are "bad girls," to a post-"sexual revolution" attitude to the effect that, since most women now have sex before marriage and furthermore work outside the home, most women are "bad girls" who deserve to be treated roughly—"they deserve what they get"—because "they gave up being put on pedestals when they went out into the 'male world.'" Chivalry, men say, was extraspecial treatment (they do not recognize the special treatment women give men—that is, listening to men's opinions as if they are more important than their own, and so forth); in some instances, as we have seen, men do not even treat women they have slept with with the same amount of respect and politeness that they would accord a business associate.

Thousands of testimonies by women on these topics can be found in the original volume, *Women and Love*.

## THE SEDUCTION SCENARIO

Women report that many men have a pattern of giving a woman attention until she is involved with them, has come to trust and enjoy them, then changing, withdrawing attention, coming and going irregularly. If a woman "complains," she may be reminded by the man, "I'm happy, why are you making waves?" with an undertone of "Now, don't start being a neurotic, clinging woman. I thought you were different." Thus, men's behavior appears "neutral"; the man is "not doing anything wrong." In fact, the man is practicing a form of passive aggression.

Do men go through this process of flirtation, seduction, saying "beautiful things" only for "conquest"? Or is it also because they want the adulation, affection, and understanding that women give?

It is hardly surprising that many women feel very angry and unsettled about these situations. While they may know that in fact it is the whole weight of the system that they are feeling, that the system is unjust, still, for an individual who has just had all her assumptions challenged, this knowledge is not comforting.

Nor is it perhaps surprising that men's commitment in marriage can look more civilized to single women than what they are experiencing. As one woman puts it, "It's all a jungle—but maybe at least if you're married, it's a private jungle."

The psychological imbalance set up in single relationships can lead a woman to ask herself, "Is everything all right with him? Does he still love me? What is his mood today?" instead of, "Is everything all right with me? Do I want this kind of relationship?" After all, women are used to men setting the rules, declaring what reality is, with women expected to adjust. Even if women realize how outrageous the situation is, they still often feel that they should stay, because of the heavy social pressure to "fit in" and "have a man."

Ironically, in nonmarried relationships it often seems to women that men have even more power than they do in marriage—ironically, since feminists fought against men's ownership of women in marriage. Perhaps this is because in a nonmarried relationship there is no public view of the state of things; these relationships can be only semivisible or "invisible."

Most men are brought up to see women as "second," fundamentally more emotional, not as "rational," and so on. Should a woman take time with a man she loves and try to get him to see her as an equal, change his thinking? Or is this a job that may take up more of her time and energy than she can afford?

More and more women are becoming restive. Individual women everywhere are asking, why does it have to be like this? *Does* it have to be like this? Isn't another system possible?

In fact it is just this thinking going on in women's lives, combined with women's growing economic self-sufficiency and happiness with friends, that is creating a new philosophical outlook, an emerging vision of what life can be, as woman after woman comes to the conclusion that there is something wrong with the system, not with her. Actually single women are doing quite well, despite it all. They enjoy their lives, being on their own—their work, their friends, some of the playing around with men.

Many women are coming to see that it is not even so much a problem with the individual men they know, but that somehow men too are caught up in an unreasonable set of beliefs that twists their lives and distorts their behavior.

Men today often feel that they have no place to turn—except perhaps to sex, through which they can at least get physical affection. In this and many other ways the gender system hurts men and closes them off from others, even while most men continue to believe in it and to defend its "values," no matter what.

### ARE MEN TO BLAME? HOW DO MEN FEEL?

"Male psychology" as we know it is as much a creation of society as "female psychology" is perceived to be. How often have you heard "women are brought up to think like that," and similar phrases? Yet rarely are men thought to be suffering from psychological brainwashing—or if they are, there is little belief that men should change their way of being in the same way that women, for the last thirty years, have worked massively to change their psyches and behavior.

Why do so many men behave the way they do toward women? Another cause might be a vague unrest men feel with their lives in general: are men the "winners" in the system that they are supposed to be? What we see (for example in *The Hite Report on Men and Male Sexuality* or in statistics on domestic violence) is men expressing a kind of fury, a nervousness that might indicate a feeling on men's part that things in general in their lives are not going well, that men are not getting the rewards they were promised by the system. Perhaps men are finding their world now somewhat frightening and unsatisfying, particularly with jobs often scarce and the future uncertain in a world where one is expected to change jobs or careers several times in a lifetime. Even the once guaranteed love from women may be taken away as men are expected to see women as equals, to "watch every little thing one says around them." Maybe men can no longer expect women to "be there," "be nice," ready to be caretakers, to make a home, and the like. No longer is there a promise that there will always be someone there, someone at "home" waiting. It is possible that how men treat women is a stage on which men are acting out their general feelings about life, themselves, and the future.

The idea of "masculinity" has undergone a great change since World War II. As Jacob Bronowski stated, "Perhaps we have dehumanized ourselves and others with World War II and the bomb."[3] Is it possible that the collective male psyche in America somehow felt uncomfortable with war, with learning to believe that it is right to fight, and dealt with its guilt by glorifying it, glorifying the tough, brutal loner, the jungle fighter—the man who could "take it," "do what he had to do"—as a way of absorbing the shock of collective responsibility for the violence and death that was the price of victory.

This style (that of the warrior or "heroic loner") has remained popular, yet not all men "buy into" this brutalized idea of masculinity. What makes them different, what keeps them safe from this desensitizing process?

### SEXUAL MISCOMMUNICATION

Women's training to be loving and giving makes dating lopsided in terms of the needs of the two parties. Alienated, unscrupulous men and boys who want to feel very "masculine," who have been taught that their "hormones" propel them to have intercourse with women, that this action makes them "real men," are aware of women's desire to love and be giving, and these men take advantage of the women by pushing for sex, pretending love.

Some men say, "Well, don't women enjoy sex too, just as much as men?" (Therefore, the thinking goes, the man is not taking advantage of the woman, he is giving her something she needs as much as he does—even if temporarily.) But while women are sometimes at a point in their lives when they enjoy experimenting and having "adventures," it is quite clear that for most of their lives, most women prefer sex in a context of feelings and respect.

Women should not have to choose between being sexual and not being sexual; nor should women have to define their sexuality under such pressure and negativity from men. Instead women and men should challenge the reigning ideology, which decrees that "boys will be boys," closing a blind eye to many boys' "hit and run" or "shopping" attitudes toward girls. This same culture looks down on teenage girls for getting abortions but does not think that the missing boys who probably pushed for intercourse are also "villains"/victims, now set up for emotional alienation and anger too.

## REAPPRAISING THE SEXUAL REVOLUTION: IS LOOKING FOR LOTS OF "SEX" "NATURAL"?

Is monogamous love and/or a desire for marriage a "natural" tendency that men have been taught to repress? Or are multiple sexual relationships "natural," and do women typically avoid them only because they are brought up to be prudes and "good girls"? (Or because people call them "sluts" otherwise?)

The presumption is usually that what men do, think, or feel is "natural," that if only women would give up their "hang-ups," they would naturally be "like men" too. The assumption since the "sexual revolution" has therefore almost universally been that women would—and should—change their values and sexual behavior to be more like men, that is, to have sex more outside of marriage and have it not mean so much. This thinking assumes that the "male" system is biologically ordained, and the "female" system is "acculturated"—that women are "held back" because of the fear of getting pregnant and for other reasons.

But is there any logical reason for believing that "promiscuity" is "natural"? Most women would say here that it is men who are conforming to an artificial ideal, men who should change and understand the connection of sex with feelings, understand that the body and spirit may not be separate after all.

## THE RIGHT TO BE SINGLE: DO WOMEN FEEL "ALONE"?

Women in my research often remark that they like spending time on their own, having time to themselves:

*I find that being single is a time I take quantum leaps in self-development. It seems to release a surge of creative energy in me. I think I am a better person for the time I spend alone.*

Although living alone is supposed to be lonely, many women say that they can be themselves when alone more than they can at any other time. Being single without a steady boyfriend is a popular way of life with women of various ages.

Women say, over and over, that they have many good women friends, sometimes friends of a lifetime, and that their communication with them is the closest of their lives. On the other hand, being single and trying out different relationships can make women feel "lonely" because of the ups and downs, the lack of stability, and constant "starting over." Breaking up or being in a bad relationship can be depressing, but being "alone" is not as "lonely" according to women. Also, more women mention feeling lonely when they are in an imperfect relationship than when single; almost no women mention feeling alone because of being single.

Most women in this study, single and married, say they would like to have more time alone. When asked, "What is your favorite activity for yourself, your favorite way to waste time?" the overwhelming majority of women chose activities that were solitary—such as taking a bath, reading a book, going for a long walk, perhaps with their dogs, or having time to just sit and have a cup of tea.

*I love to play music and dance. I love to read, I read a lot, and I love movies. I love to sit around by myself and space out, I call it. That kind of time is very important, very, very important to me.*

One woman describes her single life after years of marriage and motherhood:

*The disadvantage of blessed singleness is that I live in what I call Noah's Ark. It used to be called a "bedroom town," a place for commuting husbands to keep their wives and children, but now is a corporate headquarters town. When you go downtown at noon and the streets are crawling with squads of men in their dull business suits who practically knock you into the gutter in their arrogance.*

*Between being a suburb of families and patriarchal corporate headquarters, there is little social life for a single old woman. (I'm sixty-two now.) I have few friends. But I'm not lonely or unhappy. For the most part, I feel contented—that is, when I am not driven because I'm not accomplishing.*

*After taking the drastic, terrifying step of no longer kowtowing to my husband, I recognized him as a brutalizing monster. But at the time, he seemed better than most and everyone said to me, "You're so lucky." Romantic "love" is a myth conjured up in our society to keep women enslaved—always looking for a mate in order to feel "human." The concept is enforced by Hollywood patriarchal moguls, admen, and the like—the male brotherhood.*

*For my second job, the YWCA job counselor tore up my paper when she saw my only credentials outside of housework were the past ten years of volunteer work. No matter how I'd couch it, it would come out the same. Eventually, I had to get a renter to keep afloat. This turned out to be the biggest break for me. He moved in with his computer, and soon began teaching me with infinite patience to use it—so well that I am now doing a free-lance indexing paid job. I am enjoying this experience the most of anything since 1978. I keep thinking I should learn faster and do more. I don't know any woman with as sophisticated equipment as this, or with the knowledge that he and his friends have. It's fun knowing him.*

*After raising five children to adulthood and independence, I entered the job market for the first time at fifty-six and I am surviving—"making it"! My goals are to retain my home, remain financially independent, and start making enough money to do things like go to shows and concerts, travel and take vacations. I can see it's all within my grasp now—in just a year or two, I will have it all—and I can be proud of having done it myself.*

Finally, the stereotype of being "old and alone" is basically inaccurate: in this study, 81 percent of single women over sixty-five report that they like their lives very much (even if they could use a little more money). Most enjoy their friends, their work, their gardens, lovers, in fact all facets of life. Many women explain that they feel happier when "old and alone" than they did earlier in life.

## WHAT IS LOVE?

### HOW WOMEN FEEL ABOUT PAINFUL LOVE AFFAIRS

Is it worth having a less intense relationship, to avoid the pain of volatile ups and downs?

One woman describes her feeling of frustration, confusion, and love, all mixed together, as she experiences a great deal of ambiguity in the man she loves:

*I have a constant feeling of never being satisfied for some reason. Either he's not calling, or when he's calling, it's not romantic, and so on. . . . When I try to talk to him, really talk to him, I feel like I just can't get through—except sometimes, when he wants to talk, he'll say the loveliest things. Other times, he just won't respond and/or doesn't want to make love, and I never know why.*

*If I am unhappy a lot, and he won't talk to me about the problems or resolve the issues, should I say, "Well, everything is really O.K." because he's O.K. and he's still there and still loves me? Or should I say, "This relationship is terrible and I will leave it because be is not making me happy"? Loving him makes it difficult to leave him. Maybe I should become pregnant and solve the whole question of what will become of us (I'm sure he'd never want me to have an abortion).*

*But he keeps saying these condescending remarks, like I was a little girl or something. I found myself trying to write him a note to explain my feelings to him the other day. I wrote it late one night. The next morning I looked at it and it started out, "I know that you think of me as complicated and crazy, but I just want to explain to you . . ." I couldn't believe I had written that, and just put myself down! What a macho view he has, like* Gaslight, *the movie, to imply there is anything wrong with my thinking! You know, the movie with Ingrid Bergman and Charles Boyer, made a long time ago, where he tries to convince her she is losing her mind, by making the lights flicker and claiming they are not, that it's all in her mind? The idea is that men are the norm, I guess, and women are the deviants. But it starts subtly—I would have been outraged three months ago if anyone had implied I was "complicated and crazy"—but it happens gradually, you lose your self-esteem and belief in yourself gradually. Now all that seems apparent to me is that I want to be alone and strong again. I say that now, but. . . .*

*The problem is that first he says he's vulnerable and in love—then later he denies it or doesn't act like it, acts cold. I ask myself, "Is the goal this man at any cost?" It's almost as if someone is egging me on to go into the deep end of the pool—and then when I get there (with my emotions) and really fall in love, trust him, he says, "What? Why me?" I've been so scared all the way, thinking to myself, no matter what happened, giving him the benefit of the doubt, "Let me trust, let me trust," not letting myself believe the negative signals, thinking he was just insecure or reacting to something I had done in my own effort to seem invulnerable— I've always been so afraid, wondering, "Will somebody stay?" A relationship like ours where there is no commitment yet means anybody can pull out whenever they want—but I have tried not to believe that would be the case, to believe we are building something more valuable, more permanent, even though he has not said so.*

*Maybe this whole relationship has been a big mistake on my part. I feel less strong. Instead of working on my career, I am obsessed with our phone calls and meetings. I feel weak. Why does love have to make you feel weak? Does it? It all turns into a game of strategy. It always feels like he is in control. But who knows, maybe he feels like I am in control, he feels just as vulnerable as I do. Oh, here I go again obsessing about this relationship.*

*I am so angry at myself that I have lost myself in this love affair.*

*How to judge the situation is so hard: Is he afraid to love, or does he really not love me? It's all so one-sided, I feel sometimes. Then sometimes I think he loves me, but he would never marry me—you know the way I mean? And if he loves me, why does he leave me so often? Does he really have to spend so much time at work? If we were married, it would give me a base to know he really did care and love me in some special way; just the way we are, although he calls me every day, I always wonder and feel very insecure. Everything seems to be on his terms—he tells me when he can come and see me. I tried doing the same thing to him and being busy at work a lot, but it didn't bother him at all, it just hurt me because I missed him.*

*Why do I want somebody who is not making me happy? His low and trivializing opinion of women comes out in bits and snatches. But other times are really great, and he can be so charming and so much fun, and then say some really beautiful things. He's not that great in bed, however, I must admit.*

*My mother has counseled me the following way: She said, when I complained I couldn't get through to him about what was bothering me about the relationship, "It is easy to speak with a friend, but not with a man. With a man, you become silent. You have to find your own liberty inside—and then you can be with a man. No matter how free and strong you are, when you are with a man, you start thinking how he feels, lose any self, any center. You feel he's not completely yours—especially if you are creative. You want to be comforted by a man. Men want a woman who looks good, is brilliant, but still will be dominated." I couldn't believe she told me these things. I guess, as Laurence Olivier once remarked in one of his films, "No matter what they tell you, you really are on your own out there. Completely and totally alone." I guess this is why people become mediocre—safety in following the flock.*

*Anyway, there's something about the setup with me that's so unfair. It's O.K. if men bring up commitment, but not if we do. So—life isn't fair, love relationships with men aren't fair—but I still want one! But how do I get him??? Do I have to play a game and wait for him? Should I appear strong and independent, or do I have to seem to need him??? I feel so depressed, but there's no reason! I'm starting to be insecure, and worse, to show him my insecurities. It's not knowing what's going to happen with us, and I really care.*

One woman, after a rather disastrous experience of being "in love," decided to develop a more low-key relationship with a man she loves less but who, she feels, will be stable and with whom she can work things out:

*In the last three years, I have made a major change, removing myself from a self-destructive relationship. The man I lived with wouldn't marry me, always accused me of not really liking his daughter (who lived with us, or should I say, I lived with them). I constantly cleaned up after her, took care of her, talked to her after school, fed her, etc. Once he even hit me because she said I had been mean to her while he was out. Part of the time I lived there, I wasn't working, so I was financially dependent, and this was demeaning too. I mean, I felt like a real Cinderella. But I was crazy about him, I always liked sex with him, he was very sexy. It took me ages to leave. Even after I had gotten a degree, I still wanted to be with him, and also by that time, I was pretty low, so it was hard to get up enough belief in myself to make the move.*

*Perhaps my biggest achievement so far has been to enter analysis, and to form a different relationship, with a special friend. We enjoy a wonderful sex life together. We have both had terrible hurts in the past and run away from each other, but he is very understanding.*

*I consider myself a feminist. I think the women's movement helped me feel like I am less alone with my problems. I am still raging at the double messages in society, at discrimination, at sexism, at churches that cripple people sexually, etc. Mostly, I rage now at people who treat me like dirt. I think it's all right to rage, but I also want to learn to love—myself and everyone else.*

## PRACTICALITY VERSUS THE SOUL: MUST EVERY RELATIONSHIP END WITH THE "PERFECTLY ADJUSTED HETEROSEXUAL COUPLE"?

Is "happiness" always the goal in a love relationship? There is a case to be made for not having to have every love fit into some socially approved scheme of the perfect household and the Perfectly Adjusted Heterosexual Couple. All relationships are not tryouts for "marriage"!

Sometimes women decide to stay in a relationship because no matter how great the pain, their love is real, and feeling it, expressing it, gives them more pleasure, more of a feeling of being themselves, alive, than being stable and "normal." As one woman reports:

*I would go out of my way for my boyfriend, and love makes it seem not out of the way. This is the first time that I have felt like this. My two previous boyfriends loved me more than I loved them. I felt guilty when they would talk about our future together with happiness in their eyes and I felt doubt.*

What is a good relationship? Does it consist of getting along? Companionship? Feeling great passion? Closeness? Being there? Actually a relationship can be very unstable, or even unhappy, and still provide a kind of nourishment for the soul, or somehow open up doors in one's mind to places that didn't exist before.

As one woman puts it:

> *He is the one I want to love. Some other relationships might be easier, or more talkative, but I don't love them. I love him for the unique person he is—I love a person, not a relationship. I'm not looking for a person to give me the best relationship there is, I'm looking for a person I feel connected to.*

Being "obsessed" with love has at times been labeled "neurotic" behavior, as if only "rationality" is acceptable; and yet even the Greeks accepted "divine madness" as a good. And not even thinking in these extremes, it is undoubtedly true that people at times feel a connection beyond words.

### WHY IS "REAL LOVE" SO IMPORTANT TO WOMEN?

But are women too prone to seek after the "great love," too easily led by their feelings, too likely to continue loving when it is not "rational"? And is this thirst for love somehow reflective of a thirst for approval and love, nurturance, from a society that hardly welcomed our birth as it did those of our brothers—a society that does not give much approval or encouragement to women, except in the role of helping males?

Or perhaps our quest for love is also a hidden form of love for ourselves—we are not supposed to love ourselves, so we hunger to find a man who can love us, to certify that love—to get the love we feel we cannot give ourselves. In a way, perhaps, our quest for love is a sublimation of the spiritual ecstasy of the self, being one with that self. Is that why we may find it so hard to leave a man with whom we are "in love," even if the relationship becomes negative?

Love is still the prescribed lifestyle for women. Love can drain women incredibly, (although it should not), which has led many feminists to say that as women we should "throw off our chains" and "stop having sex with our oppressors"—reject romance with men. But feeling love is not the culprit, we are not "weak," "masochistic," and "silly"; rather, it is the cultural context, the genderizing of society, that makes love sometimes seem so masochistic.

### IF WOMEN CHANGE THEIR VIEW OF LOVE: A CULTURAL REVOLUTION IN PROGRESS

What is going on right now in the minds of women is a large-scale cultural revolution. Women, married and single, are asking themselves serious questions about their personal lives. These questions are growing initially out of their desire to have closer, more satisfying relationships with the men they are with. As their frustration with these relationships increases, many begin to ask deeper and deeper questions—finally, not only about love, but about the entire system.

As woman after woman lies in bed at night wondering, "Why did so and so not call?" or "Why doesn't my husband turn over and talk to me about this thing that he knows is on my mind, or at least that I told him is on my mind?" she begins thinking, analyzing all the possible answers. First, she may wonder, "Is it me? Is there something wrong with me?" Next she may try to figure out the psychological makeup of the man she is with, his individual psychological background. Then, to understand this, she often begins to look at his parents' family structure—and then next at the overall social patterns that made them that way—until finally, in her searching, she comes face to face with the whole system and asks herself how it got the way it is.

The pain in many women's personal lives, or the built-up frustration as they try to figure out a relationship (or deal with the loneliness inside it), leads women to a series of deeper questions about why love is so difficult—why men behave as they do, why a man can be sometimes loving, sometimes cold and distant—why? Women are asking, "Does it have to be this way?" Pondering this question, women are developing a rather clear-cut and detailed idea of what it is they really want out of relationships—what they think to be the right basis for human relationships and the society as a whole.

### WOMEN'S DISSATISFACTION: DRIVING SOCIAL CHANGE

As women think through these questions, they are causing everything to change. Recognizing the problems, thinking through the issues, women are becoming different from what they are analyzing. Having to analyze a thing so deeply removes one from it, and so women begin to feel removed from the current system, from things as they are. It is impossible to ask these questions and not change, to stop the process inside oneself. Seeing the situation, a new level of understanding and awareness takes place that cannot be undone, and so one is—whether one wants to be or not—transformed, changed forever.

The feelings of alienation women are describing here in their personal lives are leading to the formulation of a new set of political goals and philosophical beliefs, a new philosophy, based on women's traditional point of view, modified by the changes women have made during the last twenty years.

Women are in a struggle with the dominant ideological structure of the culture. As women see their relationships and their lives differently—they become different—and many are no longer content to live biculturally. And wrestling with themselves on many issues, they also discuss these matters with their women friends—comparing relationships, asking what is the best one can expect out of life, how to interpret men's actions. These discussions between women are part of a very important process of creating and maintaining a specific value system.

Finally these changes in thinking are all happening in conjunction with women's new economic position, which has been called "the quiet revolution."[4] Within the last ten years the number of women with jobs and businesses has increased so markedly that in fact women as a group are no longer essentially economically dependent on men. This is a startling development—and one whose implications have only barely begun to take hold. Although many women receive extremely low salaries (and day care is expensive), more women than ever have enough resources to make it on their own, if they have to—even with children, and even if only minimally. The 50 percent divorce rate, mostly initiated by women, and the "feminization of poverty" mean that women today would rather leave a relationship than stay and put up with a negative situation. They do not mean that they were "left" or "dumped"* but that they are seeking something better. One of the most important ways women express their values is in friendship with other women.

## THE "OTHER" TRANSFORMED/CONCLUSION

Fifty years ago Simone de Beauvoir aptly described women as the "Other"—as defined by men and men's view of the world. Now women have taken that position as Other and transformed it, turned it around, making of it a new vantage point from which to analyze and define society. No longer are women an "other" knocking at the door to be let into the society. Women now have gone beyond this point, reaching a stage where they no longer want to integrate themselves into "men's world" so much as to reshape the world, make it something better. From "outside" we are in an advantaged position to do just this: we can understand and interpret the system we are distanced from more clearly than those can at its center.

Women wish to redesign the emotional contract. Women say that subtle but extremely painful (and powerful) forms of discrimination are still built into the very structure of relationships.

The purpose here is to build a new framework for understanding these dynamics, understanding "who women are" instead of blaming women for being "masochists" or "hooked on love."

By their responses in this study women paint a picture of widespread gender stereotyping as well as a pattern of condescension from men they love. They are debating inside themselves what to do about this. The dynamics of this situation in personal life have been only cloudily seen up to now, perhaps for lack of the kind of documentation provided here. This documentation is an indictment of the traditional gender system, with its unfair emotional "contract." That contract (the still-not-eradicated psychological counterpart of the centuries-long legal domination

---

* The "feminization of poverty" is a phenomenon that has been misinterpreted; it may be caused not so much by men leaving women as by women choosing (now that they have an alternative) to be on their own, even if they have to be poor. A large number of women are refusing to stay in bad situations any longer.

of women by men) has exploited women emotionally (not even acknowledging that it is doing so), for example by using words designed long ago, such as insisting that women who "complain" have "complexes," as opposed to real problems created by a real social ideology that is negative to women. There is not "something wrong" with women. Women don't have a "problem," or a "bad attitude." There is, however, a problem with the attitudes of the social order toward women as a class.

Women now are engaged in profound active questioning about how they can go on living with this situation, what to do about it. Their personal choices seem to be to leave the relationship/marriage, to keep struggling to "get him to see," or to become less emotionally involved.

Must women have different beliefs from those held by men about what a relationship should be; must women operate by different premises and define their priorities differently? Most women believe in behaviors such as empathetic listening, trying to understand, being emotionally supportive, but they believe that men seem rather to think of a relationship in terms of "being there." Though both women and men agree that physical affection is a number-one priority, in most other ways their value systems differ. Another difference: most women note that men do not connect sex with love the way women want to.

The problem is that many men have a standard for their behavior with women that differs from their behavior with the rest of society—they operate on a double standard. Since women are "less" or "other," many men unconsciously believe that the rules are different for them. And as the pattern of men's unwitting gestures of inequality, followed by women's "bringing up the issues,"—which are often greeted with gender-stereotyped remarks—continues, women may become increasingly dissatisfied and begin to disrespect men, since it is difficult to respect someone who is unfair.

### A CULTURAL DIVIDE[5]

There is no need to posit a biological difference between "male" and "female" "human nature" to explain the two different value systems defined by women and men in my research; nor does the existence of two cultures in any way prove that they are inevitable or a product of "nature."* In fact, they are historical: two separate historical traditions that have grown up over centuries, thus giving hope that they can be resolved within a new framework. This work takes the point of view that much of how we behave is learned, including our supposedly biological gender traits.

How the transformation will be made to a new world-view, interpreting both "cultures," is one of the major questions of our time.

---

* More recent self-help books, such as *Women Are from Venus, Men Are from Mars*, stated or implied that gender differences cannot be changed. This work takes the opposite view.

## CHALLENGING THE "BIOLOGICAL DIFFERENCE" BELIEF*

As Rex Harrison sings in *My Fair Lady*, "Why can't a woman be more like a man?" So we might ask, "Why can't a man be more like a woman?"

Men, it seems, don't want to be "like women," who are considered inferior, "sissies." The general presumption is that women, to "gain equality," should try to learn from men, drop their "old values" and become more "like men."

The emotional contract reflects the general presumption of men's psychological superiority. Men have the edge in psychological power and status in relationships, just as they have higher status in the outside "work" world. Men are seen by the society as somehow more "legitimate" and psychologically "right." Men's opinions and actions are given more credibility than women's, which are more likely to be criticized or scrutinized. In other words, the culture considers whatever men do the "norm," a somehow unquestionable "reality," while seeing what women do as a "role," with inferior characteristics.

The reality is that both systems have important values—there is not one "reality" and another group of people who need to stop thinking the way they do and get in touch with "reality." The "female" system of values—belief in nurturing and putting relationships first in life—has been providing most of the love and emotional support the "male system" has been running on.

The "men are the reality, women are the role" view holds that a woman without role training (or, for some, hormones) would just "naturally" be like a man. But this contains the assumption that men are not laced with role training, and that their beliefs and behavior patterns are not just as much culturally or historically fabricated as women's. And even for many of those who agree that men's behaviors might be culturally produced or exaggerated, the assumption is still that men's characteristics are superior. But men's "psychology" or value system is just as much arbitrarily fashioned as "women's," through "role indoctrination." Men's way of life is not "natural" or somehow the bottom line of "reality" for measuring the behavior of the whole world. In fact, now, if we want to invigorate our system, we may well have to reassess what it is that our culture and political tradition are all about, what they stand for, and whether we are being true to the best parts of them.

## MEN'S VIEW OF LOVE

Let's look at this from men's point of view. How do men feel about love?

In research for *The Hite Report on Men and Male Sexuality*, it emerged that most

---

* This is true even in language, where "man" stands for "men and women" in many "humanistic" book titles and television "educational" programs; and where "he" is the "correct" pronoun to use when discussing behavior in the abstract. All this has been shown to have a profound effect on kindergarten girls and boys. It also has a profound effect on personal relationships between women and men.

men do not marry the women they most passionately love, and they are proud of this. How did they come to feel this way?

## THE SEXUALIZATION OF BOYS AND MALE ALIENATION[*]

It is the ideology that tells boys that a boy becomes a man when he first "has" a woman—that is, has intercourse/penetrates a woman—and that a man stays more of a man the more often he continues to do so. Other aspects of this credo include "The more sex, the better," "Shopping around is natural," "nature made men to disseminate their semen to the widest possible sample" (as in *The King and I*: "Bee must go from blossom to blossom"). The corollary to this kind of attitude (wherein "getting some"—that is, penetration—is still "scoring," "getting it over on so-and-so," "having her") is the idea that all women "want a man," need to "catch a man," "trap one" into marriage. So there is a built-in, never acknowledged game going on: he is trying to "get some," she is trying to "get him to care"—and he flees as if "caring" were a fate worse than death.

The psychology men have inherited from a culture obsessed with glorifying aggressive warriorlike masculinity tends to see sex as a simple biological act necessary for reproduction. Men have put an enormous amount of pressure on women to have "sex." For the most part, women find this pressure and this philosophy mechanical and insensitive, making erotic and sensual interaction almost impossible. Men have called women who say "no" to sex when there are no feelings involved "hung-up" or "Victorian" (1960s) or "anti-male," "manhaters" (1970s and 1980s).

Rather than seeing women's philosophy as just as valid as their own—a debate between two equal, differing cultural perspectives, requiring thought and analysis—many men ridicule women's point of view as nonsense.

## ADAM AND EVE AS EARLY GENDER-ROLE PROPAGANDA

Why does our society make such an extreme fetish of gender division? Many theorists have pointed to the obvious: that only through controlling women's sexuality and reproduction can men ensure that inheritance passes through them and thus maintain a male-dominated society. Without strict rules and regulations regarding gender behavior (especially for women), men could not be sure that the children women were bearing were their own, claim them as their legal property, have rights over them. This is why such continuous cultural reinforcement of "what sex is" is necessary. (Is it possible that gender division has not always been the fundamental principle of society, or that the genders were not always defined in the ways they are now?)

But there is another way of looking at the Adam and Eve story. Could it be that one of its messages—a message now unseen, but clear to those of early times—was

---

[*] See also Part 2.

to focus attention on gender division as the fundamental principle of a new social order and to establish the basic "personality traits" of these two "original beings" as the prototypes for future society? These personality traits may not have been standard for the two genders at that time. Certainly Adam and Eve are the earliest symbols known of reproduction, "sin" and the double standard toward women.*

Symbols and pictures of Adam and Eve continue to be used in advertising and design, appearing constantly all around us, reminding us of Eve's "wickedness," of the fact that she caused our "downfall," that her curiosity led to humanity being expelled from the Garden of Eden. Women were supposedly responsible for "original sin," and even today we are still reminded of our "basic natures"—thus making us try even harder to be "good," to show that we are "trustworthy," so as to be accepted by the society and loved. It is no surprise that something as old in Western tradition, in patriarchal tradition, as the dichotomy between "bad" women and "good" women[6] has not been ended by the mere twenty years of women's changing. Or even by the last hundred years since the end of women's legal ownership by husbands and fathers, since the dichotomy—and there is, of course, no such dichotomy for men—has ancient roots in the foundations of our culture.

## FUNDAMENTALIST RELIGIOUS VIEWS: THE MAN-ON-TOP STRUCTURE IN SOCIETY

There are two sides to the double standard: the playboy version—"all women are for sex, let's take them"; and the religious version—"all women should be in the home, mothers."

Has the religious revival movement made any change in the widespread male acceptance of the double standard? Not really. The movement puts great pressure on women to "realize their natural desire for children, to be mothers," and to put the needs of the children and family/father first. Women who are not married or mothers are considered "wrong or "unfulfilled," more so than men who do not have children.

While it certainly does not endorse the "playboy" mentality, the "born again" movement has produced very little propaganda exhorting boys not to see girls either as "targets" from which to get sex or as "mothers"—that is, service people—especially compared to the amount of propaganda directed at women to say "no," and stressing the values of motherhood and subordination to one's family. And most parts of the revivalist religious movement also clearly state that although husband and wife are a team, in the final analysis the man must lead—in traditional, patriarchal fashion. As Jerry Falwell put it in 1986 on television, "The man is the spiritual fountainhead of the family—the leader." In other words,

---

* Other creation stories,with some similar themes, are found in surrounding cultures around 3000 BC such as in Sumerian texts; some may be older.

the "good old days" are simply the old, unequal, oppressed days women have been struggling to escape.*

Fundamentalist movements worldwide do not challenge the double standard but tend to reinforce it. It is no surprise that much of the conservative religious movement's backbone is made up of women or that it is driven largely by women's energy—women's donated office work, organizing abilities, church attendance, fund-raising activities—since women often feel that they at least have a clear place and role in this urban system. Many women like the church because it supports them in their struggle to continue the home-family value system—as long as they stay in the home (or at most combine home with career only after their children are in school) and do not challenge that system or double standard.

## MEN AND LOVE

What is behind the "male" system that makes men emotionally distant—at the same time that it makes them need love desperately, precisely because of this emotional isolation, because they are so cut off from their feelings? Many men are wracked and torn over how to relate to the women they love, in deep anguish over their personal lives and love relationships.

Obviously men want love; they look to women for love and are angry if women are not "loving"; most men are married by the age of twenty-seven. Rarely are men the ones to bring up divorce. Men want a home and warmth, but they also have ambiguous feelings; real closeness is a threatening state of emotionality that most can't afford. Men learn that a "real man" never completely lets his guard down or loses control of a situation. A man must continually assert his "independence" or "dominance." Real closeness is forbidden to men because it makes them vulnerable.

It is often said, "It's the mothers' fault if men are macho—they bring up boys that way." But this remark is simplistic, not really to the point; after all fathers, by the example of not being home, or by their emotional distance when home, also "bring up the boys." The real problem is the ideology with which we live, the entire system which teaches men that to be "real men" they must follow "male" codes, other male examples—not create their own way.

The basic tenets of the "male ideology"† are only beginning to be understood, since for many centuries male behavior and personality and male-designed religious and

---

* Of course not all men agree with the playboy game plan regarding sex, or with the religious revival movement's version of the proper way of life for women; there is a vigorous minority of men of every political persuasion who do not see themselves either in the men-are-beasts-who-want-women's-bodies idea of who men are, or in the men-marry-mothers-only school of thought.

† It is important to point out that the "male ideology" referred to here is not something a man is automatically part of just because he is anatomically male. The "male" we refer to in the phrase "male ideology" is cultural: men who adopt the cultural style of masculinity as domination.

state systems were thought to grow out of "biology or nature," rather than being part of a belief structure that one could stand back from and analyze.

## HOW IS IT LEARNED?

One of the earliest and still repeated stories by which a system of unquestioning obedience to authority is explained to Jews, Christians, and Muslims—by which it is ordained that one must not put personal feelings of love before duty and obedience to the rules of this hierarchy—is the biblical tale of Abraham taking his son Isaac up the mountain, where God has commanded that Abraham "sacrifice" him, with no explanation given. The message is: obey and don't ask questions. As a reward for their obedience to this hierarchy men in other parts of the scriptures are promised rulership over women, children, and "nature"; women are told, "Wives, be obedient to your husbands."

Even today men are assumed in one "nature" special after another on television, and in many biological textbooks, to have a "natural" tendency (right?) to be "dominant," to rule—as part of a "natural instinct." The assumption that men are stronger and more important than women, that they have more right to be "in charge," that their thoughts are more "rational," "clear," and "objective," underlies much of the culture. In other words, the "male" ideology is still all around us and still tells men that if they follow the expected patterns of behavior of the system—if they show "loyalty"—then they will have all the "natural" rights of men to be dominant over women, children, and the planet. Thus the concept of "male pride."

The conceptualization of democratic government, as its ideas were developed during the Enlightenment and the French and American Revolutions, was in part a reaction against this hierarchical view of unthinking obedience to a ruler who was king because of his lineage and "the right of God." Men would no longer be told what they should do; now all men were thought "educable," able to think for themselves. Still, this new system of equal rights and dignity for "all" was only for men, not women (who could not vote or hold office, and the like).

## MEN ARE BLACKMAILED INTO OBEDIENCE TO THE SYSTEM

According to the "male" ideology, hierarchy and fighting for "dominance" are part of "nature"; therefore there can be no such thing as equality—"someone has to be on top." For this reason the very idea of equality with women is interpreted by many men to mean a challenge to their "dominance." A man should "keep a woman in line," keep her from her propensity to try to "run things." It is a mental construct that sees women as "the Other."*

Surely Thomas Paine in the eighteenth century could not have had in mind the propping up of the modern "macho" personality when he exalted the "Rights of

---

* The famous phrase and theory of Simone de Beauvoir.

Man." And yet this "democratic" language is being used today to support some men's insistence on being dominant. Today "freedom" in the "male" code means that a "real" man should be "independent," should not be "told what to do"—especially by a female.

But if women want equality, they have to challenge male dominance, and have to do so daily. For men who do not believe that there is such a thing as equality (since in a hierarchy someone has to be "on top"), it seems that what women are "demanding" is "dominance" or "power." And if men cannot understand equality, perhaps women in frustration will have to wind up trying to be "dominant."

The "male" ideology, based on dominance, and the "female" belief in love and nurturing thus create a tragic pattern conflicting in many individual lives. The man may become "full of his right," or condescending (even unconsciously), while a woman is trying to "talk," understand, explain, draw the man out and "demand equality"—somehow "make it all work." Often the sexes remain locked in this struggle throughout the relationship, at an unclear, basically undefined, and therefore inescapable impasse.

Many men are confused when they fall in love. My research shows that the majority of men do not marry the women that they most passionately love or desire—and that they are in fact proud of this, proud of themselves for "maintaining control." In *The Hite Report on Men and Male Sexuality*, many men report surprise and emotional confusion when (usually in their teens or twenties) they do fall in love. Many picture a really "masculine" man as being in control of his emotions (and being in love is the opposite), rational and "objective" above all else. Thus men may feel uncomfortable being "in love." There is an inherent contradiction for most men between staying in control of their feelings and loving another person, which they fear may make them "weak," "soft," and vulnerable. Although men often enjoy being "in love" temporarily, basically many are uncomfortable and say that the sooner their less rational feelings are "gotten rid of," the better.

Men's ambivalence about love involves not only a desire for "freedom" but also grows out of a fear of their own feelings flooding over them—a fear that is often reinforced by parental injunction. Boys are often advised by their fathers (or even mothers): "Don't marry the first girl who comes along just because of your sexual feelings. Others will come along later. Don't let your feelings carry you away," implying that it's "just sex," that a boy may find that his first sexual feelings will make him think he is in love. (Isn't he?)

In other words, if a "real" man should be a tough, rugged, independent loner (like the Marlboro man), how can a man accept a relationship or marriage without feeling split? If a man "should" be independent, but is not (in fact, is married, in love, or in a relationship), how can he not feel constantly torn between his feelings of love for his wife/lover and his concern that he should be asserting, as a "man," his independence? He may see the relationship as a constant test or threat. As one woman puts it, "Most single men appear to have deep fears about loving women.

They fear that loving is not 'macho.' They can let a woman love them, but try to keep their own feelings in check, hold back. It's a wonder they don't all get sick more than they already do."

For these reasons the deepest love a man feels for a woman can also bring out his deepest hate or fear, because his love is threatening to his ideal of autonomy. Perhaps he doesn't want to feel that connectedness, even if it feels good. A man may feel very conflicted if he interprets his feelings as dependency, neediness—even "weakness."

The system can trap a man, tragically, in a kind of permanent isolation and aloneness while seeming to offer "dominance," claiming that their alternative is not equality but "submission" but they must hold back their feelings, keep their emotional lives in check. Yet some men decide to go against this system and follow a way of life that feels right to them.

## TWO CULTURES: WOMEN LIVE BI-CULTURALLY

Are women psychologically different from men? What are the values of "women's" culture?

> *When I'm in love, I feel like I'm part of them—and they're part of me.*
> *If they're upset about something or if I do something they're upset about,*
> *it bothers me terribly until we can talk about it and resolve it.*

Women's philosophy (subculture) does seem to exist; it has been forged over the centuries by women's personal thoughts, by their discussions with other women about their relationships, by families, and by inner feelings of love—and by their practical experience of what it takes to make a family function. Its values include working with others (rather than emphasizing competition), valuing friendship, listening with empathy, not being judgmental, trying to bring out the best in others, nurturing, not dominating. Though some people believe that "the difference"comes from women's having a womb and eggs (female hormones?), here we are arguing that culture has created what by now is an identifiable psychology.

One woman describes the qualities in women's weltanschauung—way of looking at life—that she admires:

> *I admire the quiet work of women, their defense of interpersonal*
> *peace—doing decent things when they don't get much credit for doing*
> *anything. I want to see women move into the world and rebuild the*
> *bridge between private spheres and public works, which was destroyed*
> *by industrialization. How about the hundreds of women going to grad-*
> *uate school in chemistry? Right on! I'd like to see private morality*
> *extended to the earth; I hope that women retain some of the knowledge*

*they gained raising children and shoring up civilized human relationships when they are out in the dogfight.*

Another describes the qualities in her sister that make her feel close:

*The closest I feel to anyone is my sister—she's who I turn to in time of trouble. She doesn't try to solve my problems, just helps me sort them out and solve them myself. There is nothing I can't share with her, nor she with me. I feel good when we're together. I like best her total lack of making judgments about anyone or anything and the fact that she'll listen to anything I want to talk about.*

And one woman says what almost all women say: how much easier it is to talk to other women:

*I am nineteen, white, a college student in Des Moines, Iowa. I am creative, angry, sensual, intelligent, and a great cook. I value love, respect, gentleness. Right now there are two people that I am closest to, one a woman, and one a man. The man is my lover, and although I am living with him and try to talk to him about everything, he doesn't understand some things very well. The woman is my best friend, and we talk about everything.*

When asked what women contribute to the world, most women say that women are givers, that women take care of humanity:

*What things about women do I admire? Their marvelous humanity, their genuine caring about people, their nurturing, sharing, generosity, willingness to give of themselves.*

### DOES THIS MEAN THAT WOMEN ARE "BETTER"?

By stressing the positive, nurturing qualities that women believe in, and that they wish men to consider taking on, are we falling into the trap of saying that women's moral sense is superior to men's? No, we are not saying that women are, or have been, perfect, "saints" who love everyone, without a vicious bone in their bodies.

Although we are not saying that women are inherently "better" than men, women do have a right to be proud of their values and their philosophy—which they have worked very hard to refine. In this study women are seen as subscribing to a belief in the importance of caring about the feelings of others, a philosophical system based on the primacy of human relationships and cooperation. This system is not dissimilar to the one revealed in psychologist Carol Gilligan's study, *In a Different Voice*, in which attachment and bonding emerge as the basis of women's moral sense. Women should be respected for this system, not put on the defensive.

Women have worked out their philosophy in the area of love and family relationships because this has been the traditional area of women' s primary concern: if men have been urged to go out and succeed in the world, women have been urged to succeed in personal relationships and having a family. Women's speculations are no less dense or profound because they are focused on love or relationships instead of on "abstract" discussions of "politics." The moral and strategic issues are essentially the same.

## WOMEN'S DEEPER QUESTIONS

Women's thinking about relationships is leading women to ask deeper questions about the nature of society.

Women at this time in history are engaging in a very complex debate over whether or not they will continue to define love as their primary role in their lives in the future, whether they should stop being "overly concerned" with men and love, and whether to see the rest of life as more important.

Women are under great pressure to give up their traditional values and not be "overly focused on love." But after the attempts of the last ten to twenty years for women to "have sex like men" (not connect sex to emotions or a "relationship") and to "feel less," "love less," most women are not finding these new ways of life satisfying. Most women feel that they cannot live this way and maintain their own integrity, be true to themselves.

As women run up against the male gender system time and time again in their relationships, trying to break through, make real contact, they begin to ask themselves deeper questions about the system and why men behave as they do. In other words, the pain in their personal lives with men they love leads many women to think about why love is so difficult—and then to ask themselves a whole spectrum of other questions.*

Trying to figure out relationships, women often start by questioning themselves, asking themselves if they are doing anything wrong; then they may try to figure out the psychological make-up of the men in their lives—a man's individual psychological background. This effort often leads a woman to look at the structure of her lover's family, his parents' relationship, and finally the overall social structure, the

---

* Women's rethinking now is going on at the same time as when women are also drastically changing their economic situation. Within the last ten years, the number of women taking jobs and starting businesses has escalated so rapidly that in fact women as a group are no longer essentially dependent on men; although most women still have relatively low salaries (and day care is expensive), more women than ever have enough resources to make it on their own, even if only minimally. The consequences of this large-scale change will obviously be enormous and are as yet only in the beginning stages.

whole system and how it got that way. Asking themselves so many questions leads women to think deeply about the whole culture.

## "FAMILY VALUES": COULD THE "FEMALE" OR "LOVE" VALUE SYSTEM— THE "FAMILY VALUES" SYSTEM—DISAPPEAR?

If women give up love as a basic value (since women have carried the "home" or "love" value system more than men have), will love/family disappear as a way of life? Millions of women are now waging an inner struggle to decide whether they should do just that, motivated by the constant attack on and ridicule of "women's values," plus the fact that continuing these loving patterns, being "givers," doesn't "get them anywhere." Most media since the 1960s have been urging women to stop being so "feminine," to get "smart," be more aggressive, be more like men. If they were to do so, the change could mean the complete victory of the "male" ideology. But will men like this victory? Will it be good for the society—or will life become harsher, more unfriendly, and the world a less hospitable place? Should "women's values" become more prevalent, more, not less influential?

Will women somehow manage to keep their tradition of nurturing and warmth alive, even "underground," as a secondary culture, and thus live biculturally: acting one way when they go to work and another at home? Or will the set of values women have carried for so long be lost?

## SEEING THE WORLD THROUGH NEW EYES: THE "OTHER" TRANSFORMED

Some women are beginning to identify a new choice. The choice is not simply between taking on "male" values and keeping "female" values. A third choice is for women to keep their own value system of believing in caring and nurturing as a way of life, but to change its focus. Many women now question whether the best, the most important, expression of their loving and giving is "being there" for a man.

Some women, while keeping their belief in love, are diversifying it, shifting its focus away from individual men who don't see them as equals, and applying its emotional strength to a whole spectrum of relationships, work, and politics.

## FRIENDSHIPS BETWEEN WOMEN: A POTENTIAL MODEL FOR MALE-FEMALE RELATIONSHIPS?

Women describe their friendships with other women as some of the happiest, most fulfilling parts of their lives; 87 percent of married women have their deepest emotional relationship with a woman friend, as do 95 percent of single women. These relationships are extremely important—a frequently "unseen" backdrop to women's lives that is solidly "there" for them. Women rely on each other in moments of crisis or just for daily emotional nourishment and fun. They are alternately children, mothers, sisters, and pals to each other. There are moments of letdown, even betrayal, but despite these, women consider their friendships to be as important as love relationships with men.

In my research, covering women of all ages, 94 percent speak of very close and important friendships with other women:

> I have lots of wonderful women friends. After I broke up with Dave, I threw a "Girls' Club Party" for girls only, with champagne, pastries, and all kinds of beauty aids—facials, henna, manicures, everything. It was to thank all the great girls in the world.

> Women are the most important people in my life. My close relationships with women have kept me going where all else failed.

> Knowing her helped me find myself.

> I think close friendships turn you into a higher being. You want to excel, develop higher expectations of yourself. The worst thing that somebody can do to me is not to give me credit for what I can do (be nonsupportive). That is something that my close friends never do.

Women's descriptions of their friends brim over with warmth, admiration, and affection; the overwhelming majority of women when they describe their friends express feelings of great enthusiasm and happiness:

> We do a lot of talking and laughing. I like her honesty, and sense of the humor and irony of life. She's non-judgmental. She has helped me through difficult times, just by being there for me to talk to, by listening and caring. With her, I feel like myself. I have an identity that feels right.

> My best friend listens but does not condemn, accepts me as I am. Usually what we do together is meet for lunch or dinner, drinks, talk for hours at her house or mine. I feel her presence, comfort without words, total understanding even if I don't understand, miss her when we don't get together.

> She is my age, we are in an all-women's college. She is very supportive and a very good listener—not at all selfish, very funny and attractive. We go out for coffee, just sit and talk—or we choose some really different place to go and just do it. She is very spontaneous, and we share a lot of laughs. I always feel thrilled to see her—of all of my friends, I love and respect her the most and no matter what different paths we take—we always have things to say to each other.

*My best woman friend is someone who I know would operate in my best
interests, and support my point of view in my absence. Together we enjoy
everyday life, talking, mostly, or rehashing our views as to the nature of
this existence. We have made a pact that regardless of whether we are in
a relationship with a man, we will always have time for each other.*

*We have been friends for thirteen years. She's smart, but not academically
educated. She knows me like a book, I can never fool her. She makes me
aware of things about myself I don't even realize, she makes me think
but won't solve my problems for me. When we are together we talk for
hours. When we are together for the first time after a long while, I feel like
there is a strong bond between us, yet there are also many things that
have changed.*

*My best woman friend is vivacious, talented, humorous, full of energy,
insightful, aggressive, and interested in my well-being. We see each other
less now that she has a baby, but we still make a point of talking several
times a week.*

*She's helped me through many crises and is the first person I turn to for
support and/or advice. She is the woman I've loved the most. When we
spend time together, I usually hang out at her home so we can enjoy all
our kids together (she has four daughters). We also make a point to spend
time alone, without kids—we'll take a day and just take off—go out for
lunch, shop a little, walk around town checking out art shops and talking—mostly talking. That's what's best about it. We're able to talk about
anything and everything.*

*We have been friends for twenty-nine years. She is the mother of two
daughters and stepmother to two more, plus she has a career (finance).
She progressed from being just another paper pusher to being head of
her department. What I like most about her is her willingness to listen
when others talk. Although she has her own opinions, she hears the other
person out first, before offering her viewpoint.*

### WHY ARE WOMEN HAPPY WITH THEIR WOMEN FRIENDS?

As many as 92 percent of women state that it is easier to talk to other women than
to most men:

*We always know what the other one is feeling.*

*Women feel a common bond for each other and relate better to each other's problems. My husband takes everything like a personal threat, I couldn't tell him anything I tell my best friend.*

*It is easier to talk to women than to men. On the whole, women understand more, can relate more, and aren't squeamish about details. We offer help to each other because we can talk more easily, and the encouragement often makes us stronger individuals. We care more and love more, and aren't afraid to show it. Men can be good friends too, but they just don't seem to understand the human side of feelings by putting themselves in the other person's shoes like women do. I think the statement is both sad and true. It's healthy to have a close female friend that one can talk to about anything, but your husband should be your best friend too, someone you can share anything with. It seems those couples whose marriages last and are happy are the ones who are each other's best friends.*

*I find it easier to talk to women because men hide behind logic when an emotional response is what is needed. We all need someone to laugh with us, feel happy with us, and cry with us. If I could talk to my husband and he to me as my best friend does, we would have a super-hot thing.*

*The thing I like best about Jane is that I can talk to her about absolutely anything under the sun. Nothing shocks or surprises her. Jane's listened to me talk through tons of difficult times, fights with my folks, my sequestration from Keith—his stay in the hospital. I've helped her think through a long-drawn-out divorce, her relationship (now two years old) with her subsequent lover, and the recent death of her father. We always have a good time when we're together. We're free to be ourselves no matter how good or bad we may feel, and then all of our problems don't seem so bad.*

Women have developed among themselves a way of relating that makes it possible to share intricate inner thoughts and a large repertoire of feelings. In most cases how women talk together is different from the way women and men talk together. Women have a communication that is more detailed, more involved in searching out, listening for, and hearing the other's inner thoughts—working together to explore the feelings one is trying to express.

Over and over women say that their friendships with other women are more open and spontaneous, that it is easier to talk, that women are rarely judgmental, are good at listening and giving feedback, and that these circumstances are helpful.

Women are each other's basic support systems, whether they are single or married. Throughout their work, their achievements, their major decisions, difficult times, and changing relationships, women are being cheered on, encouraged and believed in by their friends.

Here the dynamics of women's caring and giving work to women's advantage; women do not wind up feeling drained, since the support is mutual. The giving is not taken advantage of, considered "soft" or "weak." The idea of any given conversation is to understand and help draw out the other person, not (as in some "male" interpersonal patterns) to "judge," decide if the other person is "right," or win the point. Most women are more receptive and give more "acknowledging" feedback: "I heard you and understand what you are saying."

Most men, as they explained in *The Hite Report on Men and Male Sexuality*, turn to women as friends when they need someone to talk to, not to men; 93 percent of men in *The Hite Report* stated that after they leave school they do not have a close male friend; 89 percent of those over the age of twenty-five note that their best friend is a woman or, in fact, their wife. Men rarely turn to other men for close friendship—to talk. This situation clearly indicates that where both women and men want a close companion, women's way of relating is preferred.

Why, then, is so much fun made of women's talking with their friends? Why are women put on the defensive, their conversations referred to as "gabbing away" and "girl talk"? This is merely the dominant ideology, proclaiming itself superior—when in fact the dominant ideology relies on this very talk and enthusiasm from women, counting on women to be nonaggressive, "loving," and caring—to give emotional support.

Women believe that listening and supporting the other person is one of the basic ways in which love is shown; they feel it is inappropriate to be competitive, distant, or not tuned in emotionally in a personal relationship. Many women have developed skills in observing and tuning in to the inner thoughts, wavelengths, of others. This skill is one of the great cultural resources of our society. However, this skill can be very dangerous for women individually when used in a nonequal relationship, the man "starring" in the relationship, with the woman as the non-listened-to supporting cast.

Women say their friendships with each other do not leave them feeling drained, as do many of women's relationships with men. Women's ideology works well when it is in contact with other women because, while women's "giving" is met in many men with a "men have the right to take" attitude, in a relationship with another woman the two "givings" work to mutual advantage. In other words, "giving" to other women works because most women are "giving" back.

This process can serve as a new model for men's relationships with women.

## THE STATE OF MARRIAGE TODAY

### WHAT KINDS OF LOVE DO WOMEN FEEL IN MARRIAGE?
### WHICH KIND OF LOVE WORKS BEST IN MARRIAGE?

A classic question women and men have had to contemplate is whether they want to—or can—marry someone with whom they are "in love." They may think it better to choose someone who seems to provide safe, stable companionship with less volatility, less of the vulnerability they may feel with someone with whom they are "in love."

Surprisingly there have been no large-scale studies attempting statistically to correlate types of love with the success or failure of marriages and relationships, as we will try to do here.

Women often debate with themselves the meanings of these feelings: most women—as opposed to men, who often don't even like feeling "in love," because they feel "out of control"—do like being in love but have also found it painful:

> *Being in love to me is thrilling, exciting, it's magic—but it can also turn your life upside down, and put you in a confused state of mind. It can be extremely painful and heartbreaking. I don't regret ever having been in love—but who would want to live with it???*

Women do not generally pride themselves on their "rationality" and "objectivity" in making their choice of marriage partner. For men, however, it is often a matter of pride not to have picked someone with whom they were "in love" for marriage, since, according to men, the decision for marriage should be based on more "rational," "objective" considerations.

What is "falling in love"? In fact, 82 percent of the women in this study are asking themselves why they are in the relationships they are in, what kind of love it is they feel—whether it is the "right" kind.

When women think about getting married, or when a marriage or relationship isn't going well, they wonder if it is their fault. On the one hand, if they are in an "in-love" relationship, they can perhaps think that they are "messed up," not being "rational" and "mature"; on the other hand, if they are in a "reasonable," low-key relationship, but "still not satisfied," they may blame themselves for wanting "security" too much, being "too dependent."

Are the assumptions about what kind of love works in relationships accurate? One theory holds that falling "in love" is "unreal," one is merely "projecting" onto the other person; that the only "real love" is getting to know a person over time. Others believe that a more low-key or steady love is not love at all but merely "taking care of" someone, a security-oriented definition of love, formulated to prove that one can "make a relationship work."[7]

According to the first theory, falling in love does not work for long-term relationships because it is "juvenile" (the two people don't really "know" one another, and therefore mature love is not possible). And yet just the opposite case could be made—that the relationship does not work because the two people care too much, and so their feelings are too easily wounded, and this is what creates the tension, leading to flare-ups and explosions. On the other hand, countering this argument, it could be said that while it is true that passionate "infatuation" makes people susceptible to easily hurt feelings, it also makes them care about overcoming lapses in communication and makes them want to try to scale any barriers to reach each other.

If the intense feelings of first love are transitory, why is this so?

Most of the women in this study do not marry the men they have most deeply loved. This was also true of men in *The Hite Report on Men and Male Sexuality*: most men did not marry the women they had most passionately loved. Women, as seen here, hope that by avoiding the highs and lows of being "in love," they can make a relationship more secure, if not inspired, and a better setting for living and raising children.

The assumption that "in love" marriages don't last and that more low-key love relationships are more stable and do last has no basis in statistical fact, as demonstrated here. Further, in marriages that do last, there still remains the question of level of happiness or fulfillment within the marriage. As we have seen, even a quiet love, a supposed "safe haven," can turn out to be filled with negativity or arguments. While the turbulence associated with being "in love" can be difficult, more low-key "loving" marriages can also fail. They contain the same unequal emotional contract, which is condescending to women, harasses women while also expecting them to provide love and emotional support. Low-key love, some say, can at times lead to a kind of emotional death.

In other words, the supposition that if contentment replaces passion, the marriage will be more stable is not borne out by the research of this study. Most women report that their marriages are not based on being passionately in love, and yet their satisfaction levels remain low. Therefore it is logically impossible to say that passion is the cause of instability in relationships.

This study shows that the dynamics that kill love basically involve inequalities in the emotional contract. The "emotional contract" itself must be changed before relationships can be stable and happy—whether based on "loving" or being "in love."

Statistically, in this study, marriages and relationships seem most likely to break up when the man refuses to discuss issues and problems that the woman finds important, and this situation goes on over a period of time, so that alienation grows. As the emotional distance widens, most women restructure the emotional relationship inside the marriage and the nature of their feelings. We do not know, for the most part, how relationships (whether "in love" or "loving") would fare without the interference of the unequal emotional contract.

## DEMOCRATIZING THE FAMILY: NEW EMOTIONAL ARRANGEMENTS WITHIN MARRIAGE

There are myriad emotional arrangements within marriages, but three basic models of psychological arrangements emerge from this research: (1) the emotional-intimacy model (most women say that they would prefer this type, if they could achieve more equality and closeness with their husbands); (2) the "home base" model, working on the level of "being there"; and (3) the teamwork model, in which the partners actually work together and their work/business is the focus of their life together.

In other words, first, there is the marriage in which intimacy, emotional and psychological, is the primary goal. This is the emotional arrangement most women are trying to get their husbands to adopt—and the way of life most women would prefer.

Then there is the marriage that provides a "home base" for the rest of one's life: "being there" is all that is really required. The traditional marriage, still so prevalent, is not the same as the new "home base" marriage because in the traditional arrangement the woman is providing a stable base for the husband and children to go out from and live their lives, but the woman herself has little room or time for her own life; the marriage is not a stable base for her; she is the home base for others. It is not a backdrop for her life, it is her life. In the "home-base" marriage, the emotional contract remains intact, with male distancing and harassment of women continuing—but usually the woman doesn't care so much anymore, as she has placed her primary emotional interest elsewhere.

Finally, one woman describes the team concept of marriage:

> Last winter we had saved up enough money so that we had the freedom to concentrate on our own work without having to worry about money. We worked in the studio until very early hours. Working together, with our dreams, free to use our true abilities, was wonderful.

Other women are starting small businesses with their husbands, or partners, and these team marriages are very exciting.

## HOME: LONGING FOR LOVE

What is home? Where is it? How many people have at one time or another found themselves standing in the middle of their own living rooms, being unhappy, shouting, "I want to go home!"? And how many people living in apartments instead of houses, feel, "This is not really a home, this is an apartment"? Shouldn't a "home" be physically permanent? Now at the end of the twentieth century, it is rarely permanent: we move frequently.

Much as we try, and much as statistics tell us that the stable-for-a-lifetime nuclear family is not the "norm" anymore, something in us still feels that we want "it"—and that we have failed, we are "wrong" if we do not "make it work," have that particular home. And yet, as we have seen, many women inside that kind of "home" do not always feel nourished or cared for—or even connected. Many feel tremendously lonely and angry. And men, as seen in *The Hite Report on Men and Male Sexuality*, are often angry too.

We need a new concept for the basic structure we call "home." What is our social philosophy, the overall purpose of the home? Economic production? Stable "families"? To provide a place guaranteeing the individual's right to a search after meaning, or the "pursuit of happiness"?

It is clear that women's inner questioning is part of large cultural change—one that women are playing a central role in, as those offering another perspective, alternative possible solutions to current problems. As women think through their personal lives, as they try to understand them and the men they love, they are critiquing this world and envisioning a new one. Women are going through a revolution, and they are taking the culture with them.

### A CULTURAL REVOLUTION IN PROGRESS: IF WOMEN REDEFINE "LOVE..."

Women's reevaluation of themselves and of the culture is part of a process that has been going on for some time, for over a century.* During the last twenty years this change, which could be called a revolution in women's definition of themselves and of society, has been occurring in stages.† Stage one began with women "demanding equal rights." Stage two was women trying to take a place in, join, the "male" world. And stage three, now, is women consolidating their own value system, examining and discussing the society as we know it, accepting some values of the dominant culture, discarding others—leading to the cultural struggle currently in progress.

The stage of women "demanding equal rights" was superseded by the current stage, which shows that women have attained more self-confidence. Women, as we have seen, are under great pressure to give up their traditional (even if newly redefined) values and take on "male" values (such as giving up relating sex to love). But many women feel they cannot do this and be true to their own beliefs. Women, realizing that they want to stand on their own principles, are now sifting through these principles to come up with those they want to live by and apply to the culture.

How has this happened? Women's reexamination began with "equal rights" but

---

* There have been, of course, "feminist movements" in earlier centuries as well. For example, the feminist tradition in France has been traced back five centuries to Christine de Pisan, a French writer who defended women in the 1500s. See Joan Kelly's Women, *History and Theory* (Chicago: University of Chicago Press, 1984).
† These do not refer to Lenin's or Trotsky's or Betty Friedan's stages.

has evolved into much more than this. As the historian Evelyn Fox Keller has commented, "We began by asking a few simple questions about equality, and it was like unraveling a ball of knitting; the more we looked for the beginning, the more we unraveled, until finally we are undoing the whole thing." Thus, questions women have raised about "equality" have led to discussions, examinations, and reconceptions of the nature of methodology in the social sciences, of the philosophical meanings of "truth," the various definitions of "science," and many more.

The question is: is gender ideology (and inequality) biological, "natural" (because "women have children" and because "when men compete, some are stronger and smarter"), or is it part of a historical cultural system spread by a warlike group (possibly only Indo-Europeans), which expanded out of the East in succeeding waves, between approximately 15,000 and 5,000 years ago? Have women always and everywhere been "dominated"? If we consider prehistory (history before written language), which is ten times as long as what we call "history," the answer is no.

## FAMILY VALUES AND LOVE: IS THE FAMILY'S DESIGN FIXED OR FLEXIBLE?

Do hierarchy and inequality in families keep popping up because they are "human"—or is this behavior exaggerated by ideology?

As noted earlier, one of the most important ways through which the hierarchical system of unquestioning obedience to authority (or "what is") is transmitted through the biblical tale of Abraham taking his son Isaac up on a mountain where God/Allah had commanded that he "sacrifice" the boy. Abraham is given no reason other than that the Lord commanded it, and that therefore the action was "right." From this command, Abraham learns that he must obey the system and not ask why the rules are the rules. He must show his loyalty by not questioning authority. This system, it is said, rewards men with elevated status.

Today this elevated status continues to be reinforced in men by the daily use in the English language of the pronoun "he," the adjective "his," and the generic term "man" to refer to all humans. Further, as noted, men are reminded in "nature" specials on television (and popular biology textbooks) that they have a "natural" tendency (therefore a "right"?) to be "dominant," to "rule"—that "competition for dominance" is "part of their natural behavior." But even if this phenomenon were true in some species of animals, it is certainly not true in all, and who is to say which is the "model" for our species? And even if it were "natural," would this make it "right"?

Some theorize that the idea of some people "owning" others came about when men first observed the animals reproducing and giving birth; men wanted to control female sexuality and reproduction and thus "own" their offspring. Perhaps this hypothesis is true, since men would lose control of inheritance and reproduction if women had choices of other family systems and were not forced to be focused on men, as perhaps they were not in the earliest Greek, Cretan, and other societies around the Mediterranean basin.

Most men who believe in democratic government have not applied the same principles to the family. This glaring inconsistency is not widely questioned.* In the nineteenth century many men "found" support for the idea of male superiority in "science" (or popularized science). Although as early as 1776 Abigail Adams (in a letter) asked her husband, working on the new American Constitution, "not to forget the ladies," he declined to comply.

The nineteenth-century version of "male domination" succeeded the old idea of the God-given inherited right of kings (and men) to rule, in the following way: humans, it was said, had come to dominate other animals as we evolved, because we were superior; similarly, within our species, it was claimed, males "naturally" competed with females and each other for "dominance"; therefore, if we have a social structure in which men are dominant, this fact is clearly proof that males were and are "naturally" superior—that is, stronger, "smarter," and so on. (Similarly, adherents of slavery in the eighteenth and nineteenth centuries argued that blacks were slaves because their "natures" were to be lazy and dependent, and that they were happy that way, and the like.) Darwinian competition was also used to "justify" sharp divisions between social classes in the nineteenth century, and this concept continues today as the framework for theories of "free competition in the marketplace."

Cooperation is just as "natural" as competition; many biologists and primatologists are now showing how important the cooperative forces of nature are. However, competition is central to the "male" ideology: "real" men "naturally" compete for a spot in the hierarchy, must compete (or they are "cowards" and "wimps"!). This is one of the most important credos of "masculinity."

And there is an underside to this arrangement for men too: by having to close off one side of themselves, blind parts of themselves to their inhumanity to women through the general social system, not "see," in order to be loyal to the men's hierarchy, men must coarsen themselves—deaden their sense of justice.

Men live with the internal knowledge, conscious or not, that by ruling, they are dominating women. Since they live with/have to look at those with less privilege every day, they must develop a way of not really "seeing" reality.

Research from *The Hite Report on Men and Male Sexuality* shows that most boys, between the ages of eight and fourteen, go through a stage of learning that involves forcing themselves to disassociate from, stop identifying with, their mothers. They are forced by the culture to "choose," to identify henceforth only with things "male," not to retain any "female" ways about them, for to do so would "ruin their chances" in life. (This is a choice artificially created by society, not "natural" and inevitable "nature".) This is a period of great stress for boys, who often feel guilty and disloyal

---

* Does the noble part of this tradition—the positive, outward, socially interested side of the masculine—have to include the antiwoman ideology? Can a group only define itself by making itself "special" and excluding others?

for thus "leaving" the mother; many never recover fully.* And so, boys go through a stage of first identifying with their mother, then having to break with that identification and learn to keep a distance, disassociate themselves, ridicule women/their mother, dominate them/her, and finally, reach the stage where they can rule, dominate with no qualms. This forcing of boys to choose should be ended, as this would lead to a more harmonious society. But instead, "explanations" are sought for the so-called "problems of women."

Finally, living with this knowledge of injustice built into the system can mean that gradually a man loses his ability to see injustice and to be just, to recognize justice and expect it. Because he has been so carefully educated by the "male" culture to turn a blind eye to injustice on a massive scale, idealism about life is impossible. Thus, the "male" ideology breeds negativity and cynicism, which is then blamed on "human nature."

## MEN'S FEAR OF BEING "IN LOVE"

The opposite side of the coin of a "masculinity" defined as being "tough," "able to take it," is that most men are also afraid to express emotions or be too close to women, lest they seem "weak." To put it another way, the split between love and reason in classical Western thought (with "love" decreed to be "feminine," and "reason," "masculine") makes it difficult for many men to love without inner conflict.

What does the ideology of "masculinity" tell men about how to deal with love in an ongoing, mutual relationship? Nothing. It only tells men to be dominant, to dominate relationships, and to make sure the woman doesn't "dominate" them. This explains many men's fear of being "in love" and displeasure when "overcome" with feelings for a woman. A "real man" must separate himself; assert his "pride" and "dominance" before all else.

As mentioned elsewhere, most men in *The Hite Report on Men and Male Sexuality* did not marry the women they most passionately loved, nor did they plan to; they were proud of "controlling their emotions," behaving "rationally" as "men." They experienced prolonged inner conflicts over their love relationships— but few doubts that they were doing the "right thing" when they chose in favor of "reason" and against "irrational" feelings of love and attraction. Most men believed that other men and "society" would admire them for resisting their feelings. At the same time there is a logical contradiction in this denial of emotion: men may hold demeaning attitudes to women's "emotionality," but most still rely on women's emotional support.

---

* A large part of teenage boys' "mean and nasty" crazes are attempts by them to deal with their culturally imposed guilt; that is, if one is "bad" already, one might as well glorify being an outlaw, being really tough and cruel, being "really male" (for example, as frequently seen on MTV and in children's monster or war-toy commercials) because men (by definition) can never be "good.

But change is a problem for men because to give up "dominance" may mean being seen as "unmasculine"—but to question the value of domination is the only way to improve "masculinity," or society. How can men, given this no-win situation, change their ideology?

## HOW THE SOCIALIZATION OF MEN AND BOYS AFFECTS WORLD AFFAIRS: IMPLICATIONS FOR INTERNATIONAL TERRORISM

The "male" ideology in its current phase, with its acceptance of the increasing amount of violence in the world and toward the natural environment, is seeing aggression and terrorism run riot. To be purely logical, if the "male" ideology decrees that competition is "natural," why shouldn't anyone use any means at hand to "win" in the competition for "dominance"—since power and winning are all that are respected in the final analysis anyway? In the current political situation, terrorism can be seen as a logical consequence of the "male" ideology, with its focus on hierarchy.

Every day television shows us the "news" that some nations and some individuals are very rich and powerful, while others are very poor. The poor and powerless can see the others, the rich and powerful, day after day on television and in newspapers. This reminds them/us forcefully of their/our position, reminds us that the dominant ideology only respects power—and this knowledge increases aggression, as aggression seems to be the only way to be heard. Is this true? Are disruptive acts the only way for a small state or individual to get its/his voice heard, or for a small state to make a point in a hierarchical world system?

A new system should be devised in which small countries and/or women are not driven to such states of mind, feeling that there is no other alternative than to fight or remain powerless, because those in power (or the man in the relationship) won't listen.

It is a failure of the system not to deal with all the possibilities and complexities of a very diverse world, instead insisting on dominating and trying to control a diversity that could be productive and harmonious. Valuing people and their feelings is perhaps the basis of democracy in government; can men apply this idea, valuing each individual equally, to women and their own personal lives?

## WHERE DOES OUR MEN-ON-TOP SOCIETY COME FROM?

Did this hierarchical ideology have a historical beginning, was there a time and place when this social system (as differentiated from the more egalitarian pantheon of the Greeks, the Egyptians, probably the pre-Greeks, and others) became established?

Or is "male" domination a "normal" function of male hormones—that is, testosterone levels make men restless, "aching for a fight," for a good battle or sex? Or have these hormonal influences been exaggerated by those who would wish to rationalize aggressive masculinity as "natural," to say that "male" "human nature" as we know it is "natural" and that therefore "male" dominance in the social structure is also "natural"?

Some argue that "male" domination originates not in "male hormones" but in the "biological" nature of the reproductive family; that is, as we have heard (ad nauseam), women get pregnant and "have" to stay home to take care of their children, leaving men to go out and defend them, get food. However, it has been shown that in gathering-hunting societies women do most of the gathering and that the majority of the food is gathered; therefore, women in some societies in prehistory probably provided most of the food. There is also a current debate in anthropology regarding whether the rest of the food was hunted or scavenged.[8]

On the other hand, perhaps male domination is not biological at all but the result of a historical accident—certain tribes with this ideology won key battles because of their having this ideology: an extremely competitive, combative, and warlike group could easily be the victor over less militaristic, more peaceful societies.

We do not know enough about prehistory (the time before writing, or when writing that has not been deciphered or was perishable) to trace the various strands of philosophical thought back much further than 3500 BC. But we know that high forms of art and culture existed at least as long ago as 35,000 years, as the Ice Age art exhibit appearing at the Museum of Natural History in New York, featured as a cover story of *Newsweek* in the fall of 1986, demonstrates.

The Old Testament of the Bible makes an important point of repeating, in stanza after stanza, the lineage of certain people because it wants to establish the tradition of descent through fathers, not through mothers, it seems. This practice implies that maternal descent may have been traditional for preceding millennia, as suggested by lists of female names found on clay tablets in Crete and elsewhere. The Old Testament also inveighs against the worship of female gods (who were popular in Canaan and elsewhere), thus also implying the existence of a possible important status for women, at least in religion, in other ideological systems of the time. Why did the "father-inheritance" system win out? We do not know.

Primatologists and fossil paleoanthropologists (those who study bone fragments of primates and humaniods one to two million years old) now believe that the "first families" were almost certainly mothers and children living in a clan grouping, the father being a later addition. What contribution did pre-state societies, in which women may have had a more important, or even the leading, governing role, have in forming the tradition of states seen later in history? Why did "chiefdoms" become a male-dominant system? These are new questions that have not yet been answered.

Is classical Greece one of the crossover points,[9] culturally, between earlier goddess-centered "states," such as Crete, and the warlike tradition? No one is sure; some scholars speak of invading Indo-European tribes with a warlike ideology that had invaded northern India two centuries earlier, coming then into

Greece and later Italy, pushing the indigenous populations to the south, where they continued their traditions of goddess worship (usually with many deities) up until the historical period of the Roman Empire and even later. Of course, a supremely hierarchical system must not be a multideity system, but a "one god above all" system.[10]

Archaeologists studying pre-Indo-European or Bronze Age cultures have added many more questions to the puzzle: Crete probably was not a patriarchy, and indeed, many of the civilizations around the Mediterranean basin in prehistory had long traditions of holding sacred female creation figures, or "goddesses." Ba'al, for example, referred to only by name in the Bible, was, in fact, a female deity. Archaeological sites such as Çatal Huyuk in Anatolia (Turkey, near the Mediterranean) had no walls around the city for defense; was the point of view of these societies therefore less warlike?[11] If so, this fact could disprove the "male" ideology's position today that "aggression" is a "natural part" of a fixed "human nature." In fact, contemporary society is urging men on a daily basis to be aggressive and competitive, not "soft"; if man's "nature" were to be "tough," would society need to give them these messages?

## MEN AND WOMEN: ROMEO AND JULIET CULTURES WRIT LARGE

*I want to love him and be close to him, but I just can't, the way I used to be. He can't understand what I'm talking about half the time, it seems, and when I try to insist or explain it more to him, he gets irritated. So I have to just let it go—let go of him, my dreams, love him for who he is, even if he can't understand a lot of who I am. I feel I see him clearly, who he is and how his life became what it is—but he doesn't know me the same way.*

Can one be as close as one dreams one can be? Is what's "out there" in contemporary society an atmosphere conducive to development of love relationships?

If society separates the two genders so decisively that it impedes love—a kind of culturewide version of Romeo and Juliet, the two genders educated to believe in different ways of life and to distrust one another—what is an individual to do about it?

One woman, at a very trying time in her life, wrote the following:

*I sit here in this argument, discussion, thinking to myself, surely you will say what I need to hear next, or give an opinion on this, your feelings about this . . . and yet you don't. And no matter for how many hours or days or years you don't, I can never stop listening, never stop hoping, waiting for, hearing your reply in my mind. And sometimes I think the frustration of waiting to hear your opinion, what you think, really think, will drive me mad.*

It is not that women think men are the enemy—but many women do think that men who live by the "male" ideology are the enemy. In a way, this book, besides being a redefinition by women of who they are, is a massive plea from women for men to stop living by their current rules and rethink what they are doing to themselves, to women, and to the planet.

The majority of men in *The Hite Report on Men and Male Sexuality* responded that after high school their best friends are their wives, or the women they know, because they find it impossible to really talk to other men. This statement is a clear indictment by men of their own system.

How alienated are women from a system based on the "male" ideology (in which women in the United States are not even considered for the office of president)? How far has this process gone in women's minds? Are women so dissatisfied that this is the reason for the high divorce rate? Are more women than ever now leaving marriages because they refuse to live any longer with a man or a system that classifies them as less: less important, less intelligent, less rational?

As individual women go through this process of struggling to understand what is making love so difficult, they often find themselves gradually and painfully saying good-bye—with deep regret and sadness—to their dreams of happiness with the kind of love they had wanted.

This process of leave-taking usually happens in stages. First women bargain with themselves: "Okay, so I won't ask him to do the laundry or pick up the kids anymore—it's not worth it. I love him, he's a man and you just can't expect all this overnight, but I love him and I can enjoy him—and where else could I find a better lover, or a man who loves me as well?" When even this bargain doesn't really work, next to go is a woman's belief that she is loved "well." Still she stays, because "I still love how well we know each other, what we have built up over time, and I hope he believes in this too . . .," and so on. With each bargaining chip in this interior dialogue a woman gives up one more emotional tie to the man until she realizes, finally, that she is in fact alone, living by herself emotionally.

As women struggle with this inner dilemma, questioning themselves daily about the same issue, the feeling often is, "I am giving more than he is emotionally, trying harder to make it work. Why doesn't he try harder, seem to want to meet me halfway? Does he even understand that he is not? Will the relationship ever be better? Am I a fool to continue it? Should I keep on struggling? Give less energy to it? Should I leave?"

This state of inner questioning, alienation, and frustration represents a long good-bye not only to the man in question but also to a certain society and way of life. In the process of leaving a man, whether emotionally or physically, so many women, as we have seen, go through layers of self-questioning about the meaning of love, relationships, life, the nature of family, work, what life is all about—all the basic philosophical questions one has to confront to make major decisions.

Through this independent thought, women are shifting their allegiance from the frame of reference that has for so long dominated everything.

It seems, based on this research into private life, that women today are already moving into a different frame of reference. While most are doggedly trying to get men they love to change, they are relying more and more on their women friends as major supports and primary relationships.

One woman comments on the transformation she sees in her own mind, having gone through all these emotions in relationships:

> *I think the solution is that we have to mentally transcend the whole thing. It's not a question of to be with men or without them. The real solution is when you reach a stage where somehow or another it's just not the biggest worry in your life—it's a different way that you see the world. You live in another sphere, which is to become whatever your interests are, and maybe men are part of it and maybe not, but it is not the feature. Female friendships are definitely a part of it—I don't mean that now women should give up men and live only with women and follow some feminist party line, that's not it . . . I mean you live somewhere else emotionally—love can be there and become more or less important in your life—but you don't get your identity through a man.*

### "TO MAKE A WORLD IN WHICH MORE LOVE CAN FLOURISH"—HOW?

Elizabeth Petroff correctly reminds us that we are still in the midst of a revolutionary process that is not over:

> *How much, if ever, have institutions corresponded to the imaginative ideals that women created, love as women have imagined it? How much have women really imagined what all the possibilities are?*[12]

Women in my 1980s research are questioning the human condition, noting it can be better than it is, insisting that equality and interaction as a social framework are possible, not just an idealistic dream. Cooperation and teamwork are viable ways of organizing society. Nevertheless, it is often heard that women are "too emotional" to run governments, that "women's" "soft-hearted," cooperative ideals would not work on a global level in government or international relations. And yet, how can a system that has brought us to the brink of nuclear war and ecological disaster call another system unworkable or impractical?

In large part it is the interpersonal patterns of the ideology, with its constant encouragement for men to use competition for dominance as the means of "resolving" disputes, that has led the world to the situation in which it now finds itself.

"Women's" traditional philosophy may contain other ways of resolving disputes, such as subtle negotiating. In the midst of the very real problems that society now faces—problems the current system does not seem able to address adequately—it is time to take a serious look at "women's" alternative philosophy.

The principles of mutuality in relationships, such as women use with each other, are the essence of good diplomatic skills. Confrontational situations in the world are remarkably similar to those seen in women's private lives with men. "Sticking his head in the sand," as one woman describes her boyfriend's reaction to her discussions about their relationship; in the same way some governments refuse to listen to the "demands" of disenfranchised women or small countries, trusting that the problems will "go away." These attitudes lead to more and more seething resentment, until it is too late to resolve things productively, whether in the world political situation or in the home.

Another theory of change is that revolution happens when the beliefs of some infiltrate or convert the beliefs of the many. By trying to change men in personal relationships, will women change the larger society?[*]

Sometimes the reverse happens. To make an analogy with politics: in what was termed in 1973 as the "Stockholm syndrome," a group often gradually comes to love and identify with its captor. On the other hand, sometimes a culture that is dominated by another politically and militarily does still manage to have its culture become dominant eventually. For example, the Romans were "civilized" by the Greeks after the Romans defeated the Greeks militarily. Christianity was adopted by the Romans through an imperial decree—but did the imperial decree come about because of Christianity's underground popularity? Traditions in Germany were changed by Christianity, but many of the old traditions survived simply because of their popularity and the strength of people's belief in them.

Some say women can best fight for their rights by electing political candidates: if "power only respects power," the more women become members of political groups, the more likely it is that we will see women candidates selected by the parties for major political office. "And if we vote for them, we will see them elected."[†]

On the other hand, something in the political system seems to create a tendency to select women who are as "tough as guys." The political system, as it is, can contain a built-in contradiction for many women who do not like traditional fighting. What about creating a new philosophically nonaligned coalition?

Women have a great deal of economic power—collectively, an enormous

---

[*] Of course, not all women are "just" and "kind," and many men are; it is not one's biology that creates these characteristics. However, women's shared experiences do tend to create certain understandings and ways of relating to the culture, just as do men's.

[†] The Green Party was started in Germany by a woman, Petra Kelly. The Green Party deals especially with issues of ecology and nuclear war. In Iceland, where women have been much more active than in the United States, a feminist party won 10 percent of the vote and six seats in Parliament. In Norway half the parliament has recently become female, due to women's organizing. And, as Corazon Aquino, in a speech at Harvard University on September 21, 1986, stated, "Women led the change of power in the Philippines by using nonviolent protests."

amount. Women now would be financially able to form a network to support other women and women's projects/corporations, go into business with each other.

At times in history peaceful movements have triumphed over larger forces. For example, Gandhi was able to found a movement that eventually, along with other factors, ended British rule in India. The nonviolent protests of the United States civil-rights movement are of more relevance; they have "raised the consciousness" of both blacks and whites, although blacks still suffer from lower incomes, higher unemployment, less education, and higher infant mortality rates, and no blacks are chosen as candidates for president by major parties.

Is it so simple as to say that, since women are 51 percent of the population, if women begin to see themselves as forming the core of society, the center of history and philosophy, the overall society will change.

In his analysis of the position of women in the twentieth century, written in 1972, historian William Chafe[13] describes in detail the patterns of "women's liberation" from the 1920s to the 1950s, and at the end of his argument he seems to be stating that the ideology of "women's place is in the home" (woman as second, not supposed to lead) has so far been too strong to be overcome. While Chafe is far from a radical, he (without intending to make this implication, perhaps) states over and over that only the "substantial upheaval" of World War II, and not any "propagandizing" by "feminists," changed women's basic situation. World War II brought significant numbers of women out of the home and into the work force, giving them an independent income—and this shift included women of all ages, not just, as before, mainly women who worked when they were single before they married. This financial independence, Chafe implies, brought them a certain amount of general independence and thus "liberation." But according to his analysis, it was only "compulsion" or "substantial upheaval" that forced change for women on the society.

His study would imply that women are fooling themselves by believing that any amount of talk or "consciousness changing" will create lasting, fundamental change in women's status. He has argued that patterns are repeating themselves, that evolutionary change in such a fundamentally embedded ideology is impossible. Is it?

## WOMEN'S CODE OF HONOR

### A NONVIOLENT PHILOSOPHICAL FRAMEWORK: PARADIGM CHANGE

*Women of the world, You know what's wrong—but it's wrong not only with your personal life, it's wrong in the entire system.*

So, if it is not (not only?) "power" we want, but major philosophical change as well, then the rethinking we are doing, and the devising of a clearly articulated alternative, is the kind of fighting that will make a lasting difference.

We badly need a revolution in thought and behavior patterns on every level, an important change in consciousness.

In fact, now, women have formulated new ways of viewing almost all fields of thought, including psychology, biology, philosophy, history, primatology, and anthropology, and this process is ongoing. There has been a cultural revolution, a revolution in thinking, that has caused a renaissance in almost all the disciplines, and that has perhaps hardly begun.

The interesting and important thing about this revolution is that it is not just being made by an isolated group of people; it is women and some men everywhere who are thinking these thoughts. For women these issues are pressing, since many women meet the "system" every day in the faces of men they love: the pain women experience receiving men's double messages lifts many beyond the daily routine to the highest plateaus of thought and reflection. Thus, as we have seen, it is in large part the behavior of men they love that has led to the crystallization of the level of awareness women are now expressing—an awareness that cannot be removed from consciousness.

## A NEW LANDSCAPE: BEYOND "FAMILY VALUES"

This philosophical revolution, which Jessie Bernard has named the Feminist Enlightenment, is the biggest realignment of thought in two centuries or more. It is extending democratic ideas and a different sensibility into love relationships, science, and global politics. This is not only a "female revolution" but also a general revolution, a globalization of values.

Just as the Enlightenment built upon older structures and transcended them, adding new dimensions to the philosophical framework (out of which grew the idea of democratic government), so in the same way what women are doing now is enabling society to take another philosophical step forward.

As the United Nations recognized in 1995, this struggle by women is global; though it has many aspects in many countries, 140 countries signed a document in Beijing that year stating that they believe women have rights to autonomy over their own bodies and personal/reproductive choices (see the U.N. Declaration on the Rights of Women, Beijing, 1995). These personal choices by 51 percent of the population of the world resonate politically.

Women and men are creating, on an international scale, a global critique of previous social systems and "traditional roles for women" and family. Women are questioning how social organizations, families, and governments are formed and how "leadership" is decided on; they want to contribute much more to the current changes. This profound redesign is not represented by the lurid images of "female sexual revolution" often seen in media reports, demonizing Western women in particular as "sexual and superficial."

Gender may be the basic, original split that needs to be healed to alter society, to lessen aggression as a way of life. Changing our idea of coitus and "how it should be performed" is key to changing the larger society. Sex is a metaphor, or perhaps the center of the social structure. Women are leaving behind the double-standard values of sex (in the West, represented by the images of Eve, known as the "evil sexual temptress," and Mary, "the virgin mother"). They are reviewing and reseeing their sexual identity, their ideas of female sexuality and the body, placing less emphasis on gender difference in their children and themselves; their questioning of a gender hierarchy is connected also to a questioning of other kinds of hierarchies, such as those based on race and class.

The current statistics on marriage and divorce, as noted, are strangely symbolic of the moment we are in: 50 percent of women leave their marriages; 50 percent stay, even if they are not emotionally satisfied. We are clearly at a turning point. The picture is striking—almost as if women were pausing, stopping a moment for reflection, halfway out of a door, still turning to look back, bidding good-bye to the past, before setting out on a journey.

## NOT "THE HUMAN CONDITION"—NOT FOREVER

Another world is possible, another landscape, full of a different kind of metaphorical fauna and flora, both in nature and in the human imagination—positive mental constructs not yet discernible to our "human nature as competitive" belief system. If hierarchy is the basis of all our institutions now—from religion to the state, to the family and to love relationships—this need not last forever. It is just that our view of what is possible is temporarily obstructed.

## NOTES

1   See Appendix for the *Women and Love* questionnaire.
2   See 1987 Statement by Committee in Appendix.
3   *The Ascent of Man*, hosted by Professor Jacob Bronowski, PBS.
4   So referred to by Elizabeth Dole, and later by the *Economist*.
5   For other discussions of whether or not there are "two cultures" or depictions of "woman's voice," see the works of Jesse Bernard, Joan Scott, Mary Daly, Carroll Smith-Rosenberg, Carol Gilligan, Elizabeth Petroff. Certainly a well-developed "female" culture and value system is implicit in what the majority of women are saying in this study.
6   See also Professor Wendy Doniger O'Flaherty's work for the documentation of this split in classical Indian culture in the Rig Vedas; that culture, like ours, was also based in large part on the ideology and social structure of Indo-European tribes; indeed we have an extremely important common cultural heritage.
7   Schwartz and Blumstein correlate other factors. See Pepper Schwartz and Philip Blumstein, *American Couples: Money, Work, Sex* (New York: Morrow, 1983).
8   Richard Potts, paper delivered before the American Anthropological Association annual meeting, 1985.
9   See Shere Hite and Robert Carneiro, abstracts, 1985 annual meeting of the American Anthropological Association.
10  For a discussion of the changeover in Greek mythology, see Jane Harrison, *Prolegomena to the Study of Greek Religion* (United Kingdom: Merlin Press, 1981).

11 Roundtable discussion, Institute for Human Origins, University of California, Berkeley, November 1986.

12 Petroff, Elizabeth, "Controversies over the Nature of Love," American Philosophical Association annual meeting, 1986.

13 William Chafe, *Women and Equality: Changing Patients in Amerian Culture* (New York: Oxford University Press, 1977).

# Part 4

# Icons of the Heart: Love, Power, and Sex in the Traditional Family
## (1994)

*This section contains excerpts from and further essays on* The Hite
Report on the Family, *the fourth Hite Report, first published in
1994, with the participation of over 4,000 men and women. In it,
Hite addresses such questions as "How do children, boys and girls,
grow up sexually?" and "What do children feel and how do they
develop?" The assumption had been (and continues to be) that
"hormones" make boys and girls different from one another at
puberty, when sexual changes occur: girls begin to menstruate and
develop breasts, boys begin to ejaculate with orgasm and develop
body hair as their voices deepen. However, according to Hite's
research,[1] based on the responses of over of 4,000 men and women,
puberty is more a "reproductive awakening" than a "sexual awakening"—especially for girls. The confusion of terminology, Hite suggests, probably arises from both a misplaced shyness about "speaking
about these things," and a Victorian tendency to project boys' experience onto girls (as some medical research still does: research into
cholesterol levels in humans, for example). According to Hite's
research, girls' first orgasms are not clearly linked to reproduction (as
parents also often report), as most have their first self-stimulated
orgasm before puberty. Girls have sexual feelings and orgasm from
a very early age, certainly before their menstrual cycle begins.*

*Hite also poses further questions: is the "traditional family" with
its "traditional values" the best place for children to grow up sexually? What are the special turns of mind that the family structure as*

*we know it, or have known it, contains? Is it changing? What about children in Brazil and Iraq and Africa who have no parents, their parents having died of the disease AIDS or in war? Are they creating new forms of family? Are single-parent families the wave of the future, and what does this circumstance imply for "family values"?*

# Democracy of the Heart

## A New Politics for the Twenty-first Century

### MOVING TOWARD THE FUTURE OF FAMILY AND SOCIETY
### WITH A MORE MATURE VIEW

We should give up the outdated notion that the only acceptable families are nuclear families. A more profound historical view of what is happening is needed. We should see the new society that has evolved over the last forty years for what it is, for itself, not as a disaster because it is not like the past.

The new diversity of families is part of a positive pluralism, part of a fundamental transition in the organization of society, which calls for open-minded brainstorming by us all: what do we believe "love" and "family" are? Can we accept that the many people fleeing the nuclear family are doing so for valid reasons? If reproduction is no longer the urgent priority that it was when societies were smaller, before industrialization took hold, then the revolt against the family is not surprising. Perhaps it was even historically inevitable. It is not that people don't want to build loving, family-style relationships, it is that they do not want to be forced to build them within one rigid, hierarchical, heterosexist, reproductive framework. In fact, children have often found themselves forced into situations with two unhappy parents arguing around them or abusing them, leaving the children in peril or anxious.

The movement in reaction to these changes is called "family values" or "traditional family values," or yet again, "fundamental family values." Though there is an amount of hysteria in the current political assertions that "the family" is a sacred institution, historically the family is changing; since this change will not end or lessen reproduction (if it is currently lessened, perhaps this is due to society's attempt to enforce a system based on the traditional family—that is, not implementing policies to aid those who are actually reproducing, women who are both married and unmarried), there is no reason to fear this change.

Diversity in family groupings—including groups of friends, sisters and brothers, people who love each other and care for each other—can bring joy and enrichment to a society: new kinds of families can be the basis for a renaissance of spiritual dignity and creativity in politics and business as well. Clinging to the forms of the past will only cause sclerosis of the society. Society is a living thing that changes, we need to accept that fact.

Private life is in the midst of a welcome process of democratization, which will in turn enrich, advance, and transform democracy in the political arena. Continuing this process of bringing private life into a more ethical and egalitarian frame of reference will give us the energy and incentive to maintain democracy in the larger political sphere and in international relations. We can create a society with a new spirit and will, but our inner politics will have to be transformed before a lasting transition can be made in the political arena.

One of the most useful reference points for creating new kinds of relationships in "the family" can now be found in many friendships between women. How many women remark, "I wish I could talk to him like I can talk to my best friend!" There is a vast difference between the way women see themselves with each other and the way women generally see themselves with men.

Though the economic and spiritual difficulties of the West today are often blamed on "the decline of the family" (or on "feminism" and "women"—"single mothers" are vilified in a way that, the Archbishop of Canterbury argued, would be illegal if the same attack were made on a racial minority) isn't the reality that Western democracies are not fully living up to their promise of equality for all? In fact, women have great energy and courage that are being underutilized; women nevertheless are in the forefront of the movement for reshaping personal and public institutions, endeavoring to create a more interactive democratic society.

The twentieth century proved that psychologizing the family doesn't work. Psychotherapy and its attempted analysis of the family has failed; it may have helped some people, but it does not address the underlying problem—that is, the structure of the family itself—as more and more people seek "treatment." It is not so much maladjusted individuals who are "the problem" as it is the framework into which they are persuaded. As Naomi Weisstein and Shulamith Firestone have pointed out in scholarly papers, in the early twentieth century the new Freudianism was used to "answer" the challenge posed to the social system of feminist theory, which called for equal rights for women. Of course this theory did not answer anything, but it was hoped that talking would lead to some kind of acceptance of the situation/status quo. Taking its cue from George Orwell's *1984*, the mass media has also learned the refined art of using pseudo-Freudian psychoreligious symbols of "the family" and "correct behavior" to control and direct public opinion. However, what is needed is a clear analysis of what is really going on, a courageous taking stock of what kind of world democracy and equality imply, and "going for it"! Implementing our values will bring about change in a very positive and amazingly quick way.

Diversity in families can form the basic infrastructure for a new and advanced type of political democracy to be developed within nations and among nations—a system that suits the massive societies that technology has made into one global village.

The current fundamentalist reaction to the democratization of private life is trying to return society, both the private and public social orders, to prehumanist values of earlier centuries. This type of social order has had various names: totalitarianism, feudalism, fascism, authoritarianism, and so on. Democracy is the opposite of these social orders.

Democracy needs to exist within families and in people's private lives, as well as in politics. One cannot exaggerate the importance of the current debate: fascism in the family cannot be left to exist, since it inevitably leads to a return to fascism in society as well. If we believe in the democratic, humanist ideals of our heritage, we have the right and duty to make our family system a more just one, to follow our democratic ideals and make a new, more inclusive network of private life, a new personal infrastructure for society that will reflect not a preordained patriarchal structure, but our belief in justice and equality for all—women, men and children.

Private life is in the midst of a welcome process of democratization. The family has been a repressive, authoritarian institution for too long. Those who would attack women now are trying to reimpose the unequal "holy family" model. Let's continue the transformation, believe in ourselves, and go forward with love, not fear. In our private lives and in our public world, let's hail the future and make history.

## PSYCHOSEXUAL DEVELOPMENT IN CHILDREN: REVOLUTIONIZING THE PSYCHE OF PATRIARCHY

My research on how children grow up has created a new picture of sexual development in childhood that challenges prevailing theory.

A significantly different picture of "childhood" emerges from my work than is shown elsewhere, as boys and girls describe their feelings and experiences, a spectrum of new stages appears, including inner psychological turning points not identified before.

The theory regarding childhood that has dominated twentieth-century thought is the Freudian view, with its fixation on gender. It proposed such incorrect concepts as "penis envy" (to "describe" women's dissatisfaction with their suppression and inequality); the belief that girls should transfer their feelings at puberty from the clitoris to the vagina to have "mature orgasm"; the "explanation" that if boys love their mothers, they have an "Oedipus complex" (a remarkably negative way to view boys' love for their mothers); as well as the "explanation" that men are "naturally" aggressive and desire to dominate because of "biological, hormonal changes at puberty" (which are "inescapable").

My findings challenge these Freudian and post-Freudian, "modernist" views. In fact, such ideas merely reflect the social psychological system that has been imposed on children (and on us, carrying on into adulthood)—the psychosexual identity that our social system wants us to have. Freud should have used a larger, cross-cultural sample before assuming arrogantly that his generalizations would be eternally true.

Much more interesting than such negative theories are the real, individual psychological and sexual feelings children and young adults express as they describe their childhoods, their feelings about their parents, their bodies and themselves in my research.

Based on their testimonies (many published in *The Hite Report on the Family*), I question whether "puberty" is a valid category, either for girls or boys, except in terms of reproduction: "puberty" is not the time of sexual awakening, especially not for girls, as it may not be for boys. While most boys first masturbate to orgasm with ejaculation between the ages of ten to twelve, girls usually masturbate to orgasm much earlier, almost half starting by the ages of five to seven.

Thus puberty is not so much a time of "sexual awakening" as a change in reproductive status. Freud incorrectly modeled his ideas of sexual puberty in girls on his somewhat simplistic notions about boys. Are his theories about psychosexual identity even true for boys? Many men in my research tell me that they felt sexual and had orgasm without ejaculation long before puberty; most boys go through a dark night of the soul in order to give up their closeness to their mothers and sisters and "things feminine" (cuddly bears, and the like) so they can "act like a man." And there are other oversights.

Certainly many of Freud's ideas about boys are incorrect: the change in identity demanded of boys ("Stop staying home and hanging around your mother"; "Go out with the boys and don't let them make fun of you!"; "Get interested in boys' sports like football!") is brought about by cultural pressures at least as much as by "hormones." Freud, without realizing it, seemed to follow the reproductive mores of his time, his social milieu, and his personal background, but he insisted that he had discovered "eternal verities" and that his categories were biological and therefore "eternally true."

Perhaps the most surprising information in my research is the intensity of the pain so many boys describe experiencing as they undergo this uprooting process, trying to change their identities and allegiances (from mother to father world) at puberty, as they try to learn to be rude to their mothers even when they don't feel good about doing this—to achieve their new identity, acceptance, and status in the "male world." To be fair, boys have no choice but to try their best to join the "masculine system" and adapt to its rules. However, it is very difficult for most boys to accept the idea that, not only should women be treated with scorn as objects of a different or lower status than that of men, but also women should be seen as basic objects of men's sexual desire. Men should simultaneously despise and desire women—what a confusing combo.

In short, puberty is notable because it is the time of transference of loyalty from the mothers to the fathers—that is, integrating personal identity with the social system. Puberty is when the society demands that children switch their loyalties from the mother to the father, that they become "adults."

Many people, all their lives, live out a play-enacted version of themselves, a shadow-self tailored for public consumption, displaying "appropriate" social behavior in public "life," while underneath, in private, an undergrowth of confusing feelings of joy, fear, eroticism, and pain exist, all jumbled together. How many of us live like that?

The picture of development of psychosexual identity that emerges in my research, based on its new data and new methods, reveals that the whole shape and thrust of how we see "children's" and our own identities (since we once were children) are self-servingly blind.

Who are we, before we learn to see through society's lens? Can we use these distant memories to build on?

## ORIGINS OF GIRLS' AND BOYS' SEXUAL IDENTITY[2]

The word "hormones" is often used to "explain" psychological behavior that cannot really be scientifically demonstrated to be connected to it. This may especially be true of terminology used to describe girls' behavior, and to "explain" the behavior of children (boys and girls) at puberty.

This is not to underplay the advances made in the study of hormones, nor my hope for more research.

However, as a researcher into human emotions and human sexuality (both male and female), I think it is important to take account of research done from a sociological point of view, to complement research done in the physical or medical sciences.

Therefore here I will briefly recapitulate the findings of my research regarding "puberty" in girls and boys. First, boys, since "male psychology" is less frequently discussed.

## PUBERTY IN BOYS: BULLYING AND PRESSURE FOR "MANLY" PURSUITS[3]

Boys' puberty is most often said to be caused by "hormones," and indeed, boys do experience some changes linked to the body; for example, between the ages of ten to twelve, most boys begin to ejaculate to orgasm, masturbate frequently, and sometimes begin sex games with other boys at school.

Some psychologists and others, such as Freud, link these basic facts to what they have assumed to be "natural" behavior, acting as if using the phrase "hormonal changes" ensures that the explanation or linkage is "scientific." Quite often they want to "explain" behaviors created by centuries of social tradition in this way. In fact, many behaviors we associate with "puberty" and "teenagers" are socially created or exaggerated, not "ordained" by "hormones." This approach is also often taken by the news media.

It is more helpful to consider a complex perspective on human beings, whose behavior is a combination of "nature" and "nurture."

Is the male "sex drive" a result of male hormones? There is a strong case to be made that, though men have a strong desire for orgasm that begins at the time of hormonal change around the ages of ten to twelve, it is society and not the body that in large part teaches them how to channel their emerging energy. It is questionable whether a boy growing up on a remote desert island without any human contact would automatically find that coitus was his basic means of orgasm. Remember that in classical Greece a law was passed ordering that men must have coitus with their wives three times a month, minimum; obviously Greek men at that time were not doing so spontaneously.

In my research it is clear that there are many pressures on boys that teach them that girls and women are the proper "sex objects" of their "desire," while at the same time informing them that they should keep their distance from "women" and that emotions they may feel during "sex" should not be taken too seriously or considered "real emotions"—"they are only your hormones talking." This stricture, of course, leads to considerable disappointment, confusion and feelings of deception for girls who are these boys' partners.

In fact, there is an ideology of "maleness" (for lack of a better word) that in very large part constructs "male sexuality" in boys during their teenage years, according to my research.[4]

A large part of that ideology is taught by the bullying and group behavior that is common in school at that age. As one respondent remarked, "I was called a sissy when I didn't want to play football with boys who were bigger and heavier than I—then when I did participate, I was kicked in the face and called sissy when I cried. I was humiliated and angry." What he learned was not to complain and to conform to (male) group expectations. Yet it is sometimes asserted that "men like groups of men" because "it's in their hormones."

Another man responded: "I was told, 'Be a man, not a sissy!' during sports, when I didn't succeed. I felt like a traitor." Team sport is supposedly especially "manly"—that is, playing with the group is better than "proving yourself" as an individual: "I was injured in football and had to sit out most of the season. I realized then I liked not playing, but I didn't have the internal strength to quit sports teams, everybody would have made fun of me." These are social pressures that shape behavior; these are not behaviors that emerge from "hormones" or "male nature." They are part of a long tradition of a certain form of society, and we can change these dynamics so harmful to men and boys (and later, to the women who love them).

Boys also describe pressure not to associate with girls ("You're a sissy if you play with girls"), not to have girls as friends ('Girls are for sex"), and to spend their time with other boys. As one remembers, "I was always criticized for playing with girls, I felt that playing with girls was just as much fun as playing with boys. My attitude bothered my parents." Another: "At about eleven my father blew up at me for spending the afternoon at a girl's house rather than doing something like being out playing football."

A boy who liked to cook with his mother was told by his uncle that "Boys may like to do things with their mothers, but as they get older, they find that men are the ones they really enjoy doing things with. Why don't you get involved with the other boys who have hobbies like fixing up their cars?"

It is no wonder that, with pressures like these, men so often feel uneasy and "noncommunicative" after they "grow up" when they are in love with a woman. Though they may be happy at home with her, they force themselves to stay out working even more than necessary because "this is what men do." Many men in my research did not, in fact, marry the women they most passionately loved, because this made them feel "too female," "not powerful as a man."

If boys are told repeatedly that they are "wrong" to "hang out with women," how can a man suddenly change when he is an adult to "find it natural"? (We are told that boys' and men's hormones make them look at life as they do.) This boyhood scenario is leading to many unhappy marriages and relationships, in which "the man" works seven days a week, tries not to "hang out at home," comes home very late at night after a long work day "with the boys."

These examples have been meant to give a thumbnail sketch of how boys' psychology is shaped not only by "hormones" but also very strongly by custom and practice, handed down from generation to generation, masculinity being taught by "older boys" to "younger boys" through the often winked-at system of taunts and bullying.[5]

## GIRLS AT PUBERTY: WHAT IS PUBERTY IN GIRLS?

There is a large amount of data in my research about girls' development of sexual identity and experiences at puberty. Basically, the data show that girls have much more of a "reproductive puberty" rather than a "sexual puberty" or "sexual awakening." At puberty girls become able to reproduce; as their menstrual system begins, they develop breasts and ovulate monthly, discharging an egg.

However, most girls can orgasm via self-stimulation from a very early age, many from the age of five or six, and their desire for orgasm does not become exceptionally different at "puberty"—not to mention whether or not they have a desire for coitus, as discussed above in relation to boys.

Based on my data, I offer a critique of the social construct of the female "sex drive"; since this critique is multifaceted, I will here pick one of these facets to discuss in brief detail.

## PSYCHOSEXUAL IDENTITY AS DEVELOPED BY DAUGHTERS
## WITH THEIR MOTHERS

There is an unidentified taboo on sexual intimacy (communication) between mother and daughter at a very early age, according to my work.*

There is a significant moment relating to the body between mothers and daughters, one that occurs early but influences women psychologically all their lives—a "moment" that has not been previously identified. The psychology set in motion by this situation is too often presumed to be "natural," referred to glibly as a product of "the body and its changes."

The phenomenon of girls becoming irritable and cross with their mothers during their early teenage years, just after "puberty," is well known. Where does that anger and alienation begin? Is it simply a product of "hormones" or "the changes" that "make girls want to differentiate themselves from the mother"? This view, the theory of "separation," assumes that separation or differentiation from the mother is good because "nature needs it to happen."

However, does nature or culture wish mother and daughter to be at odds, "rivals"?

The estrangement begins, in my analysis, with early sexual taboos between mother and daughter that have not previously been identified.

Mothers know a lot about sexuality, it appears to daughters, but usually don't share much of this information with their daughters. Sexuality seems to children to be the mother's privilege and secret, something they should not ask too much about; that is, they should not ask the mother what she feels and experiences sexually. One girl describes being fascinated by her mother's body while knowing that touching it or asking any direct questions was off limits: "I remember looking at my mother one day when I was about ten. She was wearing a thin blouse, you could see the shape of her breasts in her white lacy underwear underneath. I remember staring at her full chest, her torso, and thinking it was astonishing, magnificent—so big! Not like mine . . . I wonder if I felt I could never look as sexual and powerful as she, that I was much smaller? Of course, I had no breasts yet. Did I think of myself as always the thin one, the smaller one—was my identity set at that time?"

Most daughters feel uneasy: at the same time that they learn they cannot ask the mother about her own sexual feelings, cannot know what the mother experiences;

---

* Puberty in girls has been generally misunderstood, based on little research at all, simply generalized from an understanding/misunderstanding of boys. Based on my investigations, it appears that girls have a reproductive puberty, but not a sexual puberty. In this way, girls' puberty may be significantly different from boys'. Most girls can orgasm via self-stimulation from a very early age, many from the age of five or six; their desire for orgasm may or may not become notably stronger at "puberty"; they do not manifest "a new desire for coitus" (nor masturbate vaginally). There is a large amount of data about girls' sexual identity and experiences at puberty in my research reports; here I am presenting a theory about the expression of female sexual identity, based on that research.

most girls also know that they themselves are sexual, that their own bodies have sexual parts that feel good. Still, they cannot directly see "those parts," since they are located in a part of the body that a girl would have to use a mirror to see. This circumstance is different from the way boys grow up, since boys can look down and see/touch their penis and sexual body easily; they can also see other boys' and men's sexual anatomy in public urinals and at home in the bathroom; thus boys feel much more comfortable with their sexual identity than do girls, who must learn about that part of their bodies, most often via having a sexual experience.

Could girls learn more about their bodies from their mothers? (This is not to say that a mother "should" open her body to her child; the point here is to look at what is in fact occurring, thus becoming more objective in understanding the development of girls' sexual identity.)

Most mothers hide their own lives, setting up a climate in which they clearly do not expect to be asked "private questions" by their daughters, such as whether they masturbate, how often they have sex, how they achieve orgasm, and so on. Most daughters are given a book and told, "Ask me any questions about what you don't understand."

Simply because some mothers say "Ask me anything," or "Feel free to talk to me whenever you want about whatever is troubling you" doesn't mean that there is real dialogue, according to girls. The fact that the mother usually does not give details about her own sexual experiences and means of orgasm, both during masturbation and with partners, leaves a feeling that the subject is not really "okay." The daughter often feels that the mother could tell her, could help her, could give her information, but doesn't; the girl feels that her mother is hypocritical, perhaps even stupid. ("Doesn't my mother know about orgasm? How does she have them? Does she live on another planet??")

Another girl reacted to her mother's silence by thinking that her new, developing body was "not her" and tried to get rid of parts of her body that were feminine—reminding us of the problems of anorexia: "I dreaded the moment my mother would discover I had breasts. I was disgusted when I developed hips. I decided I'd better diet to get back to my real shape, my boy shape, my 'normal' shape. At my all-girls school, big breasts were considered tarty; small were better. Having your period later was better too. We were part of the anorexia cult, we were all so thin we began menstruating very late. I desperately didn't want to become like my mother. I wanted to stay a child, a young girl, forever—not become one of those hated women."

Why are many mothers so coy with their daughters about sexuality? Why can't a mother show a daughter her vulva, for example, why "must" it be hidden? Boys see their fathers' penises—giving them a sense of normalcy and self-acceptance. Why not girls? Would it be wrong? Yes, mothers do have rights too!

If mothers must pretend to daughters that they have no sexual life, the daughter wonders: is it bad for a woman to be sexual? If not, why must my mother pretend her sexuality doesn't exist, that she has no sexual life? Why doesn't she talk to me about it? Or why has she decided not to have a sexual life? Does this imply the daughter should have no sexual life either?

All this sets up a climate of distrust and suspicion, a wariness about someone you live next to but do not know intimately, and who refuses to share anything with you. Does this mean that in order to feel closer, daughters and mothers have to become "sexual," be "lovers"? No, it simply means that they have the right to relate as complete and honest friends and companions. The rift or problem that occurs between mothers and daughters is not inevitable.

This early closed door results in a series of closed doors in the mind later.

## WHY DO GIRLS HAVE ORGASMS BEFORE THEY CAN REPRODUCE?

Believing that the institution we know as "sex" is fixed or eternal presents many problems, not the least of which is the question of where the female orgasm fits into "sex": if the female orgasm is not connected to conception/reproduction (it is not necessary for a woman to have an orgasm in order to become pregnant), then why "bother" with female orgasm at all? Why should it exist in nature? Primatologists at times still argue this position in "animal research"; it was common to hear asserted as late as the 1970s that the female orgasm did not really exist in humans, or that it was a faint, "residual reflex." This idea was disproven by the laboratory work of researchers such as Masters and Johnson, and M. J. Sherfey.

The inequality of the scenario known as "sex" is historical and cultural, not fixed biologically. We are currently in a period of transition, when many women and men are attempting to change and challenge inequality in "the sex act."

## BEAUTY AND FIGHTS BETWEEN MOTHERS AND DAUGHTERS

It used to be thought that girls "naturally" fight with their mothers around the time of "puberty" because they need to separate, find themselves as distinct individuals. In fact, women's rivalry is a problem with deep social roots that are intended to divide (and conquer) women, keep them apart in a society in which they are supposed to remain second class.

According to my research, the disruption in the relationship begins early; when it is unanalyzed, it gradually becomes more and more pronounced, especially at "puberty." The alienation has various layers.

Of course, on the simplest of levels, the conflict is over "beauty" and "sex appeal"—women's "looks." In our culture sexual rivalry is encouraged between daughters and mothers: mothers are seen as "older women," while their blossoming daughters are called "Lolitas" and "sexpots"—more fun and "desirable." Older women are not regarded as beautiful, their power is seen as negative and "domineering," their self-expression "demanding" and their sexuality "bawdy."

If younger women are considered "more beautiful" than older women, does the daughter automatically push her mother into second place in terms of power? An incident brought this home to one young woman: "The guy at the supermarket checkout started flirting with me. He was winking and asking where I lived and so on. He was completely ignoring my mother, which might have been okay except that when she went to join in the conversation he acted as though she was invisible. When she paid for the shopping he hardly looked at her—quite the opposite of how he was behaving with me. I liked him, but felt uncomfortable for my mother. On the way home, I could feel that some distance, some tension, had grown up between us. We had dinner but there was something unspoken going on, we couldn't look each other in the eye. I felt disloyal, compromised. As though I was attractive but my mother wasn't."

Though she hadn't "done anything wrong," a signal from "the world" had managed to put her at odds with her mother, to distance the two and cause tension and fighting to break out. Too bad they didn't feel comfortable talking directly about what had really happened.

The topics of beauty and age are taboo between most mothers and daughters, the social pressures are so intense—and painful. Fortunately a climate is growing in which women can more freely express admiration for each other's beauty—"young" or "old," traditional or original—can take pleasure in this beauty, rather than seeing it as a threat involving competition and rivalry.

Yet, all too many daughters find themselves feeling a mixture of shame and pride for being seen as "prettier" than their mother (while mothers feel under pressure to dress "less pretty," "not act too young"—"Don't be feminine and flirtatious, lest people laugh at you,"—cut their hair, and so on), so that the situation escalates: while girls feel shame and resentment (for the unchangeable situation), mothers feel jealous of and irritated with their daughters, yet guilty and self-blaming for these feelings.

Based on my research, I believe that "beauty" rivalry is just a symptom of why mothers and daughters fly apart, the exterior wrapping of an alienation between them that starts earlier. Both mother and daughter can happily and easily overcome their feelings of resentment by understanding this deeper layer, even when years of "trying to be reasonable and understanding" have not succeeded.

The estrangement begins, in my analysis, with early sexual taboos between the mother and daughter. Although mothers know a lot about sexuality, they usually don't really share much of this information with their daughters. Sexuality seems to children to be the mother's privilege and secret, something they should not ask too much about. For example, mothers have interesting underwear (different from a young daughter's), do private things in the bathroom, stay up late, sleep with another adult—they have a whole area of life that is hidden. Each girl wants to share this adult mystery—wear female perfume, shoes, lipstick, and "do the same things in the bathroom."

Most daughters feel uneasy: they learn that they cannot discuss matters sexual (or even anatomical) with their mothers—that is, at least they cannot know what the mother experiences; most girls also know that they themselves have sexual feelings.

What a pity that under the family system we have, most girls feel guilty and ashamed about their sexual feelings. Most quickly learn not even to wonder if their own mother masturbates—for if she did, wouldn't she have told her daughter? And if not, WHY not?

Many girls wind up feeling paralyzed. The block between them and their mothers about acknowledging the body and sexual feelings—just because some mothers say "Ask me anything," or "Feel free to talk to me whenever you want about whatever is troubling you" doesn't mean there is real freedom for a two-way dialogue—creates a strange barrier between them, which casts a pall over the rest of their relationship. The daughter feels the mother *could* tell her, *could* help her, *could* give her information, but she doesn't trust the daughter enough, doesn't see her as a full person with full rights. She feels that her mother is hypocritical, perhaps even stupid. ("Doesn't my mother have sexual feelings? Doesn't she know about orgasm? Does she live on another planet??")

While mothers think they are doing the right thing, very young daughters, finding that they cannot pierce the mother's veil of secrecy (and should certainly not try to touch her!) feel shut out and rejected. And, each daughter wonders, "Why is she closing me off this way?"

Since sex in most families is hidden, girls grow up developing their sexuality as a secret self. Most daughters, as a result of the mother's silence and guarding of her sexual knowledge, are left believing that when she does act or feel sexual, she may be disobedient, "wild" or "rebellious." She may feel reassured when she meets boys and men who will, at least in some ways, give her "permission" to be a sexual being and share their own sexual information. Thus most girls develop a "good girl" persona for the home, and a more secret "I'm really sexy" persona for other situations—even today reinforcing the old double-standard mind-body separation in women.

This double-standard idea is reinforced by the mother's (and father's) attitudes. Again: why can't a mother show a daughter her vulva, why "must" it be hidden? If boys see their fathers' penises, this familiarity gives them a sense of normalcy and self-acceptance. Why not girls? After all, their reproductive organs are the same as those of their mothers; they need to know (and see) more about the adult female body, but the mother believes that she shouldn't talk about those experiences she herself has had—and definitely should not show her vulva to her daughter! She believes she should teach her daughter to be modest. Thus, both daughter and mother wind up being terrified of seeing each other's bodies, being "too intimate."

While there is some cultural acknowledgment that boys might see their mothers as erotic (Oedipus is "normal," in the sense that "normal men desire women"—though not, supposedly, their mothers), or notice that she is erotic to men her own age, there is little understanding that there could also be an erotic recognition and appreciation between mothers and daughters. Mothers and daughters are not supposed to "see" the sexual side of each other. This part of their identity is supposed to be invisible, visible only to men. Of course the result is that both women must pretend, deny to each other and themselves that they "see" or notice that part of the other. Feeling uncomfortable, they live with a lurking sense of dishonesty and distrust of each other.

Does this mean that in order to feel closer, daughters and mothers have to become "sexual," be "lovers"? No, it simply means that they have the right to relate as complete and honest friends and companions. It is possible to have an appreciation of someone else's sexual beauty without acting on it or denying it to oneself.

The rift or problem that occurs between mothers and daughters is not inevitable. It does not arise "because women are natural competitors" but because mothers and daughters are under the spell of the invisible handwriting that decrees that women must not form a deep-seated alliance (since that would "overthrow" the position of "the man" in "the family" and society); superficially, "women cannot share sexual secrets" or "mothers cannot tell daughters about their own sexuality." Alienation and distrust grow out of this situation, so that women learn to regard each other as competitors rather than primary relationships, as important as men.

If women's relationships as mothers and daughters were allowed to develop "naturally," would their bond lead to a different social order?

One of the biggest changes to come in the near future could be the reassessment by women of their relationships. Women have already radically changed their relationships with men; now they may be beginning to address their relationships with each other.

## GIRLS' AND BOYS' PSYCHOSEXUAL DEVELOPMENT IS DIFFERENT: SEEING THE PENIS BUT NOT THE VULVA

There is a basic fact of anatomy that Freud—and everyone else—has completely overlooked. This fact has probably created reverberations inside your mind that you may not be aware of, whether you are female or male.

The difference visually in terms of the male body and female body has a fundamental impact on how boys and girls (and we) grow up to see their bodies and sexuality, and define themselves psychosexually.

Its importance is so central and obvious that, once noticed, it is a wonder no one has commented on it previously; perhaps this mysterious silence originated because society considered it impolite to speak about sexual anatomy, especially in girls and women.

Specifically, boys have a different relationship with their bodies and "sex" because their anatomy puts them in daily contact with their "sexual organ," or penis. Boys need only look down, and they see their penis, since it is there on the front of their bodies. But girls cannot see their "sex" or genitals at all, without bending down in a very awkward position. Girls can feel their genitals, but they do not see them; furthermore, girls are instructed not to touch themselves intimately when wiping themselves in the toilet. They are inhibited from even trying to look at this part of their bodies, for example with a mirror (not to mention looking at another girl's) by a sotto-voce message that subliminally tells them that "nice girls don't look at it."

Boys in the course of normal life touch their penis when they urinate: they hold it and see it. They see the penises of other boys and men at the school public urinal or in the shower; boys' toilets at school, for example, or in train stations, are constructed openly, so that men normally see the penises of other men. In other words, the penis is not a "thing apart" or "strange" to men and boys. Boys grow up feeling comfortable with this part of their body.

Girls grow up feeling much more alienated (and even intimidated) by their own sexual anatomy. Many are even informed by their families that they should not use a tampon inside themselves until they are married . . . mysteriously. Thus, the only real way most girls and women have of knowing their own sexual vulva and vagina is through their first sexual experience with another person! Is it surprising then that women are much more likely to accept the comments that men and society make about "what it's like down there"? Men cannot be told a complicated mythology about the penis and how it functions that is not realistic, but women have few defenses or information built on such a long and daily personal acquaintance with their bodies, so that when they hear via social clichés that "it's dirty down there" or "looks bad," they have few quick retorts. These comments and clichés about their sexual bodies have a serious impact on most girls and women, making them feel much more ambiguous about sex than men.

Can men even imagine what it would be like if they had bodies in which they never saw their penis, if it were hidden behind them, for example, or inside them? Men should try to imagine what it must be like for a woman. A woman can almost "see" her clitoral area or pubic mound; that is where the hair begins to grow at puberty, and is at least an identifiable location visible when standing in front of a mirror undressed. But in order to see the vulva directly, not to mention the vaginal opening and inner lips of the vulva, a girl or woman must stand in front of a mirror and spread her legs in a highly uncomfortable position (hoping no one comes into the room at that moment) in order to catch a quick glimpse of at least the exterior portions of her anatomy. Men are used to seeing their penis erect, nonerect, and in various stages in between. This is not the case for women.

I hope that my pointing this out will be of help to people as they begin to rethink their ideas about "male sexuality" and "female sexuality." Female sexuality is not "dirty down there"; anyone who looks at the vulva will find astonishing pearly pink-beige flesh, perhaps more beautiful than the skin anywhere else on the body.

## THE REDEFINITION OF PUBERTY IN GIRLS

Somehow over the decades references to girls' "puberty" have gone unresearched, with few people noticing on what little information references are based.

Freud and others lumped together boys' and girls' development under the category "puberty"; however, closer examination in my research shows that this is a simplistic category that should be reviewed.

It seems doubtful that "puberty" is a valid category for girls at all. While most boys first masturbate to orgasm with ejaculation between the ages of ten to twelve, girls usually masturbate to orgasm much earlier, almost half starting by the ages of five to seven, according to my research. Puberty is not so much a time of "sexual awakening" for girls as a change in reproductive status. Freud among others incorrectly modeled his ideas of puberty in girls on his notions about boys.

Freudian theories regarding childhood dominated the thinking of the last century; it appears that Freud simply projected his view of how boys develop their sexuality into girls, imagining that "if boys cannot orgasm fully before puberty, neither can girls." As is well known, Freud was incorrect about many or most of his theories about girls and women, proposing such incorrect concepts as "penis envy" (to "describe" women's dissatisfaction with their suppression and inequality); proposing that girls should transfer their sexual feelings at puberty from the clitoris to the vagina to have "mature orgasm"; proposing that if boys love their mothers, they have an "Oedipus complex"—a remarkably negative way to view boys' love for their mothers; and other generally antifemale matters.

In fact, as my research surprisingly reveals, many of the changes seen in boys at puberty can be ascribed to cultural factors put in place by boys' fathers and other older boys at school, as well as television programs; boys go through a long period of inner turmoil over the issue of whether to "betray" their mothers, which society demands they do in order to join "the man's world"—although there is no real reason to force boys to make this choice. Thus my theory of "Oedipus Revisited" differs significantly from Freud's "Oedipus" theory.

Freud relied on a hypothetical biology (less informed than that available to his contemporaries in other countries, such as France) to prop up his theories about female sexuality; in reality his theories were actually ("unconsciously") modeled on preexisting social institutions, as various scholarly books have demonstrated. Viewing various social institutions as "biological" (thus "universal" and "eternal") enabled him to imply that his theories were true for all people in all cultures and historical periods. While it is true that sexuality plays a more central role than had previously been accepted "scientifically," and that we must thank Freud for pointing this out, his further interpretations of how the sexual dynamic operates were filled with damaging cultural clichés and assumptions.

The picture of psychosexual development that has emerged from my research demands a rethinking of the whole shape and thrust of how we see children's and our own psychosexual identities. Listening to testimonies from thousands of girls and boys, as well as women and men remembering how they grew up, a new map of childhood development emerges, illuminating inner turning points not recognized before.

Girls may experience a turning point significant for them during their first orgasm—a turning point that is as significant for them as the (usually) later changes they experience in their body's reproductive capacity and physiology (such as the growth of breasts, body hair, and monthly vaginal bleeding or menstruation).

My research would indicate that girls have a reproductive puberty, not a sexual puberty (or "sexual awakening"), since they can masturbate to full orgasm many years before puberty. Just as women can orgasm perfectly well after "menopause" (the end of reproductive ability), just so girls can masturbate and orgasm frequently before supposed "puberty" (the onset of reproductive ability). Female "sexuality" in terms of orgasmic pleasure and excitement is not linked to reproductive sexuality in women.

Girls in fact are forced to develop a split identity growing up, as their sexual feelings (and even later their reproductive changes, such as the onset of menstruation) are not positively acknowledged or welcomed into the society (menstruation, for example, is not celebrated in most countries with a family party congratulating the girl). Via this silence, girls are subliminally "informed" that they should be ashamed of their blood (via the way in which their first menstruation is hushed up in the family). Thus when most girls do begin menstruating, they absorb negative messages about it from the culture around them: it should be hidden, people should not know, no one should talk about it or refer to it, the father "doesn't need to know" (most fathers are not told when their daughter begins menstruating), the blood is "dirty" and "smells bad," a girl should "try to keep clean"—especially boys should not know: "It is embarrassing for boys and men."

Girls also absorb from the society around them the message that girls are less welcome into the world altogether than boys. On birth the joyful exclamation "It's a boy!" is heard much more often than a shout, "It's a girl!" International agencies point out that many infant girls are killed or "left to die" at birth because a boy is preferred; in some parts of the world today there is a marked statistical tilt increasing the number of adult males. Whereas usually around the world the proportion of females to males is 51 percent to 49 percent, in at least one large country (China) it is now 46 percent to 54 percent—what happened to the missing percentage?*

Furthermore, in the society's icons of the traditional family—Mary, Jesus and Joseph—there is no daughter. Girls today love to read books such as *Little Women* and *Alice in Wonderland*, watch the Disney film of *Cinderella*, because these provide rare

---

* The shortage of women in China is well-known and well-documented. Due to China's "one-child policy," many couples abort their female offspring, or allow them to die, in favor of trying again for a male offspring.

chances to see a young female heroine in action. This may also be one reason why the young-woman doll Barbie is so popular. (Other "dolls" are generally infants, which girls are expected to hold in their arms "like a real baby," not teenage "role models.")

Society would benefit from rethinking its view of girls and recognizing in a positive way that girls are developing their sexual identities much earlier than most parents believe.

## THE NEW ALICE: IF JESUS HAD HAD A SISTER

It is odd that there is no daughter in the Christian holy family. The Holy Family is composed of Mary, Jesus, and Joseph. This, the model on which we in the West are supposed to build our lives, has left girls in an awkward position. Who were they supposed to be?

Lurking in the background of our culture was the character of Eve, the unmarried girl-woman who, by being sexual, supposedly caused the downfall of "mankind."

Thinking about *Alice in Wonderland*, I nominate Alice for iconic status, along with other questioning youths in our psychological pantheon. It seems to me that Alice, with her intelligent irreverence for a (from her point of view) topsy-turvey world, is an apt archetype for the identity of girls at puberty

Were all the little Alices of this world supposed to identify with her? Is this why single women are constantly being asked, "Are you married yet, dear? And do you have any children?" Only when Alice becomes a mother, "Maria," can she stop being questioned about her identity.

Freud's naming of young men as "Oedipus," facing heroic struggles, follows along the Holy Family model, in that the son is seen as a great protagonist, dealing with serious issues, worthy of notice. Yet Freud's naming of girls "Electra" was not successful. In fact, most of his theories about women have turned out, with time, to be false; Freud understood very little about women. For example, one of his now-disproven theories was that at puberty girls should change the stimulation they need for orgasm from the clitoris to the vagina.

Similarly, he seems to have believed that girls have puberty in the same way that boys do. Somehow I had also assumed it to be true. However, my own research now indicates something entirely different.

While girls may have what we could call reproductive puberty, they do not usually have puberty in the sense that boys do—that is, a sexual awakening. Most girls can orgasm completely long before they are able to reproduce, through self-stimulation.

Many parents tell me they have noticed their small daughters masturbating and had to tell them, "Please don't do that, or only do it in your own room." The implications for psychological revision are startling. This suggests a history of childhood that is totally different from Freud's. Girls reaching puberty lack an Oedipus figure to give guidance; they need an alternative.

In other ways, too, as Alice could tell you, girls are seen through a distorting lens by much of psychological theory. Girls are given few or no models of girlhood or young womanhood; the only proper role for females, it would seem, is to "grow up" and become "full women" by getting married and becoming mothers, performing motherly functions; heroic activities are slated, still today, for boys' futures.

There are many examples of boy heroes, young unmarried men as important protagonists: neither Jesus Christ nor James Dean had to get married to "prove himself." Yet when young women are active or challenge authority, they are often labeled "angry," "neurotic" or "maladjusted"; conversely, if they are loyal and "serving," they can be labeled "masochistic," even "self-destructive."

I propose a more positive, new idea: Alice. With her intelligence and clear-eyed questions and observations about the status quo and its rules and regulations, she speaks for many girls.

It is unfortunate that traditional psychology presents the family as a biological given, rather than a political or social institution, with pros and cons—an institution one can choose or not.

The traditional view has allowed the "family" to assume the proportions of a sacred, mythological, never changing reality ("biology"), putting the burden on the individual to "adjust" to the institution, rather than allowing individuals to build flexible families of all kinds that suit them. The overly rigid family system causes problems for both boys and girls, perhaps particularly for girls.

Sexuality is an integral part of the personal identity that girls must try, in this not-so-friendly-to-them context, to formulate. This is made harder by its being denied or silenced, not "seen"—or, as noted, frequently declared "bad." One thinks of the oft-repeated maxim, "Good girls keep their legs together."

The symbol of society's denial and negativity toward female sexuality is the silence and gloom surrounding menstruation. Even today there is, at the onset of girl's menstruation, generally no thought of giving her a celebration or a special dinner to welcome her into a new phase of her life and celebrate the changes going on in her body In very few families is the father even informed. A celebration would do much to alter the negative atmosphere that has hung over female sexual identity for centuries, an atmosphere that has labeled menstruation "the curse," female sexual feelings "wicked," and sexual appearance in women as "cheap" and "whorish."

There should be a new movement of support and respect for girls to take pride in their bodies and their sexuality—in a different style than that we have seen so far with either Madonna or the Spice Girls.

## WHAT IS "THE HYMEN" AND FEMALE VIRGINITY?: IS THE "FIRST TIME" LIKE GIRLS IMAGINE?

*I loved dating. I loved showing off my boyfriends. I only dated hunks. My first kiss was sweet and tender, I remember it vividly. I was 14. The first time I made out with a boy, I was 15. He was very aggressive and horny. I remember feeling so horny myself! I loved all of that time, the touching, the kissing, the air of suspense and possibility: what will we do? My body was just ready for it all, I was so turned on.*

When girls imagine their first sexual encounter, they dream of it with great pleasure. Many girls base this fantasy on their experience of "petting" and erotic affection, although later it may turn out that they find "petting" more pleasurable and exciting than coitus.

Most girls, even today, go into their first experience of intercourse, thinking that they should have "more pleasure than they've ever had," that the pleasure should be much greater than during "just petting" or masturbation. But they are often used to having orgasms during these activities and are shocked when they do not have orgasms easily during coitus—and find the feelings different from the clear-cut orgasms they are used to.

*The Hite Report on Female Sexuality* first demonstrated that it is not the "norm" for women to orgasm from simple coitus, but rather from exterior or clitoral stimulation—and that this stimulation should become a standard part of sex. The Report also showed that many women were faking orgasms during intercourse, feeling terribly guilty and "abnormal" if they did not have them, never daring to tell their partner, but instead going into the bathroom to masturbate privately for orgasm after sex.

With the continued depiction of women in videos and movies as "coming" from intercourse, in the same way and (often) at the same time as men, the reality of most women's need for clitoral stimulation to orgasm has begun to be obscured, and girls (who have little information from their mothers and rely mostly on magazines, films, and their sexual partners) are again having to go through sometimes several years of experimentation and worry before feeling confident and comfortable with their bodies' way of having orgasm (usually not from intercourse, but from some form of clitoral stimulation).

My research demonstrates, quite surprisingly, that most girls do not experience pain or bleeding on first coitus; the percentage of those who do is quite low. In fact, even more surprisingly, it may not be anatomically "normal" for girls to have a painful-to-break hymen. Those who are "supposed" to know—gynecologists and pediatricians—in fact have no particular expertise in this area, since (1) gynecologists usually do not see very young girls, and (2) pediatricians usually don't do in-depth or detailed vaginal examinations. Therefore, is the assumption that "normal girls" have hymens simply based on hearsay or "learned" in medical textbooks? On what body of knowledge and investigation, if any, are these texts based? According to my research, only 18 percent of women felt any painful tearing or saw any blood on first intercourse or at any time earlier in their lives. This fact would imply that a belief in the prevalence of a full hymen in girls is a myth, and a dangerous one at that, especially for women in cultures that punish women if they are not virgins on marriage.

We may be doing a great disservice to girls and their families, causing them needless worry over this question, by letting this assumption continue unchallenged. In the worst-case scenario, it can cause parents to take their daughters to doctors to be "checked" and "sewn up" before marriage, especially in cultures where hymens are a fetish.

Many men (husbands and boyfriends, or gynecologists) simply assume that if the woman or girl has no hymen, she "must have done it," or has "fallen off her bicycle," or they may admit, "Well of course, there are variations in human anatomy."

Doctors should inform parents and girls themselves that, while some girls may experience bleeding, this is not by far the "average" case; most girls do not. Sex education and information for girls and boys should be taken seriously. It will improve their relationships as they grow and mature.

## WHEN DO GIRLS BECOME SEXUAL?

Most girls begin masturbating quite early, and many before puberty, according to my research; 45 percent of girls begin masturbating by the age of seven, and over 60 percent by the age of twelve. I am unaware of any other large-scale study addressing this question, remarkable as that may be.

Girls almost always discover masturbation alone, by themselves, secretly. A few girls try masturbation because they have heard it is possible, but far more commonly, they simply discover it by listening to their bodies or finding one day that something they do feels very good.

The downside is that so many girls learn to associate shame and guilt with touching themselves and with sex in general. Feeling guilty for feeling pleasure . . . all too often, the messages become inextricably intertwined. Later the guilt and "danger" can become part of the fun.

According to my research, while almost 60 percent of boys in my sample have masturbated in the presence of another boy, only about 9 percent of girls have done so. The beginning of menstruation could be a magical and fascinating moment in a girl's life. Instead there is a kind of hush-hush atmosphere, a denial and hiding. Seventy-two percent of girls and women report that they feel inadequately prepared for this event, so minimal is the discussion, even today. Only 12 percent of fathers discuss menstruation with their daughters. Not even 10 percent of girls are given a celebration to mark the occasion.

It would seem that girls are not supposed to feel any pride in their maturing adulthood and bodies. In some more "liberated" families there is a reaction as, "Well, it's normal and healthy, so what? Don't let's get carried away and make a big deal out of it." The family should clearly recognize the daughter's body as good. Instead, the onset of puberty and menstruation are greeted with the cry, "Be a good girl," according to 97 percent of those I studied. In other words, parents become preoccupied with restraining the daughter sexually, often wanting to make sure that she remains a "virgin."

Wrote one respondent: "'Be a good girl' was like a religious chant in my house. It meant to be whatever they wanted me to be at the time. It meant be a little Christian, be virginal, be obedient, be passive, be a little mother to my dolls, be a cook, be a homemaker." Anger and any sign of rebelliousness are definitely not a part of "femininity," although rebel boys are often praised and received with respect. While "boys will be boys," girls must not "throw tantrums," must not "dress like a prostitute," must not go out and "make a spectacle of themselves," and so on.

Most mothers and fathers participate heavily in this genderizing system, but they do so frequently in covert ways that they do not fully recognize. Like mothers and fathers in Africa who force clitoridectomy on their daughters, these Western parents truly believe that they are doing their best to bring up a proper, charming, and socially acceptable individual. Girls who fight back are simply termed "rebellious," and (the parents believe) need even more to "be tamed." As one daughter describes: "My family's—and especially my mother's—depiction of me was always as someone who had a 'wild temper,' someone who was 'likely to explode,' and they used to rag me about it. I don't think it was true." How mothers and fathers deal with daughters' sexuality and desire for "freedom," is very troubling.

Thousands of little flowers should be blooming, but instead girls are still raised to have complexes about their bodies—complexes all too clear when schools today have to worry about girls becoming anorexic and tending to bulimia. Fortunately countercurrents are surfacing, and we see new kinds of young women growing up proud of their bodies, becoming Olympic gold-medal athletes and sexual pioneers.

## SPANKING: THE ROOTS OF SEXUAL MASOCHISM?

For many children, especially after about the age of five or six, the only intimate physical contact they have with anyone is with their parents when they are punished: when the parent actually lays hands on and takes physical power over the child's body, touching it and moving it about in some way. At the same time the parent is usually showing a (gratifying?) degree of emotional agitation, passion, and involvement.

When asked, "Did your parents touch and cuddle you?" many people answer, remembering back, "No—only through spanking."

The majority of children have been hit only once or twice, as this girl describes: "Apparently I was just about a model child. I was only hit once in my life. I was about four and ran out in a parking lot and narrowly escaped getting wiped out by a car. My mother spanked me for that." Infrequent and relatively nonbrutal spankings such as this are less traumatic than are repeated violent abusive eruptions, often premeditated, as other people describe. But almost all spankings are still very much remembered.

Girls and boys are struck with equal frequency, according to my research, but in different ways. Girls tend to be punished by the mother, usually in a more spontaneous "slapping" or hitting way. If a father punishes a daughter, this act is more likely to be nonspontaneous ("Go to your room and wait for your punishment there") and to involve spanking or lashing with a belt on the buttocks.

A father's punishment is usually more severe and more feared; he seems bigger, more overwhelming and frightening, his authority more unquestionable. It is much more frequently fathers who strike boys, although the fear is always there for girls too, in such warnings as, "Wait until your father hears about this!"

"I was very young, maybe six, when I first masturbated to orgasm," one woman in my research wrote, "It was on my own, with a lot of guilt. Until I was twelve, I fantasized about being spanked while masturbating, rubbing against a pillow. Then I stopped feeling guilty and used my fingers. At the same time, I stopped fantasizing about being spanked."

Another reported: "We used to play house. I was the mummy and my brother was the daddy. I would fix dinner and then we would do dishes. Mummy would complain that Daddy wasn't putting the dishes away. He would say, 'If Mummy isn't nice, I'm going to have to spank Mummy.' Then he would put me over his knee and spank me. I wouldn't cry during the spanking (it didn't hurt), then we would say, 'OK, now it's time for bed,' and lie down together (on the floor or ground) as if we were in Mummy and Daddy's bed, to go to sleep. I wonder if we wondered what they did there."

Spanking and beating give a strong unspoken message connecting power, violence, and sexuality. Spanking especially is an invasive "sexual" experience that defines the child's body and connects the buttocks and genitals with violence and sometimes pleasure.

The aim of physical punishment, according to many child-care books, is to break the child's will: the child must learn to obey unquestioningly. This effect is more important than actual physical pain. Thus, to be most effective, the event must be set up in advance—say, fifteen minutes or so,—during which time the child is told to "wait" in his or her room for the spanking. After the event, the child "should ask to be forgiven," thus reinforcing the "deservedness" of the punishment.

These are also basic elements of sadomasochistic activity. The teaching of these connections between power and genitals often creates a strong love-hate, fear-intimacy bond with the abusive parent or person. It has been suggested that sadomasochistic sex may be a way for some people to reenact these scenes (emotionally and psychologically reexperience them) but make them come out with a different end result.

Other interpretations of sadomasochistic sexuality stress that such activity is not "harmless" or (even less) "therapeutic" in any way; it merely demonstrates how deeply people have been imprinted with horribly deformed definitions of "love" as hate, fear, and submission—or aggression and control—and so can only "love" in this way. In particular, it is notable that in heterosexual sadomasochistic pornography it is almost always the woman who is made to experience pain and domination of her body. Sadomasochism is a statement about the power relationship between men and women, and sometimes an incitement to men to abuse women. Yet its erotic appeal in our culture cannot be denied.

How exactly might the connections be made in the child's mind between the parents' power, the private violent invasion of the body, the "rule" that the child cannot resist or fight back—and possible simultaneous sexual stimulation? When a child is hit on the buttocks, blood rushes to the area, causing a tingling in the genitals. Girls, according to my research, seem slightly more likely to be hit on the buttocks, while boys are hit on the back, or the back of the legs. More of girls' sexual anatomy is exposed in the bent-over position than is boys'; although the scrotum is vulnerable in such a position, the penis remains in the front of the body, while the vaginal opening, toward the back of the vulva, is nearer the buttocks and nearer the blood-flow brought on by the blows.

This kind of violent touch can be sexualized in the child's mind, not only because of a real flow of blood into the genitalia, but also because of a longing for intimacy with the parent: if painful physical touch is the only fulfillment of that longing, then this can "feel good."

This is a problem in many countries. Five European countries—Sweden (1979), Finland (1983), Denmark (1985), Norway (1987) and Austria (1989)—have outlawed the physical punishment of children, and other countries have organizations working toward legislation.

In these situations, children are generally forbidden to act/react appropriately and effectively to defend themselves from assault and invasion. Indeed, if they try to defend themselves or fight back, the punishment may be more severe, they are told. The "best thing" for them is to submit. Thus the association of love, fear, and pain begins early and remain embedded in the unconscious mind for life, unless it is removed.

According to author Philip Greven, citing sociologist Alice Miller, "Spanking, whippings and beatings are the painful origins of much adult sadomasochism. The astonishing absence of studies of sadomasochism in our history and culture is evidence of the denial that most people experience concerning the long-term consequences of physical punishments both for the psyche and sexuality. It is the early fusion of pain and love and the eroticization of coercion through the assaults upon the body and the anus that often shape the creation of sadomasochistic feelings, fantasies and behaviors in adults."

If spanking and physical punishment are widespread in a society, it is logical that sadomasochism will also be. It may not be an aberration; it can be inherent in any culture in which children suffer from painful physical punishments and humiliation that come from more powerful authorities.

## GIRLS AND THEIR MOTHERS: ADORATION AND CONTEMPT[6]

*I don't want to be like my mother.*

Daughters often reserve their strongest emotions for their mothers.

> *I felt secure in knowing my mother loved me beyond all else; I believed she even loved me more than she loved my father, my sister or even herself. I thought she was the most beautiful mother in the world.*

> *I admire strong women, intelligent women, independent women. My mother was a wimp.*

> *A perpetual sense of guilt, that's what I feel about my mother.*

> *The woman I have loved the most in my life is my Mum. She is supportive—strong, intelligent, beautiful and creative. She taught me everything from how to make cookies to inspiring me to have a career. My mother is the greatest woman I have ever known. She did everything for me I ever needed. I can only hope to become half the woman she is.*

When I began investigating mother-daughter relationships in the 1970s, I found a large number of girls and young women absolutely despising their mother, yet all thinking that they were individually and uniquely reaching this conclusion about "her."

Today a majority of young women describe positive feelings for and experiences with their mother, even though they still have a large number of complaints. Fights are by no means a thing of the past, nor are feelings of conflict, nor is the old saying, "I hope I'm not like my mother." But there is definite, palpable change.

Though things are changing between mothers and daughters, still most daughters react almost with horror when asked the question, "Do you want to be like your mother?"

> *If I grow up to be like my mother, I'll put a gun to my head.*

Women of varied social classes, races and backgrounds vehemently state that they don't want to be like their mothers. Why? Explained one respondent: "I am afraid of being anything like her, even to the point of hating myself for looking similar to her. I hate the thought of old age because I think I will get to look more and more like her. Psychologically, I am working to separate from her upbringing of me and find my own identity."

What is this fear we have of being like our mother? Is it really that we don't want to be like her or look like her—or is it fear of being "one of those women," second-class, not important, not counting? Of developing subservient behavior? Or is it fear of being considered "unattractive" and "old"? Or all of these? After all, mothers are frequently the butt of jokes, depicted as "nagging," being no fun and too "demanding."

Many girls and women muse over how much they *are* like their mother: "In many ways I am very much like her. I worry about things like she does, and like her, I try much too often to please everyone." Another remembered, "I didn't like it when my Mum tolerated stupid people or went along with things they said. I worry when I see myself now being a mirror of this sometimes."

The relationship that is most necessary to disrupt and destroy in patriarchy (the social order that is now dissolving) is that between mother and daughter. Any natural feelings of bonding, physical closeness or desire, love, had to be stamped out, forbidden, lest women become "too strong" through a belief and trust in each other. Thus, through centuries of indoctrination women arrived at the place where they now would consider it "unnatural" and unlikely that daughters would ever be emotionally or sensually attracted to their mother. Or vice versa.

Yet it was considered "normal" that fathers and daughters would at least notice each other sexually. The separation of mothers and daughters was in part enforced by "jokes" and allusions to the dreaded taboo, "lesbianism."

If daughters grow up to see mothers as number-one figures, as powerful as men, society will change enormously.

## TEENAGE GIRLS WITH THEIR BEST FRIENDS

Fortunately most girls have a "best friend" in whom they can confide. As one respondent put it: "We talk on the phone every day for hours, about everything. Some of our most open talks are at 3 am. We spend hours on the phone or out on the beach under the sun, especially when the guys are there. We also have lots of fun roller-skating. We discuss how to ask a guy to wear a condom and how to get out of taking drugs guys offer us without looking uncool."

Another reported: "My best friend was even closer to me than my boyfriend. We talked every night on the phone about guys, sex, and being fat—although we weren't fat! We baked cookies at least three times a week and gossiped over the bowl of dough. We were inseparable: we snow-mobiled, skied, swam, explored the woods, drove, sunbathed and got drunk together (when we had a crisis, like flunked an exam, dented the car, had to make a trip to the dentist). It was wonderful."

Most girls, describing their relationship with their best friend, explain that with her they feel important, self-confident, and able to express themselves fully—express themselves more than at any other time.

Of course girls' friendships are not always a bed of roses. Sometimes there can be painful betrayals and break-ups, but at other times there is a gentle drifting apart—that is, when one or both of the girls feel subtle pressure to choose between a "boyfriend" and the "best friend." Why is it necessary to make a choice?

It is notable that many of the things girls enjoy doing with their best friends are pleasurable because they are very sensual. This includes trying on clothes together and looking at each other in them, sewing clothes together and talking about where they will wear them, sampling make-up and putting make-up on each other, fixing each other's hair, talking about their "weight" (their bodies), and their skin—almost the same things that their mothers often enjoy doing with them during the years of close physical intimacy of late childhood.

These are some of the few ways women are "allowed" to touch each other by a society that is terrified that women might "like each other too much."

In their friendships, it could be said that girls, in a way, share even sensuality and eroticism—that is, girls together can share vicarious sex by discussing their dates, how it felt to kiss and touch a boy, how it felt when he touched them or explored their body ("how far"), what he said and how they felt.

As one girl describes it: "It was a wonderful time when I first began getting attention from boys. I was very happy. My friends and I spent hours talking about clothes, experimenting with make-up and going places where we knew we'd see boys. . . . Those were my favorite relationships. I'm always trying to get one back."

Should girls break off their friendships with their best friends in order to focus on boys? The assumption is that "mature" women should turn their allegiance and love toward men exclusively. Yet why should women break off these marvelous relationships with each other?

My research suggests that there is no specific "heterosexual sex drive" that asserts itself at "puberty" separately from the strong social pressures to direct one's sexual feelings in that direction. Many times this pressure has a happy result: it is not that these feelings are false or "bad," rather that they are a response to social demands—sexuality is being directed in a certain way. It could be more fluid; if we were living in a different "social order," it very well might be.

My research demonstrates that there are a multitude of affections, sensualities, and personas latent in almost all children and adults, but that to fit the social system, these feelings are directed and channeled, especially at "puberty," to fit the patriarchal (father-ownership) model of the family and society. In psychological terms this channeling means that all eyes must be trained to focus on the male; all emotional, psychological, and sexual attention must be fixed on the father, with one exception: boys must be made to see girls as sexual (and reproductive) objects of desire. Girls "cannot," therefore, put each other first any longer.

Statistically it is quite rare for girls as best friends to become lovers, while it is relatively common for teenage boys. One young woman describes having had a sexual relationship with her best friend: "I had a best friendship in high school which turned into a sexual relationship and lasted about two years. Over the years, we have managed to keep in touch on rare occasions. She is a lesbian, and I am not. At one time, this part of my past disturbed me a great deal, but now I consider it a fairly usual, but private, part of growing up."

We have seen that the great majority of teenage girls have a best friend with whom they share their feelings, experiences, and plans for the future. Although it is a small minority who have a physical, sexual relationship, these are usually very loving friendships that can mean a lot to the girls involved.

## IS SEX BY DEFINITION "IMPURE"?[7] ARE GIRLS "IMPURE" AFTER PUBERTY?

"Sex is dirty" we are told. Words for sex, "four letter words," are often also used as swear words, including "cunt," "cock-sucker," "jerk," and "slut." Sexual love has long been considered impure, while traditionally "real love," family love (seemingly asexual), is seen as better. People claim that, "sexual love is lust, an "animal feeling" that will not last, that is not as worthwhile as "the other kind of love," which is "more noble, more pure."

There is an idea that runs through Christian culture, as well as through Islamic culture (they are, after all, branches of the same tradition), that female sexuality is "dirty," that women who are sexual may be "linked to the devil," "temptresses" of men, not expressing their own desires and feelings! In fact, "male sexuality" is also seen as "bestial"; one popular euphemism is critical of a man because "he thinks with his dick." This metaphor means that his thinking is influenced by his sexual urges—therefore he is not rational. Not only is the sexual body seen as stupid and animallike, it is also "impure" (it confuses and "tempts" the mind into irrationality and the spirit into impurity). In fundamentalist Judaism, women were and are required to take a ceremonial cleansing bath, a *mikvah*, after each menstruation, before being allowed to have coitus again with their mate. To view mind and body as separate in this way, to posit this basic bipolar idea, is the source of much of our inability as a society to cope with the AIDS epidemic, for example, but these views were not always historically present. The concept of "impurity" has been used as a way of marginalizing women and making many men fear "female sexuality" and the vulva.

Purity is now, in this age of back to basics, increasingly a focus. Traditionally "purity" has been seen as "close to god," using the mind and spirit while denying the body, "things of the flesh." Spending time on sex is/was considered "sinful" and "polluting." Having a lot of sex (especially nonreproductive sex, anything other than coitus, for example oral sex) "sullies" the person who "indulges" in it. People should try to resist "the sins of the flesh," "carnal desire," in order to remain "pure," according to this view. Or "rational" in the twentieth-century version.

In some ways the Western view of sex—though the West is certain that today it is the model of openness and "tolerance" (even "going too far," many feel)—is not dissimilar to views held by fundamentalists in parts of the Islamic world, where female sexuality is seen as "impurity" and that therefore women should be covered. While the West may "tolerate" miniskirts in the young, it is generally believed that "serious business women" should not wear them, nor probably "somebody's mother." (This is not to say that miniskirts equal sexual freedom; read on.)

## SEX, PURITY, AND THE FAMILY

Most people grow up with parents who do not betray any trace of sexual emotion or physical passion in front of "the children" or others; parents usually do not speak to others, even family members, of their orgasms! They behave as if they do not have sex together. Thus people learn that sexuality is not a part of proper society or family/home, that if we really want to get "sexy," we should "find someplace else to do it," "get a motel room" or do the deed behind closed doors and never refer to it.

Why this negativity? There are many kinds of love, most of them good, including sexually passionate love; however, we are warned over and over again "not to confuse sex with love," not to let sex take control of our thinking or "let sex get the better of us." We are told that ecstatic feelings during sex are not ecstatic but base lust, desire is "animal," "not on a higher plane." The social order, it would seem, wants us to believe that sexual pleasure is a lesser form of experience than is spiritual meditation, that our bodies are less important than our minds. Is this "wisdom" true? Or are they linked (would they be linked easily for us, without the imposition of a bipolar ideology) physically, mentally, and emotionally?

Scholars have puzzled over the origins of the idea that sexuality is "impure" for decades, never finding the answer. Many today believe an idea such as sexual impurity to be out of date, yet many still unconsciously continue to believe remnants of it. For example, no government in the world speaks out against the imprisonment of the entire female population of countries such as Saudi Arabia, which uses sexual clichés (claiming they are "religious") to claim that this repression "protects women," ensuring that their society remains "spiritual" as part of their "religious tradition" (yet if men were forced by an all-female government to wear black and cover themselves from head to toe, were not given education or jobs, would people consider this way of life "religious"?). In other words, such societies seek to claim and "justify" their actions as part of "religious purity" and "custom." People in other countries would be wrong to accept this "explanation," since these are not cultural matters: they are the persecution of women. The West, on one level believing that sexy miniskirts are "impure" ("You wouldn't expect a woman to wear one to church, would you?"), shows a misplaced respect for the politics of governments that repress women.

The prejudice that claims spending time on sex is not as "legitimate" or worthy as focusing attention on the soul or mind is part of the Christian Virgin-birth worshiping belief system, which decrees that the saints are "pure" because they "denied the flesh," didn't "indulge" in the "pleasures of the body." The Christian tradition falsely sets up an opposition between love felt in the body and spiritual love, insisting that "love" in its best form must be asexual ("beyond animal lust"), focused primarily on "unselfishly" taking care of another (that is, spiritual love, as it is called in our limited vocabulary) or on God, the most abstract love. Today, we continue to think that love is most "pure" when it is "above the sexual urge": a mother's love, for example, is more "pure" than a single woman's love for a man that includes sex.

This vast oversimplification has created a sea of troubles, leaving many of our feelings either invisible, unexplained, or declared illegitimate. Love, including intense sexual intimacy and experimentation, is a pure and spiritual experience for many—perhaps most—people.

## ICONS OF THE HEART: DEMOCRATIZATION OF THE FAMILY[8]

One constantly hears that "the family" is in trouble, that it doesn't work anymore, and that we must find ways to help it. That we must "preserve family values." But let's look closely at these seemingly obvious statements.

If "the family" doesn't work, what does this statement mean? If the family doesn't work, maybe there is something wrong with its structure. Why assume that humans are flawed and that the family structure is fine and good?

We see constant headlines in the press such as "Divorce Statistics on the Rise," or, "Alarming New Statistics on Children Suffering Abuse," or "Battering and Violence Against Women in the Home." Many conclude that these statistics reflect "the breakdown not only of family but also of society and civilization" and that if we would only put "the family" back together we would end all our problems, and "once again" have a peaceful and prosperous, perfectly harmonious society.

Yet, is this belief true? Statistics on violence in the home were not gathered during the supposedly blissful 1950s, that golden age of the nuclear family. Society preferred to push its "personal problems" under the rug or send them to the psychiatrist's couch. Today if people are leaving the traditional family, as the statistics seem to imply—whether through divorce or changing the composition of the family, the style of family life—who are we to say that they are making "the wrong decisions"?

People today are concerned about the quality of their marriage or personal partnership. Rightly, they want to live in a way that makes them happy and makes others around them happy as well. They want acceptance from the society around them, but at the same time they want their relationships to reflect qualities they can be proud of, such as honesty, equality, and mutual respect.

Today people are creating a social revolution by applying the ideas of democracy and justice to their private lives. Many people are torn in their personal lives between doing "what they should do" and what they feel is right—between following the form of "family" and appearing "normal" and gravitating to the relationships that are working for them.

I believe that this conflict inside people today is caused by the ideas of democracy and justice, so praised in public life and government for the last two hundred years, now penetrating people's consciousness about their personal lives; not only do people feel that they have the right to think for themselves about voting and decide whom they elect to government, but that they also have the right to decide the shape of their personal lives.

"The family"—that is, human love and support systems for raising children—is not in danger of collapsing; what is happening is that finally democracy is catching up with the old hierarchical father-dominated family, that the family is being democratized. We are all, most of us, taking part in the process: almost no one wants to go back to the days before women had (at least in theory) equal rights in the home, before there were laws against the battering of women (who are no longer property, but individuals with their own inherent rights), before the freedom for men and women to divorce if they can no longer form a loving unit with the other person . . . all these things are advances over the old "traditional family."

And yet, current "back to family values" reactionary rhetoric strives to end this positive development. "Traditional values" hype attempts to legitimize women's old status as "servers" by romantically labeling it "family values," while denigrating the gains women have made, improvements in the family which clearly also benefit men and children.

What we must decide is whether the "family," as traditionally defined, is in deep trouble—or whether we are in a productive process of change, a process of democratizing and revolutionizing the family for the better.

I believe that the statistics showing the extent of battering, domestic violence, and children suffering abuse, for example, reflect, not the moral breakdown of family and society, but society's becoming more moral today, taking more interest and care for the problems than it did before. These were problems society did not want to see before, problems making it impossible for many to live the dream of closeness, warmth, and happiness promised by "the family" concept. In other words, what we see is a progressive and positive trend expanding the idea of "family" to the larger society, not a moral collapse.

## WHAT DOES THE PHRASE "TRADITIONAL FAMILY" MEAN?

When we think of "family," images of 1950s advertisements float through our heads—Dad smiling, Mom staying home, washing and ironing, surrounded by their clean and obedient 2.2 children. Or, reflecting an earlier image, we think of the archetype of the Christian "holy family," which we see especially at Christmas with crèche scenes.

Our perception of "the family" is filtered through the model of the "holy family," with its reproduced icons of Jesus, Mary, and Joseph. The family as we think of it is one of a mythological archetype, based on hierarchy and reproduction, the ideal father a nice "king in his castle." Surely, you might comment, in this day and age people no longer think like that; the modern family is not a religious one, most people are not Catholics—and most of the families (in the United States and the United Kingdom especially) are not of the old, nuclear variety. Yet the images linger on in our minds, and we measure ourselves (or find ourselves being measured in newspapers) against the three leading icons of this "traditional family" archetype, held up to be the only "right" kind of family, every other family being flawed or wrong-headed, tragic.

The icons of the "holy family" surround us in some of the most glorious art and symbolism of Western history. In the sumptuous images and colors of great paintings, in intricate works of architecture and music, the story of the "holy family" is told and retold. Artists such as Titian, Raphael, and Michaelangelo were commissioned by the church to create masterpieces out of biblical themes, as were composers such as Bach and Handel. The church was the primary sponsor of art for centuries.

No matter how beautiful (especially in its promise of "true love"), this family model is an essentially repressive one, teaching authoritarian psychological patterns and a belief in the unchanging rightness of male power. In this hierarchical family love and power are inextricably linked in a pattern that has damaging effects, not only on all family members, but also on the politics of the wider society. How can there be a successful democracy in public life if there is an authoritarian model in private life? And the emotional spectrum we have come to believe represents an eternally fixed "human nature" reflects this background; in other words, it is historical and culturally shaped, it can change.

Now that families are becoming different, we are seeing people question things in their upbringing that for centuries have not been questioned. We are beginning to see people ask themselves exactly what "love" is, and try to build families based on love they find that does not exactly fit into the system or follow the old models of "right living." Yet most people feel unsure, even guilty, about the new lives they are constructing.

Whether or not most people's lives fit into the "traditional" hierarchical holy-family model archetype, most people feel a certain admiration and nostalgia for the symbols. Why? Why do the icons hold our hearts? So used have we become to these symbols that we continue to believe—no matter what statistics we see in the newspapers about divorce, violence in the home, mental breakdown—that the icons and the system they represent are right, fair, and just. After all, we are told, the "holy family" is a religious symbol, so who can criticize it? We assume without thinking that this model is the *only* "natural" form of family and that if there are problems, it must be the individual who is at fault, not the institution.

We cannot even begin to imagine that our beautiful family system, the object of all those magnificent paintings and symbols, might not at heart be good or right. What is "reality," we wonder—is it the icons, or the violence in marriage we read about? And what *should* "reality" be? Shouldn't it be a "harmonious family," like the icon? Aren't we flawed as individuals if it is not? And if it doesn't work, who is to "blame"?

Yet, it seems to me, the statistics we are seeing do not represent a "decline" in the family or a collapse of civilization. What is happening is a transformation of the culture, not a collapse. It may be one of the most important turning points of the West, the creation of a new social base that will engender an advanced and improved democratic political structure.

## WHAT IS DEMOCRATIZATION OF THE FAMILY?

The democratization of the family means two things: that relationships within the family are becoming more equal, that all members—especially the woman and man—make decisions equally, and that both give each other equal emotional support.

It also means that now people can choose the kinds of families they form; families today need not only be of the reproductive type, they can also include networks of friends, and they can consist of "single mother" families or dual mother families as well.

Naysayers cry that these "other families" are perverting society. They even accuse single mothers of creating "criminal children." Statistically, while there may be a connection between children's criminal behavior and poverty, there is no link between one-parent families and "criminal psychology" in children. In fact, my research shows that children who grow up with only their mothers, especially boys, can turn out to have much better relationships with women later in life.

Not only do single mothers not cause "criminal children"; if anything, the connection between crime and single mothers is the reverse; that is, if violence is increasing in society, then it is increasing in the home too, thus causing more and more women to leave and so *become* single mothers. To blame them (they are usually experiencing financial hardship) is simply scapegoating women for the problems in family and society—nothing new!

Throughout the course of history, individuals have challenged institutions, and for the better: Martin Luther challenged the church officialdom of his time, Gandhi challenged the British government on behalf of Indian citizens, and Martin Luther King challenged the United States government on behalf of African-Americans. Individuals have the right to challenge the official idea of the family and to find improved ways of living their lives. Why should we think that institutions, including ideological, "religious" institutions such as the "traditional family," are "good" and the individual who disagrees with them is "wrong"?

Too many people, all their lives, live out a play-enacted version of themselves, a shadow-self tailored for public consumption, displaying "appropriate" social behavior in public "life," while underneath, in private, an undergrowth of confusing feelings of joy, fear, eroticism, and pain exist, all jumbled together.

This situation is beginning to change. Most people today have discovered in their own lives that trying to copy one archetype of how to construct their personal lives does not permit them to relate honestly to the people around them or on the level they would like. So they are seeking in their own lives to find what does work, thus leading to the diversity of choices we see today and to the new government statistics on changing lifestyles all over the Western world.

What we are witnessing now—and participating in—is a revolution in the family. The way we live our lives, with whom and how, is being questioned and debated in a groundbreaking and important revolution. The fundamentalist reactionary forces that are calling for the "preservation of family values," opposing this democratization, are wrong to insist that the revolution is causing harm and have no statistical base for such claims. This is an excellent revolution, one that has been needed for a very long time. The problems we are seeing in "the family" are caused by its antiquated authoritarianism, not by the humanizing and equalizing process of democratization now going on in family and private life.

We should have faith in ourselves, believe in our own experience and history, not be afraid but continue with confidence to the future.

## EXPLODING THE NUCLEAR MYTH: DIVERSITY IN FAMILIES[9]

What's wrong with mother-headed families? Are children disadvantaged by having "only one parent, female"? Or is every family a "normal family"?

Many people today in the Western world are opting out of the institution of "the family" as it has been rigidly defined and are creating their own forms of families.

The percentage of those still in a "traditional family" (father at work, mother at home with the 2.2 children) is, according to European Union statistics, only 7 percent. In most of Europe today half of the population is unmarried, according to German, British, French, and Italian government and other surveys.

Many people feel guilty about revolutionizing their lives. This feeling indicates a profound social transformation, one that is taking place furtively, defensively, even guiltily, as the mythology persists that one is not quite "normal," has not quite "made it," if one doesn't achieve nuclear-family status.

Western publics are made to feel that it is important for a political candidate or a head of government to be married and have children—that is, to be "normal." The subtext seems to be that people should respect, worship, and elect the candidate with the family most resembling the "holy family"—the Jesus, Mary, and Joseph model.

Why do we feel guilty about the creative ways we have begun to live our lives? Those who would have us conform to just one sort of family are the same people who see nothing wrong with authoritarian forms of government, those who do not believe people are entitled to govern themselves and make choices.

Every family is a "normal" family, no matter whether it has one parent, two children, or none at all. A family can be made up of any combination of people, heterosexual or homosexual, who share their lives in an intimate (not necessarily sexual) way. And children can live as happily in an adopted family as with biological parents. A family doesn't have to have children in it. Women are under a great deal of social pressure to have children, but a woman is in no way diminished if she chooses not to have children. Wherever there is lasting love, there is a family.

People make institutions, not vice versa. The fact that individuals are changing the family is a sign of a healthy society. Democracy in politics and education has given society increased vigor as more and more individuals feel that they have the right to think for themselves.

Many single-parent families are headed by women. There is an unruly debate going on today in most Western countries about women's right to change the family. It is claimed that by doing this women are ruining children and society—never mind that men have opted out even more completely by leaving women and children, whereas women are "only" leaving men. Women are taking up the combined work of earning a living and looking after children, and making a valuable contribution to society.

To put the controversy over single parents into some historical perspective: in the United Kingdom, for example, marriage was a private matter until legislation in 1753. Rates of cohabitation and "illegitimacy" rose until 1900, when motherhood as synonymous with marriage was firmly established. The turn of the century saw a revival of legal marriage, peaking in the 1950s.

Dr. Susan McRae states: "It may be the single-earner, high-fertility family of the 1950s (against which lone parents and the cohabiting couple are often measured and found wanting) which is at odds with history."

There are very few statistics about the effects of these kinds of households on children, although during World War II, for example, a large number of families were without fathers for several years without this situation being frowned upon. It was "excused," no conclusions drawn, since this family formation was "a temporary circumstance due to war." Yet how the family functioned then is relevant to us today.

Today the assumption of much popular journalism is that the two-parent family is better for children, but there is no real foundation for this belief. The data here show that there are beneficial effects for the majority of children living in single-parent families. It is more positive for children not to grow up in an atmosphere poisoned by gender inequality.

In my research with men and boys, I was surprised to find that boys who grew up with their mother alone were much more likely to have good relationships with women in their adult lives; 80 percent of men from such families formed strong, lasting ties with women (in marriage or in long-term relationships) as opposed to only 40 percent from two-parent families.

This does not mean that the two-parent family cannot be reformed so that it provides a peaceful environment for children. Indeed, this is part of the ongoing revolution in the family in which so many people today are engaged.

The great majority of single mothers, whom fundamentalist groups try to put on the defensive, can indeed be proud of the excellent job they are doing in bringing up their children, often despite financial hardship.

As we have seen, the one-mother family enjoys a long and great tradition in the early mother-child icons of prehistory; and as one mother has astutely pointed out, since most fathers leave child care to the mother, all mothers are single mothers!

Do girls and boys who grow up with only their father have a different kind of emotional and sexual identity? Single-parent families are mostly single-mother families, yet there is an increasing number of single-father families too. Is it true that most single fathers don't take much part in child care, but instead hire female nannies or ask their own mothers, sisters, or girlfriends to take care of the children?

Men can change the style of families by taking a greater part domestically and by opening up emotionally, having closer contact with children. My research highlights men's traumatizing and enforced split from women at puberty. Healing this rift is the single most important thing we as a society can do to end the distance men feel from "family."

Do girls who grow up with "only" their mother have a better relationship with her? According to this study, 49 percent of such girls felt that their childhood was a positive experience; 20 percent did not like it; and the rest had mixed feelings. Mothers in one-parent families are more likely to feel freer to confide in daughters because no "disloyalty" is implied to the spouse. Daughters in such families are less likely to see the mother as a "wimp"; she is an independent person. Boys who grow up with "only" their mother experience less pressure to demonstrate contempt for things feminine and for nonaggressive parts of themselves.

We should give up on the outdated notion that the only acceptable families are nuclear families. A more profound historical view of what is happening is needed. We should see the new society that has evolved over the past 40 years for what it is, for itself, not as a disaster because it is not like the past.

The new diversity of families is part of a positive pluralism, part of a fundamental transition in the organization of society, which calls for open-minded brainstorming by us all: what do we believe "love" and "family" are? Can we accept that the many people fleeing the nuclear family are doing so for valid reasons? If reproduction is no longer the urgent priority that it was when societies were smaller, before industrialization took hold, then the revolt against the family is not surprising. Perhaps it was even historically inevitable.

People do want to build loving, family-style relationships; however, they do not want to be forced to build them within one rigid, hierarchical, heterosexual reproductive framework.

Diversity in family forms can bring joy and enrichment to a society: new kinds of families can be the basis for a renaissance of spiritual dignity and creativity in political life as well.

Private life is in the midst of a welcome process of democratization that will in turn enrich, advance, and transform democracy in the political arena.

Continuing this process of bringing private life into an ethical and egalitarian frame of reference will give us the energy and moral will to maintain democracy in the larger political sphere. We can create a society with a new spirit and will, but politics will have to be transformed by the use of an interactive frame of reference; families must continue democratizing, to provide a firm foundation for this process.

## BULLYING OF BOYS, SEX, AND SOCIETY

It is "politically incorrect" to have sex that includes ideas of power—but how could we avoid such ideas, growing up in the culture we do? We should, however, know what it is we are doing and why, as opposed to referring simplistically to "hormones" and claiming that we have no choice but to live as we do.

Pressure on boys to express disdain and contempt for "girls," at the same time that there is pressure to begin being "sexual" toward women, together cause a traffic jam in most boys' minds and fuse the two together, connecting sexual desire and violence or rejection of the female forever ("He's a sissy" becomes a feared epithet).

Clearly, men do fall in love with women; still, they usually continue to put "masculinity" before love, and prefer to be "one of the boys" than to work on a relationship with a woman.

This "value system" could be changed by banning the taunting and bullying of boys (no more shouts of "He's a mama's boy," and so on).

Banning bullying, with less emphasis on men in packs, would have a positive effect on society.

## BULLYING

Implementing the theory of Oedipus presented here[10] could lead to a more permanent "world peace," it could change our idea of "human nature": by ending the bullying of boys, it could bring about a more positive, more "tolerant," and diverse emotional landscape for society.

Endless articles are written about "how terrible" the wars and terrorist bombings of the last several years are—and they are. So let's ask: what is the cause of the terrible killings and bombings? They have gone on for a long time, not only in the Middle East, but also in other parts of the world, for example, between the Irish and British, between ETA and the Spanish government, between the Tamil Tigers and the Sri Lankan authorities, and between the Mexican freedom fighters and the Mexican government.

One of the causes of the atrocious "modern wars" we are seeing today is the increasing glorification of "being tough," the increasing social permission for bullying of boys at puberty.

Most boys are traumatized as they grow up because they have to learn to "leave" their mothers and her value system, leave "the female world" and join "the world of men"—where they have to "'prove themselves" in front of the other boys by "never showing weakness" and being "tough as nails"—otherwise they will be marginalized or excluded from the group, labeled "a sissy" or "a wimp."[11] If we would ban the bullying of boys, make it an offense, we could change the mentality of masculinity, and therefore of the culture.

## "ISN'T IT STRANGE TO THINK OF YOUR PARENTS HAVING SEX?"

Does love include sex and the body? What definition of love do children learn from the way their parents relate physically?

Finding their parents in any kind of physical embrace comes as a fascinating shock to most children, as these testimonies from my research demonstrate:

> My parents were rarely affectionate, at least in front of us. They just pecked each other when my father came home from work. But I remember seeing pictures of them with their arms around each other, which fascinated me, since I never saw them that way.

> My folks were only affectionate once that I can remember. We three girls gave them an electric blanket at Christmas, and my dad put his arm around Mum and hugged her when they opened the present. We all commented about this afterwards, that's how unusual it was. They often argued, especially after they'd gone to bed.

> My parents never kissed in front of me. When I was about thirteen they linked arms when we were out shopping. I was amazed. I sometimes wondered whether they've ever slept together or had sex together!

> Once I was passing their bedroom door and I saw them in Dad's bed holding each other. I was very surprised and embarrassed—I was about fifteen. It was like, wow! They really do that.

> They were seldom affectionate in front of me, though I have a lovely memory of seeing them dancing on the front porch and kissing. Once they saw me they stopped.

As many as 83 percent of children in my research reported that their parents seemed completely asexual—in fact, this may be true of some (but only some!) of the parents, while other parents may be having sex lives apart from each other (masturbation for orgasm, or sex outside the relationship); most, of course, are simply hiding "sex" from their children's eyes, thinking that they are doing the right thing.

But there are degrees of indicating a physical connection, and it is important for parents to "let children in on" a bit of their physicality.

If parents hide their physical love for each other and never, for example, kiss each other on the mouth passionately in front of the children, then children quite logically draw the conclusion that "real love" is never sexual, perhaps not even physically affectionate. But isn't affection a great part of what love is? It feels like that to children when their parents hug and kiss them. However, if the parents don't hug and kiss each other, is the definition of adult love different? And if so, what is it? All of this is quite confusing for children.

Why do parents feel that they shouldn't touch each other in front of the children? Because the children would be jealous? Because it would give the children sexual feelings and ideas? Or do many parents really not want to touch each other? The questions children have are many: "Is it that our parents really want to be affectionate, but have to hide it in front of us? Should no one, including us, see them touch—why???" Conclusion: "It must be shameful or embarrassing somehow." Or, "Maybe they don't really like each other—maybe what I feel is wrong."

Children also wonder: if parents don't want to be affectionate, then why exactly are they together, especially if they argue much of the time? If they are only together "for the sake of the children," this puts an awfully big burden on the children to be "worth it" or to "make their parents happy" and so on, thus confusing the definitions of love even further.

Girls especially find gender inequality in the family mixed with love hard to understand, confusing, even terrifying. This is, of course, because for girls seeing this reality means vowing that "my life will be different" or coming to terms with the position of women in the world, either despising their mothers for "letting it happen" or "understanding." Girls in such families wonder: Can they avoid being considered lesser beings when they become women? How can they love a father who represents such a system? Or a mother who lets herself participate in it? What can love mean for them?

Do these questions have anything to do with so many girls' wishing to put off "womanhood," even to the point of becoming anorexic in an attempt not to "have hips like a woman"?

Boys also learn damaging ideas of love from the traditional family structure, as they are taught to associate love for women with guilt—since a real man should "keep his distance" and "not need a female." Or boys may discount love that includes sex, since they have learned that sexual attraction should not be taken seriously or counted as "real love." But where did they learn that?

To begin to see love clearly, to recognize our emotions, we must gain distance from our near-obsession with "family membership."

Perhaps we can begin by looking within ourselves, for we each hold the key to understanding these feelings.

## A NEW FRAMEWORK FOR GROWING UP/BRINGING
## "FAMILY VALUES" UP TO DATE

We should give up the outdated notion that the only acceptable families are nuclear families. A more profound historical view of what is happening is needed. We should see the new society that has evolved over the last forty years for what it is, for itself, not as a disaster because it is not like the past.

The new diversity of families is part of a positive pluralism, part of a fundamental transition in the organization of society, that calls for open-minded brainstorming by us all: what do we believe "love" and "family" to be? Can we accept that the many people fleeing the nuclear family are doing so for valid reasons? If reproduction is no longer the urgent priority that it was when societies were smaller, before industrialization took hold, then the revolt against the family is not surprising. Perhaps it was even historically inevitable. It is not that people don't want to build loving, family-style relationships, it is that they do not want to be forced to build them within one rigid, hierarchical, heterosexual, reproductive framework. In fact, children have often found themselves forced into situations in which two unhappy parents were arguing around them or abusing them, leaving them in peril or anxious.

The movement in reaction to these changes is called "family values" or "traditional family values" or, yet again, "fundamental family values." Though there is an amount of hysteria in the current political assertions that "the family" is a sacred institution, historically, the family is changing; since this will not end or lessen reproduction (if it is currently lessened, perhaps this change is due to society's attempt to enforce a system based on the traditional family—that is, not implementing policies to aid those who are actually reproducing, women who are both married and unmarried), there is no reason to fear this change.

Diversity in family forms—including groups of friends, sisters and brothers, people who love each other and care for each other—can bring joy and enrichment to a society: new kinds of families can be the basis for a renaissance of spiritual dignity and creativity in politics and business as well. Clinging to the forms of the past will only cause sclerosis of the society. Society is a living thing that changes, we need to accept that truth.

Private life is in the midst of a welcome process of democratization, which will in turn enrich, advance, and transform democracy in the political arena. Continuing this process of bringing private life into a more ethical and egalitarian frame of reference will give us the energy and incentive to maintain democracy in the larger political sphere and in international relations. We can create a society with a new spirit and will, but our inner politics will have to be transformed before a lasting transition can be made in the political arena.

One of the most useful reference points for creating new kinds of relationships in "the family" can now be found in many friendships between women. How many women remark, "I wish I could talk to him like I can talk to my best friend!" There is a vast difference between how women see themselves with each other and how women generally see themselves with men.

Though the economic and spiritual difficulties of the West today are often blamed on "the decline of the family" (or on "feminism" and "women") "single mothers" are vilified in a way that, the Archbishop of Canterbury argued, would be illegal if the same attack were made on a racial minority—isn't the reality that Western democracies are not fully living up to their promise of equality for all? In fact, women have great energy and courage that is being underutilized; women nevertheless are in the forefront of the movement for reshaping personal and public institutions, endeavoring to create a more interactive democratic society.

The twentieth century proved that psychologizing the family doesn't work. Psychotherapy and its attempted analysis of the family has failed; it may have helped some people, but it does not address the underlying problem—that is, the structure of the family itself—as more and more people seek "treatment." It is not so much maladjusted individuals who are "the problem" as the framework into which they are persuaded. As Naomi Weisstein and Shulamith Firestone have pointed out in scholarly papers, in the early twentieth century the new Freudianism was used to "answer" the challenge posed to the social system of feminist theory, which called for equal rights for women. Of course it did not answer anything, but it was hoped that talking would lead to some kind of acceptance of the situation/status quo. Taking its cue from Orwell's *1984*, the mass media has also learned the refined art of using pseudo-Freudian psychoreligious symbols of "the family" and "correct behavior" to control and direct public opinion. However, what is needed is a clear analysis of what is really going on, a courageous taking stock of what kind of world democracy and equality imply, and "going for it"! Implementing our values will bring about change in a very positive and amazingly quick way.

Diversity in families can form the basic infrastructure for a new and advanced type of political democracy to be developed within nations and among nations—a system that suits the massive societies that technology has made into one global village.

The current fundamentalist reaction to the democratization of private life is trying to return society, both the private and public social orders, to prehumanist values of earlier centuries. This type of social order has had various names: totalitarianism, feudalism, fascism, authoritarianism, and so on. Democracy is the opposite of these social orders.

Democracy needs to exist inside families and in people's private lives, as well as in politics. One cannot exaggerate the importance of the current debate: fascism in the family cannot be left to exist, since it inevitably leads to a return to fascism in society as well. If we believe in the democratic, humanist ideals of our heritage, we have the right and duty to make our family system a more just one, to follow our democratic ideals and make a new, more inclusive network of private life—a new personal infrastructure for society that will reflect, not a preordained patriarchal structure, but our belief in justice and equality for all—women, men, and children.

The family need not be a repressive, authoritarian institution. Those who would attack women now are trying to reimpose the unequal "holy family" model. Let's continue the transformation, believe in ourselves, and go forward with love, not fear. In our private lives and in our public world, let's hail the future and make history.

## NOTES

1 See Appendix for the *Hite Report on the Family* questionnaire.
2 This paper was originally delivered as a lecture entitled "Origins of Psycho-Sexual Identity in the Traditional Family: Questioning the Connection Between Pubertal Behavior, Formation of Sexual Identity and 'Hormones'" given to the British Society of Pediatricians, Obstetricians and Gynecologists, London, 2001.
3 See also "Oedipus Revisited," Part 2.
4 This research is presented at length in *The Hite Report on the Family* and *The Hite Report on Men and Male Sexuality*.
5 Please also see Part 2 of this volume for a reinterpretation of the Oedipal theory regarding boys at puberty.
6 First published in the *American Journal of Nursing*, 1985.
7 See also Part 6.
8 Part of this article appeared in the *Washington Post*, Outlook section, 1996.
9 Parts of this article appeared in the *Sydney Morning Herald*, based on excerpts from *The Hite Report on the Family*.
10 See Part 2.
11 Ibid.

# Part 5

# Lesbianism, Homosexuality, and Gay Rights: To See the World Differently

## (1976, 1981, 1987, and beyond)

*In the following section, based on research published in 1976, 1981, 1987, and beyond,[1] Hite poses and addresses such questions as "Are lesbian and homosexual relationships and partnerships working?" The result is documentation by women and men of all ages about their sexuality, their sexual relationships, falling in love, their families and long-term relationships, and how they see themselves and the world around them. Based on research done in the United States from 1972 to 1989, as well as research done in Europe between 1990 and 2004, this section includes the testimonies of women and men of all ages, backgrounds, and points of view, in often exquisite and moving personal stories of love gone wrong, love beginning, sexual doubt, and sex of all kinds.*

# Are Homosexuality and Lesbianism Natural?

Why do some people prefer gay sex? Why do they fall in love with members of their own sex romantically?

Traditionally, what is called "sex" has been an activity that, by definition, was heterosexual: it "obviously" had to be done between two people of the "opposite" (opposing?) sexes (because otherwise it would not lead to reproduction—and would not be "natural").

While some people experience the "desire to make love" as a desire for heterosexual coitus, others experience other feelings. In my analysis I want to "go beyond" expanding our "tolerance" to "accepting lesbianism and homosexuality"; I want to make "sex" much more diverse, to include a much larger spectrum of choices.

It is not "abnormal" or "perverse" for people to create their own idea of sex, including having sex with someone of their own sex.

In the 1870s two German "sexologists" came up with the term "homosexual" to label and categorize same-sex activity; prior to that time, this special term did not exist. "Lesbian" is also a relatively recent designation historically, although it refers to the Isle of Lesbos in ancient Greece, where Sappho the poetess, supposedly a lesbian based on her lovely poems, lived in ancient times. Lack of designation implies that sexuality contained a wider diversity of behavior than we today expect.

Our society assumes that "sex" is "natural behavior" that consists of "foreplay," followed by "penetration" and intercourse, best had in a context of reproduction within a family; the further assumption is that no matter how sexy, sex should still "naturally" culminate with "the act" (of reproduction—that is, coitus) as the full, "natural" expression of "the sex drive."

Alfred Kinsey brilliantly explained fifty years ago that he believed the words "homosexual" and "lesbian" should be used as adjectives only to describe activities, not to label people—especially since people have the capacity to change their sexual orientation during a lifetime (sometimes more than once).

Heterosexuality became the dominant form of sexuality only about 4,000 years ago (despite what many think—that is, that sex has been "forever" the same, it has "always been like that"). Before that time, eroticism would seem to have been seen and expressed quite differently; clichés referring to "the world's oldest profession," as if women had always "by biology" been ordained to "provide coital services" to men as men's basic source of pleasure, are ahistorical clichés used to prop up the dominant sexual ideology.

Too much of our natural eroticism has been channeled by the social order into reproductive rites—rites we are urged to repeat over and over with a partner (either within marriage or in the context of singles who "meet and mate"). Although traditional heterosexual sexual activity can be beautiful, why should it be the only good way people can relate? Or the only way "civilization can continue"? People have lived and reproduced in various kinds of societies; think of the ancient Greeks (who had a completely different conception of sexuality and eroticism and morality), or civilizations from Polynesia to Brazil to Africa and South America that existed without insisting that only one definition of sex was correct and good or that only one was morally correct. (In our society's view not only is there only one way that physical sexuality should "appropriately" be expressed, but additionally, not to do so is to be "immoral"; only one way of having sex is seen as "moral," "right," and "good.")

Our concept of sex was created to support our social system, channeling our erotic expression into reproductive-style activity; a more "natural" spectrum of behavior would be broader, with a variety of ways in which to express oneself.

There are or could be various conceptions of "sex" that are all equally good—without an implication that one is the main way. I wish to expand our idea of the sexual/erotic so that "a thousand flowers bloom"; to speak against the oppression of women in the traditional institution of "sex," and to show how heterosexuality or any kind of sex can be conceptualized in a new way.

Neither male nor female sexuality is limited by "genital geography," and it has been one of the greatest public relations victories of all time to convince us that it was. The very naturalness of lesbianism (and male homosexuality) is exactly the cause of the strong social and legal rules against it. The basing of our social system on gender differences should be replaced by a system based on affirmation of the individual and clear support for all life on the planet.

## LESBIANISM

### WHAT PERCENTAGE OF WOMEN ARE LESBIAN?

It is impossible to know how many lesbian women there are in the United States, since, because of the fear of persecution, there are few reliable statistics. Kinsey estimated that perhaps 12 to 13 percent of women had "sexual relations to the point of orgasm" with another woman at some time during their adult lives. In the 1970s Dr. Richard Green, of the University of California (Los Angeles) Gender Identity Research Treatment Program, commented that there may now be an increase in bisexuality and/or lesbianism among women "partly for political reasons"—as one of the ways women can "disassociate themselves from the extraordinary dependency they've had on men all these years."

At the same time it is important to note that preferences can change during a lifetime or can change several times; what is called "gender identity" is not so cut and dried as the preceding statistics might imply. As Kinsey explained, there are not two discreet groups, one heterosexual and one homosexual.

Many women express interest in having sex with another woman: "I have been married for twelve years. I've never had a physical relationship with a woman, but I feel it would be more satisfying than with a male. I don't know how to relate to another woman physically, as I've never had the opportunity to do so. There is a woman whom I'm attracted to and feel is the same as me but I am afraid to approach her." Another: "There are times when I feel such a warmth from my best friend that I experience it sexually and almost desire her. But I have never let her know I have this feeling, because it might make her afraid of me."

## WHAT IS SEX BETWEEN WOMEN LIKE?

What is "different" about sexual relations between women is precisely that there is no one institutionalized way of having them, so they can be as inventive and individual as the people involved.

Perhaps the two most striking specific differences between lesbian relations and most heterosexual relations are that there are generally more orgasms, and sex is longer ("sex" is not over when one of the partners has orgasm, since most women do not find that orgasm ends their sexual arousal).

The higher frequency of orgasm in lesbian sexuality has been noted by other researchers, going at least as far back as Kinsey. Lesbian sexual relations also tend to involve more overall body sensuality.

## WHAT DO WOMEN DO TOGETHER SEXUALLY?

*The basic difference with a woman is that there's no end, where you have orgasms and then end—it's like a circle, it goes on and on.*

*We hug a lot and kiss and caress each other, we masturbate each other with our hands and fingers and orally, as well as combining both. Also, mutually masturbate, with other parts of our bodies . . .*

*Sometimes I think I could go straight from deep mouth kissing to clitoral stimulation to have orgasm. It depends on my state of "readiness." I like also to have my lover touch me very lightly, with her tongue and hands, all over my body, especially my buttocks and lower abdomen—when she uses her mouth it's different than her fingers. Sometimes I like her mouth at first and then her finger, and the other times, just her mouth. Either her tongue gently flicking my clitoris, or her mouth sucking me hard, or her finger moving right above my clitoris in an increasingly rapid up and down movement, usually makes me orgasm. Sometimes she pushes her mouth hard against me and shakes her head rapidly from side to side— I orgasm this way also. No one way works best all the time; different ways at different times work marvelously well. One thing, I guess it's easier for me if we start love-making with our clothes on and do not have more than a minute's interruption for removal of clothes. Otherwise I get a little self-conscious.*

*Sex is slow with long preliminaries and explorations, conversation, gentle mutual stroking and then clitoral stimulation in unison. Great! It's great to do and feel the same done to you.*

*She's soft and gentle, knowing exactly how to rub my clit and what pressure to use—taking as long as we want coming—coming—coming.*

*The women I've been with have kissed me and I them, we have hugged and gently touched each other; just having our bodies together and being warm sends a fire surging through my body. One woman sat on my pelvic area lightly, with her back to my face, and stimulated me vaginally/clitorally with her fingers, very gently, taking her time and not at all concerned with getting me excited but more exploring—which releases me to take my time and do the same. I enjoy all of them very much and hope to see that I make women a more active part of my life. I am doing this by seeking them out by going to womens' and lesbians' activities and putting myself in a position to meet them for the conscious purpose that I want to make love to a certain kind of woman that I love.*

*Love-making with a woman is always more variable than with a man, and the physical actions are more mutual. While the same places are kissed and touched with a man, the whole feeling is heightened for me when the lover is a woman, and it is so different because of all the psychological and emotional factors involved. The touches become different, the kisses different—the whole aura is different.*

*Sex with a woman includes: touching, kissing, smiling, looking serious, embracing, talking, digital intercourse, caressing, looking, cunnilingus, undressing, remembering later, making sounds, sometimes gently biting, sometimes crying, and breathing and sighing together.*

*To relate to another woman physically, you just caress her body the way you like to be caressed and/or the way she indicates she likes. You explore love-making together and find out what works. I don't think there are any "cookbook" approaches that work in all situations—thank goodness. For me it comes more naturally than it ever did with men.*

*Technically, women together do what male and female together do— touch and kiss and caress one another, except there's no penis. (And I've yet to meet a lesbian who uses a dildo. I think that is one great big male porno trip.) Sometimes it feels good to put my nipple into her vagina, or vice versa. Cunnilingus is beautiful too. When I perform cunnilingus, I like to not only stroke the inner lips and edges of her vagina with my tongue, but I also like to suck her clitoris. This excites me very much and my partners always seem to enjoy it. I also enjoy tribadism, holding each other very closely, our thighs pressing against one another's genitals; or lying diagonally with each other, our legs in a "V" sort of scissors around each others torsos, our vaginas warm, moist, happy, touching, our hands holding.*

*I like women's bodies, I feel as though women are natural sexual partners. Breasts are beautiful, all is beautiful. I like women's soft skin and softer feeling of muscles with fat over them, finer fingers, smaller joints. Because I had a woman lover (and because I'm a woman), I recognize more parts of a woman's genitalia than clitoris, vagina and vulva—I know and love intimately every fold, every texture and variation of sensation. I often masturbated with my woman lover (we wouldn't have even called it that, but there's no word for what we did). We just did what felt best, and if one of us couldn't make the other come, she'd take over while the one who'd been rubbing or eating touched some other part, kissed her breast or lay close and pressed against her. Often I'd rub my own clitoris while she fucked me with her fingers—of course, the other way around, too.*

*Sex with a woman for me involves kissing, feeling one another completely, and basically humping—pressing mound of Venus against mound of Venus or each other's leg. Also cunnilingus and manual and even anal lingus! Pressing against her backside, riding her, which feels good.*

*It's most stimulating to be in a sitting position facing my partner. She also sits and presses her hand gently into me. This way I can determine the speed and intensity of the movements. And we can see each other, kiss, talk, and feel each other's breasts.*

*My best sexual experiences were with the first woman I ever loved. I had been married for a thousand years and she was a total virgin. We didn't even practice cunnilingus, yet they were powerful sexual encounters for both of us because they were a dream come true emotionally. We were mad for each other.*

*We like to stimulate ourselves and neither of us minds this or feels embarrassed. Sometimes, usually, if she comes before I do, she keeps making love till I come but if she doesn't then I masturbate and she holds me while I do and it's just the same as making love. I must be lying face down to have an orgasm. I must be rubbing my clitoris against a part of my lover's body or a soft object. (Before getting in this position, I like my breasts to be sucked. I like that the best. I also like manual clitoral stimulation and oral.) Then I get in a face-down position. Sometimes my lover lies on top of my back and I rub against a pillow or soft blanket and sometimes (usually) I lie on her back and she stimulates herself manually and the feeling of the waves in her hips and legs and my thighs and clitoris moving against her brings me to orgasm.*

*I like non-genital sex just looking at her face and body in the moonlight. Or I like it when she lies on top of me and looks down into my face. She looks loving and proud. Once my heart had an orgasm when she was hugging me and looking at me and saying how she loved me. It felt like it just jumped up and had a wave like my body does when it comes. I like smelling a lot. The first woman I was in love with (when I was twelve) had a smell like wild woods and autumn leaves, and I loved it. I like to smell my lover's hair and her breast and her melt. I like to suck her breasts and I like her to suck mine. She does all kinds of new and wonderful things to me. I never felt like I do with her.*

*Being together with a woman is one of the most beautiful things on earth. Recently, on the giant New Year's Eve Millennium celebration, I booked a hotel room and invited my girlfriend. It cost me a bit, but then what the hell. . . . We checked in (or I did, not sure about their gay-friendly policies at posh hotels (she came along later), washed up and settled in, then went down to dinner in their lavish dining room, but by 11 p.m. we left to go up to the room. We gazed out the window at the stars, then kissed very deeply and declared our love (mostly she declared her love to me), and I carried her to bed. (I lift weights.) I undressed her slowly, playing with each part of her body and telling her what I was going to do to her, while she moaned and pretended she didn't want anything so violent. . . . I told her I was going to rape her, and she would have to just take it, no matter what I put inside her nor how hard, that she was lucky to be fucked by me and should keep quiet. This made her moan all the more (what I wanted) and I tied her arms together above her head (while she protested). This gave me free access to her body, to touch it and look at it any way I wanted. I went down on her and kissed and licked her crotch until she couldn't take it any more and begged me to make her come with my hand. I ignored this and started to pull and tug at her nipples (I know she loves it), then she yelled at the top of her voice demanding I fuck her with the candle I kept holding and showing her—so loud I had to put my hand over her mouth and "threaten" her with "punishment" if she tried that again. . . . Soon I couldn't resist coming so I stood up and made myself come in front of her, then fell on top of her . . . anyway, this gives you some idea. I love her a lot.*

*I'm pregnant and I'm living with a woman. Everyone asks me, doesn't she mind that you're going to have a baby? They don't realize, of course I didn't have sex with him! It's all done outside the body, he's just a friend (for a long time). She's keener than me for the baby, it'll be our baby not "mine." It'll have two mothers. I feel fine, I'm just like I normally am, just that I have a bump in my tummy. Sexually, I don't have any problems either, no big ups or downs and I like sex as much as I normally do with her. It's so beautiful to explore her body and feel her exploring mine, with all the changes. The other day she was lying with her head on my stomach when we were in bed, her fingers inside me, I was coming and she was listening to see if the baby could feel our happiness. We are very close.*

*The first time she held me down and more or less raped me with a big dildo, also using a bottle in my ass, I didn't know what was happening. I was on my back looking up at her, I felt incredibly turned on. I came and came and came. Another time she pinned me down holding my arms with one hand and clamping her other hand over my mouth while wearing a dildo that she fucked me with. . . . She was looking down at me daring me to scream or cry out. I didn't but my mouth was open and gaping. She can really get me going!*

Women who previously had sex with men explain the reasons why they now choose to relate sexually to women.

*I have been relating sexually to women for over four years. I have always had strong, warm, loving relationships with women—ever since I can remember. My feelings of sympathy, compassion, and understanding have always been more strongly directed towards women. In other words, women have mattered and do matter to me more than men, and even though I've had more sex relationships with men in the past, they have not compared in depth emotionally to my relationships with women, sexual or non-sexual.*

*I had my first feelings of sexual desire for another woman eight years ago, when I was fourteen. We both got scared after that (terrified would be much more accurate) and tried to convince ourselves we were heterosexual. In that next three and a half years I slept with seven or eight men but never was very satisfied with the relationships emotionally, sexually, etc. They weren't satisfying because I just don't feel the complete relationship—emotional, spiritual, etc. Besides, I like women's bodies much more. When I was nineteen I fell head over heels in love with a woman and realized that I couldn't kid myself any longer. I knew then that I was a lesbian. She was much more afraid than I (this was the first time she had realized that she felt this way about another woman), and our sexuality was not expressed with each other very frequently for that reason. I was in love with her for almost two and a half years. About a year ago I saw my first lover again (from freshman year in high school) and we began to sleep together. In the year since then I slept with two other women before I met my present lover. We've been living together now for three months and we both expect it shall be for a long, long time. We are extremely comfortable with each other in all ways. Neither of us wants to sleep with anyone else (at least right now). I am now twenty-two, she is twenty. She has been out since she was thirteen though she too slept with some eight or nine men in the first few years of her sexual experience. Neither of us would ever get married, even if we weren't lesbians. The political implications are too large and damaging. We live with two other women and really enjoy collective living.*

*After thirty-four years of marriage I tried a woman and loved it, so I got divorced. I think I had always been attracted to women. In junior high and high school I had "crushes" on girls, but I was too young and stupid to know what was going on and what to do about it—information regarding lesbians was practically non-existent then. I used to say, during my marriage of thirty years (married thirty-five years, no extramarital experiences, only had intercourse with one man ever, though I am very enterprising and very resourceful, and run a business of my own), quite sincerely, that yes, I had orgasm almost every time. Almost no one is willing to admit to not having orgasms—what, me frigid? But then, taken by surprise in a lesbian relationship, I experienced real, buffola total eclipse orgasm for the first time. Wow! I'd never felt anything like that before. The rather pleasant, generalized sensations I was accustomed to feeling with vaginal stimulation were in a class with sensuously warm oatmeal. No wonder women have never made such a big thing out of sex—it's nice, really, but one can do without it. I believe that most women who claim orgasm without having experienced the clitoral detonation are speaking in ignorance.*

### LISTENING ON ANOTHER FREQUENCY

*I think this is a window on a world that most women have no conception of whatsoever.*

#### ORIGIN OF THE TABOO

The general villainization of homosexual contacts in our society has a long history, as Alfred Kinsey has explained in his famous reports:

*The general condemnation of homosexuality apparently traces to a series of historical circumstances. . . . In Hittite, Chaldean, and early Jewish codes there were no over-all condemnations of such activity, although there were penalties for homosexual activities between persons of particular social status or blood relationships, or homosexual relationships when force was involved.*

*The more general condemnation of all homosexual relationships (especially male) originated in Jewish history in about the seventh history BC upon the return from the Babylonian exile. Both mouth-genital contacts and homosexual activities had previously been associated with the Jewish religious service, as they had been with the religious services of most of the other peoples of that part of Asia, just as they have been in many other cultures elsewhere in the world. In the wave of nationalism which was then developing among the Jewish people, there was an attempt to disidentify themselves with their neighbors by breaking with many of the customs which they had previously shared with them. Many of the Talmudic condemnations were based on the fact that such activities represented the way of the Canaanite, the way of the Chaldean, or the way of the pagan, and they were originally condemned as a form of idolatry rather than a sexual crime. Throughout the Western Middle Ages homosexuality was associated with heresy. The reform in the mores soon, however, became a matter of morals, and finally a question for action under criminal law.* [2]

Kinsey (who was originally a biologist) also tells us that other mammals and other animals routinely have lesbian and homosexual relationships:

> *The impression that infra-human mammals more or less confine them-selves to heterosexual activities is a distortion of the fact which appears to have originated in a man-made philosophy, rather than in specific observations of mammalian behavior. Biologists and psychologists who have accepted the doctrine that the only natural function of sex is repro-duction have simply ignored the existence of sexual activity which is not reproductive. They have assumed that heterosexual responses are a part of an animal's innate, "instinctive" equipment, and that all other types of sexual activity represent "perversions" of the "normal instincts." Such interpretations are, however, mystical. They do not originate in our knowledge of the physiology of sexual response, and can be maintained only if one assumes that sexual function is in some fashion divorced from the physiologic processes which control other functions of the animal body. It may be true that heterosexual contacts outnumber homosexual contacts in most species of mammals, but it would be hard to demonstrate that this depends upon the "normality" of heterosexual responses, and the "abnormality" of homosexual responses.*[3]

Kinsey mentions that lesbian contacts have been observed in such widely sep-arated species as rats, mice, hamsters, guinea pigs, rabbits, porcupines, marten, cattle, antelope, goats, horses, pigs, lions, sheep, monkeys, and chimpanzees. And, he adds, "Every farmer who has raised cattle knows . . . that cows quite regularly mount cows."

The argument over whether homosexuality is biological or psychological in ori-gin (the origin of the "problem," as it is usually put) is still raging in some quarters,[4] but the "answer" hardly matters anymore. Homosexuality, or the desire to be phys-ically intimate with someone of one's own sex, can be considered a natural and "normal" variety of life experience. It is "abnormal" only when you posit reproduc-tive sex as exclusively "normal" and "healthy." (Discussions of why one becomes heterosexual would come to the same nonconclusions.) To consider all nonrepro-ductive sexual contact "an error of nature" is an extremely narrow view.

One of the best descriptions of how we more or less "unconsciously" select our sexual partners on the basis of gender (and screen out those of the "wrong" gen-der) has been given by Pepper Schwartz and Philip Blumstein. They explain that given a state of physiological arousal for which an individual has no immediate explanation, "he or she will "label" this state and describe his feelings in terms of the cognitions available to him . . ." They continue:

> [T]he sources of arousal are likely to be more diverse than the sources to which it is attributed by the most astute laymen, [and] the greater the confidence in, or need for, a heterosexual identity, the more likely that ambiguities will be resolved in a heterosexual direction. But when one has taken on gay identity, the interpretation is likely to go in the other direction.
>
> In other words, homosexuality—like heterosexuality—becomes self-fulfilling.[5]

With specific reference to women, Schwartz and Blumstein write that women often do not recognize sexual attraction towards other women for the following reasons:

> Women have a different arousal system from men. Their arousal is a total-body response, rather than a genital one. While some women may feel sexual tension in the genital area, or lubricate during an exciting encounter, these signals are less visible than their counterpart in the male. To put it simply, a woman can reinterpret her excitement; a man cannot miss noticing his sexual arousal and labeling it as erotic. . . . If a woman has sexual tension in an inappropriate environment, she has more freedom than a man in how she can label that excitement.[6]

In female-female relationships the cues that a woman receives from another woman are more subtle than the cues men give each other. Two women do not have to explain away an erection should one of them get excited while they were having a tête-à-tête and talking about their sex lives. If they are getting excited, and they want to communicate sexual interest in one another, they have to rely on eye contact, intensified attention, and other kinds of interpersonal connections to convey their meaning. However, these kinds of cues are confusing; they may be interpreted as merely friendly or nonsexual affection. Women may be afraid to believe—even if they want to—that another woman is giving sexual cues to them.

Because of this—and because women are not used to being wooed by other women—women rarely activate erotic responses and may not realize or admit to themselves that they have been in a sexual encounter, because of the passive aspects in the female sexual tradition. Since women have been taught to eroticize people who eroticize them—that is, interpret their worth and sexuality by the way men "turn on" to them—many women discover their own sexual feelings when they are approached by a man. When they see someone sexually aroused and interested in them, then they decide that they might be sexually interested in the other person. To some extent this seems to be true for both sexes—people start to get sexually aroused when someone begins to show sexual interest, begins aggressive moves, and makes the other person feel desirable. Sexual tension begins to build, and soon the two people must acknowledge its presence (even if they choose not to act on it). With women this sexual tension may not get a chance to build because each person may initially be embarrassed, unpracticed, and unsure about the validity of the encounter as a sexual experience.

## IS LOVE BETWEEN WOMEN ANOTHER WAY OF LIFE?

Is love between women different? More equal? Do women get along better with each other than they do with male lovers? Is there a difference in the way women in gay relationships define love, compared with the types of love they describe with men?

The question, as one woman in her twenties asked, "Are women better? There are women I meet who are like 'soul sisters'—and then there are those who are just like most men—cold, distant, unable to communicate, using people, not taking other people's feelings into consideration. Have a lot of us been co-opted by male views of power—power as necessary to make a relationship attractive? We don't have many alternate models. Still, intense and maybe over-analyzed as they have been, I think my relationships with women have been closer and more rewarding than any relationship I have ever had with a man. Maybe we're not perfect, but we're definitely onto something."

And another: "The conversations with Anne-Marie would be so complete and involved—like 'Oh, this dinner we're going to, I have really mixed feelings about it. How do you feel about it?' And then we would speculate on our thoughts, talk about it. Or if we were having a fight, one of us would say, 'You're really taking advantage of me,' and then the other would say, 'Tell me why—explain to me how you feel about that—tell me what you mean, in depth,' and then she would listen to me for five or ten minutes—she might complain about what I said, but still she would listen. That's the relationship I had with her. I think that your identity develops through these discussions. Even though when you have two women together who are extremely introspective and always examining what's going on, it can be really too much, the constant questioning—still, it's great."

## 1987 STATISTICS

As many as 11 percent of the women in this study have love relationships only with other women. An additional 7 percent sometimes have relationships with women. One of the most surprising findings is the number of women over forty, most of whom were in heterosexual marriages earlier in their lives, now in love relationships with women for the first time; 16 percent of women over forty have love relationships only with other women, and 61 percent of women over forty now living with another woman, as lovers, were previously married. Of the total "gay" population, 31 percent are in relationships, 52 percent are living together, and 17 percent are single.

## HOW DO LESBIAN WOMEN SPEAK OF LOVE?

*How do I love her now, after ten years? I love her mind, her body, her abilities. She's very brave and strong, exceptionally brilliant, and a beautiful woman.*

*Our love feels like a stream that flows on and on, growing ever stronger and deeper, giving me a sense of peace and center. Her sense of humor always makes me laugh; her constancy and the knowledge that she is eminently dependable give me strength; the wonderful sparkle of my passion for her—the sense of joy in her just being there—is a daily joy for me. We live near each other, we sleep together, bathe together, wash each other's hair, and rub suntan lotion on each other. I love the warmth and intimacy of that. We sort of roughly share money, whoever has some shares—we're both poor. We generally tell each other everything—intimate things, memories, dreams. We are monogamous.*

*When we make love, she makes me feel as though I'm the most beautiful woman in the world. She plays with my long hair and tells me how sexy she thinks it is. She tells me she loves the shape of my breasts. I especially love it when she whispers, "You are so soft."*

*My lover is the one I live with twenty-four hours a day, and go on holiday with. She is a spark strange to me. Close, but from far, far off, like no light I've ever seen. A sound that constantly catches my ear, and sets my mind reeling. I am in love with her comfortably, vigorously, and for a long term. I love her too. She is my lover, my soul mate; the one I think about when I see a certain smile, when my heart sings—a sister I have known from centuries ago. We were together once, and it was easier or more difficult than it is now—but someday, some life, it will not be hard; it will be as natural as it feels. I'm in love with her depth, her sparkle. It makes me secure to know I'm deeply loved.*

*My lover is beautiful, courteous, intelligent, well read, and attentive. Her political and spiritual views are important to her and similar to mine. I feel happy when we are together, we have a lot of exciting adventures. For example, she had an idea of how we could start a business and get rich, and we are working on that now and have a good chance of succeeding. We live together and have a pleasant lifestyle. We don't fight but we do argue sometimes. As time passes things are working out. Our biggest difference is opposite tastes in silverware design—that and a few more serious issues! I have a greater fear of intimacy, which is slowly diminishing.*

*I work too many hours. I neglect her sometimes and she suffers in silence. She is developing her assertiveness, and I am becoming more attentive. We share very well.*

*I am twenty-five years old, black—in love with a thirty-two-year-old woman. She's all I think about, I can't sleep, can't think straight, she's just constantly on my mind. I would like to settle down with her and be comfortable, also financially. My lover feels the same for me. When she first kissed me and told me she wanted me too, I was so happy. Being in love with her is a challenge—it's joy, pain, frustration, hurt, learning, happiness all rolled into one. My favorite love story is my own.*

*I like to be married. The best part is the constant love, and the worst is the fights. We're wife and wife. We got married. It was originally her idea. She proposed. We decided to get married because we were terribly attracted. It wasn't a hard decision—it took me one night of thinking. I felt very good, elated, and my feelings for her didn't change.*

## ARE WOMEN IN GAY RELATIONSHIPS MONOGAMOUS?

While 94 percent of women in lesbian relationships believe in monogamy, one-third have had or are having sex outside their relationships:

*I was having an affair with another woman while I was with my present lover. The affair grew to be very serious and I started to feel love for her. But I was, and still am, very much in love with my present lover. I was very confused and felt guilty. But still my feelings grew for the other woman. Eventually, my lover found out and we almost broke up. I still have strong feelings for the other woman, but we are not having an affair anymore. I think it's better that way because I still have the one I really love.*

*I love women. I love to flirt. I love the seduction. I've never slept with other women when I wasn't sleeping with my primary relationship. That doesn't seem at all sporting.*

*When I was younger, I cheated occasionally, but I do not like feeling deceitful. I think monogamy is preferable if you have a close relationship with one person.*

*The affair is/was not serious. It was with a close mutual friend. It fulfilled a need in me for adventure and passion, but this need is not as important as my need for my more comfortable primary relationships. The sex outside my relationships was/is basically fun and is not something that is absolutely necessary.*

*I was seeing someone, but finally I stopped. It made me sad. It was with a man I had been seeing before my relationship with the woman began. The affair was not serious. It was the revival of a long-ago connection. It had more to do with sex and more to do with youth and the past.*

*First, I was bugged by her fidelity (suffocated)—and then I was bugged by her infidelity (betrayed).*

The percentage of gay women involved in sex outside their relationships is much lower than that of married women or women in long relationships with men. More gay women know about their lovers' affair than do heterosexual women.

Is the possibility of contracting AIDS now changing the patterns of monogamy or casual sex in lesbian relationships? While gay women, as other women, discuss AIDS, there is little lessening of sexual activity because of this possibility in the gay female community. However, transmission may be most likely when a woman is menstruating. Many gay women do have themselves tested often.

The agonies of being jealous are universal and can happen to anyone in love, as this woman 's story shows:

*We were out at a disco. I got jealous about the amount of women who went up and talked to my girlfriend. I was feeling insecure because she seemed very happy to talk to people, and I didn't see her half the night.*

*The next day, I felt really bad about it, and I started to think, "Why am I acting this way? What's wrong with me? I have to get a handle on this." I wanted to explain to her, and say, "Look, I'm really sorry, it's just my own insecurity." So I talked to her on the phone, and she said, "Listen, I've got to get out of the house tonight, let's go to a movie or something." And I said, "O.K., O.K., great, let's go have dinner—we'll talk, and then we can go see a film," and she says, "O.K."*

*So I get home from work, and she's in there putting her makeup on, and she says, "Let's go out to the bar." And I said, "To a bar?! I don't want to go to a bar. I really want to talk to you, we need time together. I don't want to go to a bar again, O.K.?" She was very insistent. "Let's just go for a while." Finally, I said, "Look, I really feel like we have to talk." I'm freaking out, and she's saying, "I just want to go out to a bar. I don't want to talk, talk, talk, being heavy all the time, being so serious all the time! You don't want to have fun!"*

*Then my response became: "O.K., all right. You want to go out? We're going to go out. Boy, are we going to go out!" I decided to go out with the idea of getting totally obliterated-drunk. That was the way I had to deal with it. I didn't feel strong enough emotionally to say, "Well, you go out and I'm staying home"—although I do that now. I knew that I was wrong, essentially, the night before, so I didn't want to create a whole other compounded issue on all this.*

*It started out, we were hanging out together, kind of moping, 'cause we were still annoyed. Then we started hanging out with other people. I ran into this girl I knew and started talking to her, so this made my girl-friend very happy, 'cause then she can just go and do what she wants. She stayed outside, talking to the people outside the door. Then she comes running over to me and says, "Isn't this wonderful? We both are having a great time at different parts, and we're still together. We can still have other friends and meet new people and still be together. Isn't this like a mature relationship, right?"*

*So I'm saying, "Yeah, yeah, yeah," and meanwhile I'm drinking rum. We ended up hanging out till I don't know how late it was, and I just kept on drinking. I got completely drunk, got like thrown into a cab, taken home, put into bed. I mean, I don't even know how I got home. It was one of those nights where the next day you're told everything that happened to you, everything that you did.*

*The next day, I woke up in a complete panic, because I woke up and she wasn't there. She was not in the bed. I started to flip out. I'm thinking, "Did I come home with her last night? I can't remember." So I get up and she's not in the house. I panic. Then she calls and I say, "Were you home last night? Did you sleep with me last night?" And she's really pissed off, saying, "I slept with you." Now, I become a complete lunatic at this point, right? An utter fool, drunken, crazy, insane, a schizophrenic person, all due to insecurity from previous relationships. She had left the house at seven in the morning. She couldn't sleep and she was upset from the night before because all I kept talking about in my drunken state was responsibility and finances and "somebody has to do the laundry." All my resentments were coming out.*

*I went through four days where I was totally sick to my stomach, couldn't eat, couldn't function, couldn't do anything, and that's when I ran to see my therapist. My feeling was that I'm not going through this all over again. I'm going to work it out.*

Being the "other woman" in a gay relationship is eventually traumatic, according to most women:

*My present lover was in a monogamous relationship when we met. We had a "stormy" affair for one and a half years before she finally broke up with her. It was hell. I wanted her to leave, we had periods of not seeing each other for weeks or months at a time, then we'd get back together when we couldn't stand it anymore.*

*I was in a relationship with a married woman for two and a half years. I minded that she was married but I was getting out of my masochistic phase and put up with her stuff.*

*I was in love with her. It was painful. I knew she needed me but I knew I couldn't give her the day-to-day stability that her lover gave her. Our affair inspired her, gave her something she needed, gave her strength. Her own relationship grew from it. I was never resentful, because I wanted the best for her and I knew we could never live together.*

*My first relationship was with a married woman. I was twenty-one years old and didn't know what I was getting into. She had cheated on him before. I did want her to get divorced, but not for my sake—for herself. Unfortunately, she did move in with me and it was the worst hell (one of them) of my life.*

Most women, finding out about their lover's affair(s), are very upset:

*My last lover was a woman of forty-one with two children. I went out with her for two years. I took the relationship seriously, and fully expected it to continue. I felt totally dedicated to her, in a way that surprised even me with my non-monogamous leanings! She, however, mistrusted my feelings, and began playing all sorts of mind games with me. Seeing how far she could go, what she could get away with. Of course, I let her, explaining it all away to myself as: It's something she needs to do, it's important that I let her follow her needs, etc. And she did. Took the ball and ran with it. Going out with others, trying to make me jealous. I rationalized it away. It eventually got quite terrible, and we broke up with a gigantic fight.*

*The first time I broke up with my girlfriend was spectacularly draining. She is very important to me. I'm definitely the closest to her of anyone, but I'm not sure I'm in love anymore. This is why I just moved out. I love her but I don't think I'm "in love" anymore. I don't think she's happy either. She is a horrible philanderer and always has been. I put up with it for three years. We lived together two years. I finally decided I didn't need that bullshit, so I moved out. I still see her and sleep with her, but I sleep with other women too. After all that time of watching her go out with others, I decided to try it too—now I like it and I'm not sure I'm basically monogamous anymore either. I think I wanted to see what my lover liked about it and maybe to get back at her—not get back, but catch up. Feel even. I was terribly angry and she was away a lot. Being with another woman in another city, I did it once—I liked it, did it again, had some one-night affairs, and I'm now on my third "relationship" outside the relationship. None have been serious, but the one I'm having now may become so.*

*I started therapy because of the awful time I had dealing with my breakup with her. It helped immensely. I was horribly jealous when she was cheating on me and I wasn't. She constantly lied about the other women. I read her diary. Now I don't give a shit. I'm very independent. I went on with her when I shouldn't have. But breaking up is awful. It's as bad as divorce, of course. I try to get over it now by having lots of sex and plenty of fun. It's odd, I've had the best sex of my life with this woman I see on the side, she's also a delight in bed. I'm afraid I'm going to lose even that sex link with my girlfriend. We (my girlfriend and I) have great sex. Very physical, very verbal. She talks dirty to me. She tells me how excited she is, she tells me what I look like. We moan, we coo, etc. So, my relationship has become peripheral. I want to leave it. I think we'd make better friends and that's what I want. I've hated her at times. We've had violent fights where I've hit her and been hit by her or some lover or other of hers. She has done things to me I never thought I'd swallow, but I came back for more abuse. I had to work my tail off to keep this thing going for three years, and now I want out. In fact, I am out.*

A few are more philosophical about whether a relationship is monogamous or not:

*In her past she's been pretty innocent. She only got into some heavy petting with one boy. How do I feel? Everybody goes through it. I'd like her to be monogamous but I'm not possessive enough to try to force her to be that way if she doesn't want to.*

One young woman believes that there is too much sexual intermixing or affairs among friends in her group because of the small size of the gay community in her area:

*This kind of stuff goes on all the time. The groups become really incestuous, one person sleeping with one person's ex-lover and then the other one, and everybody knows what everybody else is doing. If we had affairs with strangers no one knew, that would make it easier, probably—but the gay community is such a close-knit group and the numbers are not that big—so you wind up sleeping with lovers of ex-lovers and mutual friends, and it's very painful sometimes. That goes on continuously and there are no scruples. Nobody has any morals about anything, it seems.*

*I think that this has to do with women subconsciously thinking that we obviously have no morals to begin with, to be having a gay relationship in the first place. Therefore, why should we put any confinements or restrictions on ourselves? Also, if you're gay, then you're living an "alternate life," and why should you conform to what society says is morally right? We're not conforming in any other way, so why are we supposed to conform in this way, to monogamy? Monogamy is something that's been institutionalized, set up.*

*That seems to be a lot of the mentality. Although the ones who talk about it in an existential way have generally ended up being the ones who are screaming the most when their girlfriend is screwing somebody else. They say that this is all right, this is the way things are, and then when it happens to them it's a whole other story. I watched that happen with two friends, who sat there and told me and my girlfriend, "Oh, yeah, well, it's O.K. to have affairs. We handle these exterior affairs. I have mine, and my girlfriend has hers. We just cope with these things, because they're inevitable, and it's going to happen." Then, when it actually ended up happening inside their relationship, the one who had been talking the most about how they could handle it was totally losing her mind! Meanwhile, listening to them, my girlfriend gets the idea that this all could work out, that this could be O.K. . . . .*

But most gay women are and always have been monogamous:

*I find it difficult, in an emotional sense, to maintain more than one sexual relationship. I would like to be able to handle more than one affair at a time because I think I would grow from it and I like to experience new feelings. It is possible that I would have sex outside of the relationship in the future and I would tell of my intentions before the affair started. I know my partner is not having sex with anyone else. I trust her and would not want her to be monogamous. It is very important to me that my partner and I communicate to each our feelings about monogamy. We are currently at the same place in our feelings but that could change in the future.*

*I would not have sex with anyone else while involved with her—there is absolutely no reason to. Yes, I want her to be monogamous and I want her to tell me if she is not.*

*It was a terrible weakness in her to go after women. You can find your friends charming, but why do you have to act on it? There are women that I'm extremely attracted to, but I have different kinds of relationships with them, because I've channeled it into another way.*

## COMING OUT IS HARD TO DO—BUT MOST WOMEN SOUND VERY HAPPY ABOUT IT

Women coming out can be very shy:

*Just recently, I have begun to include women in my choice of sexual partners. My relationship with my friend has grown much more important. We have made love. When we made love, she stared into my eyes and whispered my name. We masturbated each other. With her I loved sex. This is especially significant because, in the past few years, I have not enjoyed sex very much. I love to touch her body. it is so thrilling.*

Most women under twenty-five who have recently come out feel good about their lives, but often are told by others they are "doing something wrong," "making a big mistake":

*I am twenty-two years old. I recently informed my mother that I am lesbian. She took the news horribly!! She believes the only way I can be happy is to marry and have children. This really shocks me, as she is very miserable with her life. Although she is usually quite understanding about most things, she could not deal with the fact that I was a lesbian at all; to her that represents total failure!*

*On the one hand I feel that I have certain bisexual tendencies, but on the other hand I don't. I love making love with a man but I just have this curiosity about women. There, that's it. It doesn't sound like that much of a problem, but it bugs me. I have alluded to this "problem" with my fiancé but we really haven't talked about it. I feel I am accepted and understood by him, I guess, but I still can't reveal a few thoughts and feelings to him because of my own insecurities. I began to tell him something a while ago . . . but I couldn't. I hinted. The reason it's weird is because it has to do with sexuality and we both are open about that. But this specific aspect of myself cannot be shared unless I am comfortable with it myself. I guess I'm not. It's not that he wouldn't accept that aspect of me—or understand it—I don't accept it or really understand it myself. (How's that for being vague!)*

The period before coming out is often filled with agony, inner doubts, and a feeling of loneliness, caused by trying to make oneself "fit in" to heterosexual "norms":

*I wasn't gay in high school and knew no one who was. I should say, I didn't know in high school that I was gay. I didn't like high school. I was lonely, never felt like I fit in, didn't date. I felt like being intelligent was boring and lonely. I started dating boys in senior year in high school, had a few sexual experiences, and then came out to myself at nineteen—so my heterosexual career was short-lived. (I have, however, had a few heterosexual "interludes" since.) I wanted to be with boys so I would feel normal, but still didn't feel normal—the sex I had was to be tolerated and rarely "fun." It was much better with girls (at twenty and later). But even then, even with girls, it took me a while to become really sexual— the excitement was still unusual for me and transitory for a long time.*

*In high school I became aware of my attraction to other women, but I quickly forced it out of my mind, telling myself, "Everybody has these feelings, it's O.K. if you don't do anything about it!" I never considered that I might actually be a lesbian, since lesbians were obviously sick and deviant and I was neither.*

*High school was rough for me. With boys, I was nervous, I liked them, even liked kissing some, but found them very aggressive and not very attractive physically. Being with a girl was ecstatic. Although I was gay, I didn't really know what to do with it, so I was pretty much in the closet. I didn't like feeling abnormal. I was loneliest my whole life before I came out. My parents never knew I had sex at fifteen, but I came out to them as soon as I came out to myself. My mother was more upset than my father, who accepted me regardless.*

*When I was in high school (five years ago), I felt ugly, fat, left out, and weird. I think it was related to my emerging lesbian sexuality and my realization I was not about to fit in. I then transferred to an alternative, open-concept school where most of the kids were outsiders—super smart, gay, or from unusual parents, etc. I felt happier—like I fit in most of the time—but still I had problems. My mother was stricter and I had an earlier curfew than my friends. They all laughed at me. I was always between things—my mother's wrath if I arrived home late or my peers' laughter.*

*I dated boys from fourteen to sixteen. I felt it was a social necessity, but it always made me feel sad and alienated because I knew I was gay. (I fell in love with another girl at age twelve and we shared some physical affection. I was unable to admit to myself at sixteen that I loved her far more than any boy.) My first straight sex was at eighteen, and my first lesbian sex too. But my parents were proud when I dated boys. They never noticed my women lovers. I felt awful about that because I knew I was a fake.*

*Leaving home was splendid. I wanted nothing more than to live freely and openly as a lesbian and explore all the other wonders of life. And that's what I'm doing!*

But when the decision to "come out" is made, the picture changes and the amount of enthusiasm and pride expressed by almost all lesbian women is remarkable: 94 percent feel only positive about their decision to "come out."

*I "fell in love" in my last year of college with a classmate. I was floored when I realized what was happening to me emotionally. I said to myself, "You're in love with another woman, you are!" I was shocked, surprised, and very pleased to at last have "fallen in love." I was shocked because I knew that falling in love with another woman was not considered normal, surprised that I was doing something considered abnormal by society, since I'd always been a very popular girl, dated the star basketball player in high school, a summa cum laude in college. But with those boys I had not fallen in love, and very in love I was with Jane. She was my first love. I always liked sex, but after Jane I preferred women and sought them out, while men sought me out. I wonder if my aloofness from them, untouched emotionally, increased their pursuit; if it did, that didn't impress me.*

*I came to be a lesbian when I was about twenty. I kind of knew all along as an adolescent that I had homosexual feelings, but chose to date boys to cover up my feelings. When I was sixteen, I had a terrible crush on a cheerleader that I worked with in a restaurant. After a time, we became friends, and about four years later, lovers. The entire relationship lasted nine years and was very intense and passionate.*

*Sex with women is much more of an emotional feeling and a closeness that I just haven't found with men. It's much more than a different physical touch, it's an inner intensity that can't be equaled. There are no rules or expected sexual behaviors involved. It's the freest kind of love I know.*

*By the way, my mother thinks my lesbian lifestyle is great! I like my mother very much, I admire and respect her and think she is one in a million. I can't think of too many seventy-year-old mothers who think their daughter's lesbianism is great and support her lifestyle. I think I am very much like her—enthusiastic about life and always running in high gear. I like my mother's enthusiasm for life and her open-mindedness.*

## WOMEN OVER FORTY: BECOMING GAY FOR THE FIRST TIME

One of the most surprising findings in this study is the number of divorced women in their forties and fifties who are having love relationships with women and finding this a comfortable—in fact, excellent—way of life.

Amazingly, 24 percent of the gay women in this study were having a lesbian relationship for the first time after the age of forty; this figure represents a definite departure from past statistics. The following woman, previously married and with children, describes this change in her life:

*Throughout my life, my women friends have been strong, courageous, beautiful people whose friendship has meant more than nearly anything else. But never in all of my forty years had it occurred to me that I might love a woman in a sexual way. I have hugged and kissed woman friends, we have wept and laughed together, struggled through our respective marriages and divorces together, worked together. But never did I realize that I would feel physically attracted to a woman. It did not occur to me that I might have the ability to love a woman. I have engaged in conversations in which I espoused the theory that human beings would be bisexual if social barriers had not restricted their thinking, etc. But those conversations were intellectualizing on my part.*

*Now suddenly, a new world has opened up to me. I've asked a thousand questions, with dozens yet unasked. I have learned and experienced so much joy and dazzling pleasure that I find it difficult to understand why I didn't discover it before.*

*Two years ago, I moved to this state to take on a new job. Since I was here, I had been celibate the entire time. My job was so time-consuming and full of pressure, I had little time for myself My daughters are older and require attention from me in the evenings. After weeks also of evening meetings and late nights at the office, I preferred to be at home with them, rather than looking about for men.*

*About this time, through some gay friends of mine, I happened to meet a very special woman. In the beginning, I had no intentions of looking for anything other than female companionship with her—we had mutual interests and would share records. This turned out to be the most wonderful relationship of my life so far. It has literally revived me, and brought me back into the world of feelings, happiness, relaxation—inti-macy and love. My daughters think we are just friends—that is all I am prepared to cope with with them right now.*

*I still think of myself as single, and probably always will. I treasure my singlehood almost as much as I treasure my self-identity. I love being single. The happiest times in my adult life have been when I was single. My lover wants for us to live together and make a long-term commit-ment, but I am not interested in giving up my freedom. I doubt I'll ever give it up.*

*All of her touching excites me. My breasts and nipples are the most sen-sitive, and she can bring me the closest to orgasm this way. But it is the clitoris which holds the magic. I'm tempted to say that orgasm is the best part of our sex. However, I did orgasm with my husband and it was not as exquisite as it is with my lover, it is the quantity and quality of hold-ing and affectionate touch which I share with my lover that makes it all so different, so wonderful.*

Another woman, age forty-two, describes the "magical quality" of her life now—in contrast to life with her ex-husband:

*I'm a relatively well-adjusted, happy, healthy, loving middle-aged woman, deeply in love, probably for the first time, and closest to my lover—another forty-two-year-old woman.*

*There's a glow—a magical quality—to being "in love" which gives all of life's experiences more joy and delight. It may not be necessary for everyone, but I wouldn't have missed it. We have compatibility on every level—physical, mental, emotional, and spiritual—which has been the key. In the past when I loved someone, my husband and two other men, we only ever connected at one or two levels.*

*My love and I have lived together for two years, and we had known each other at work for four years before. Companionship, total intimacy (including exquisite sex), and economics, all are considerations in our partnership. We've been able to save money, make major purchases jointly, and share our house while renting the second. We have taken all our vacations together, including a study tour of Europe and trips to visit relatives and friends. Our physical intimacy and passion is more tender and gentle, slower but deeper and more powerful. We fall asleep every night with arms and legs intertwined.*

*For the first time, the loving seems equal—I have always felt that I gave far more than I received. Now I feel totally loved and secure—and so does she. We enjoy everything about our life together—cooking, dishes, garbage—are all easy and effortless—not the power struggle of* my married years. Going to bed at night or for an afternoon nap is our favorite activity—just for the snuggling, holding, and sweet talking.

Talking is relatively easy and equal. She's learning to ask for what she needs—knowing that it's finally O.K. to ask—that happiness is not related to total self-sufficiency as she had thought. We are both sharing all parts of ourselves—without withholding, judging, or criticizing. Years of therapy and growth experiences before we met had prepared us for a close and deep relationship—but we hadn't found a partner with the same background and expectations until now.

When I got married in 1961 at eighteen it was because I hated dating and living at the dorm or at home. I found a sweet, sensitive, sophisticated man and decided I'd do better if I were married. Although we eventually divorced, I believe that my choice was good—I have yet to meet a man with his strengths and qualities.

Yet later, when my son was an infant and my marriage was very unsatisfying, I cried myself to sleep frequently. I didn't see divorce as a possibility because I took the vows "deadly" seriously. I was the loneliest when my son was young and we lived in the mountains with no neighbors and I commuted forty miles to a job with no kindred souls.

For most of our marriage I was the primary wage earner and it was a problem for his ego. The decision making was "equal" but the earning wasn't and I was always reluctant to veto his wishes—not wanting to "emasculate" him with money. We always lived on the edge of financial disaster—we overspent and had no savings.

Most men forty and over are very threatened by the women's movement—feeling that if women gain something, men will have to give up something. My husband had very mixed feelings. Intellectually he supported women's issues in church, school, and work settings—but at home he was hostile about helping with housework, cooking, and other "women's work." His head and his heart were not together.

At two points during my twenty-year marriage I experimented with affairs. One was with a friend's husband (they had just separated). But the sex was no better and he was no more capable of intimacy than my husband.

My current partner is the most important relationship I've had. This is the happiest and closest I have ever been. It's almost too good to be true—beyond any dream or fantasy I ever had of marriage or life with a man. It's the first relationship that does not require "working at"—it's been effortless for two years. In addition, I've had several deep and lasting (ten-plus years) friendships with women.

To women today I say: love yourself first and don't eliminate women as possible partners in life!

## WHERE IS THE DIVIDING LINE BETWEEN GAY AND STRAIGHT AFFECTION FOR A FRIEND?

*My best friend is the reason I answered this. I love her, she's helped me through some of the lowest points of my life. She's encouraged me to be the whole person I am today. We probably had an affair without sex. I can't ever say how much of the happy, healthy me of today I owe to her. She helped me to find out what I want and who I am. When I'm with her things are great. We enjoy each other. I love her the most of any woman in my life.*

*As I've grown up I've had many crushes on women—some of which have turned into good friendships (nothing sexual). I believe women can be attracted to women sexually as they are to men. Usually I find this physical attraction dies as soon as I get to know the person well and become friends.*

*My best woman friend and I are compatible and feel very comfortable around each other. She is very honest and open, very accepting, and doesn't try to change me. She lets me be. We communicate so well. Our love for each other has been very strengthening. We have both helped each other with difficult situations to make major moves in our lives. We also have been sexually attracted to each other, but decided not to act upon it. We have used it to become closer emotionally. I love her and hope that we remain close throughout the years. We have even talked about being the "life mates" of each other. Why do people have to be married or lovers to spend their lives together? I feel that two friends can make that commitment.*

*My best friend and I have hiked together, traveled, read philosophy, Zen, and holistic health together, worked, talked, played together for six years, and developed a deep (but non-sexual) love for each other which we were sure would last forever. We spent most of our time together though I was married (she was alone). She is very intelligent, funny, beautiful, and we went through so much pain and pleasure together. My relationship with my current lover ultimately destroyed our friendship, the intrusion of another woman was too much.*

### LESBIANISM CAN BE POLITICAL

Besides the increased affection and sensitivity and the increased frequency of orgasm, some women felt that sex with another woman could be better because of the more equal relationship possible, that sex with women should be a reaction against women's second-class status in society:

*Is sex political? Of course. When I quietly parted from my last male lover (for women) I suddenly, for the first time, moved into my own space, my own time zone, and my own life.*

*Because of my own tremendous conditioning, which I believe is almost universal, it is almost impossible for me to have a truly healthy sexual relationship with a man—probably for any woman.*

*Sex is a form of comfort and to have sex indiscriminately with males is to give them comfort. I think it should be seriously considered. I see lesbianism as putting all my energies (sexual, political, social, etc.) into women.*

Janis Kelly has had some interesting things to say along these lines in "Sister Love: An Exploration of the Need for Homosexual Experience":[7]

*All heterosexual relationships are corrupted by the imbalance of power between men and women. In order to maintain superiority, males must feed on the emotional care and economic servitude of women. To survive in a male-supremacist social order, women must cripple themselves in order to build the male ego. Due to the stifling effect of this culture and to the damaging roles it enforces, women cannot develop fully in a heterosexual context.*

*Love relationships between women are more likely to be free of the destructive forces which make [these] defenses necessary. Institutional norms and the restraints of a power-oriented culture have, of course, also influenced women; nevertheless, the domination-subordination patterns women sometimes bring to lesbian relationships cannot overshadow the essential equality of the persons involved. In addition; many of the responses nurtured in females are extremely conducive to non-exploitative interaction. Sensitivity to the feelings and moods of others, care-taking, and gentleness are among the qualities more encouraged in women than in men.*

*Because men occupy a superior social position and are schooled to covet power over others in order to maintain that position, they can rarely accept others, especially women, as equals. Human contacts must be arranged hierarchically, and women must be on a lower level. Tension is inevitable when a woman refuses to accept this position and must be "put in her place." In contrast, women are able to start from a foundation of equality and devote their energy to growth and creativity rather than to struggling to maintain identities against the destructiveness of the traditional female role.[8]*

It is important for women to recognize their own potential for having sexual feelings for other women. We need to learn to love, respect, honor, be attentive to, and interested in other women. This effort includes seeing each other as physically attractive, with the possibility of sexual intimacy. As long as we can relate sexually only to men because they are "men" (and as long as men can relate only to women because they are "women"), we are dividing the world into the very two classes we are trying to transcend.

Any woman who feels actual horror or revulsion at the thought of kissing or embracing or having physical relations with another woman should reexamine her feelings and attitudes, not only about other women, but also about herself. As the feminist columnist Jill Johnston has written: "[U]ntil women see in each other the possibility of a primal commitment which includes sexual love they will be denying themselves the love and value they readily accord to men, thus affirming their own second class status."

## BEING WOMAN-IDENTIFIED: A VALID ALTERNATIVE

Many women still do not feel that they can find permanent security with another woman. Yet, as one woman puts it, "There are a lot of qualities women assume they can get only from men that they can get from a woman too, if they just tried."

## ANOTHER WORLD, ANOTHER CULTURE

There is a feeling here of looking in on a special culture, another way of life, breathing a different air. The existence of this world is a great cultural resource: it provides a place of strength and beauty to draw on, opening up for all the pleasure of diversity and new ways of seeing things, being together.

Why should anyone have to defend lesbianism as a way of life? In fact, as historian Carroll Smith-Rosenberg has written in her study of women in nineteenth-century America, one can see things just the other way: in fact, "to see heterosexuality as an artificial construct imposed upon humanity (would be) a revolutionary concept."[9] Who is to say which is more "natural": to love the opposite sex or one's own? Greek men of ancient times would certainly have been hard pressed to give an answer. Perhaps it is even more important here to ask why it has become so taboo for women to hold hands even in friendship, or to demonstrate physical affection as they did in Victorian times. Once again it seems imperative for us to review our entire concept of sensuality—as well as our priorities in terms of friendships and feelings for other women.

Many women here have expressed the deepest feelings of love, joy, passion, and sorrow for the women they love, feelings that reverberate with the deepest longings of all our hearts.

## SEX AND LOVE BETWEEN MEN

*In our society you can go to war and kill a guy, but God help you if you're caught in bed with one.*

There is still a great deal of prejudice against homosexuality:

*I have known for a long time that I have homosexual tendencies. This used to worry me until I fell in love with another man for a while. And it was just that. I wasn't gay or some screaming faggot, I just fell in love with someone and that person happened to be male.*

*I see no real reason for homosexuality to be taboo. But like a lot of other things, it just did not fit into the society (openly, of course) that we were forced to enter (by birth). Last century mentally retarded children were kept in hiding from the public eye. When these children were big enough to cause a lot of trouble, they were taken to the insane asylum (as it was called then) and some of them were never seen again. A homosexual was considered the same as mentally retarded except worse.*

*Homosexuality is sick and disgusting. It's against the laws of nature. It's not what God intended—no way.*

*The Bible speaks against it and a Christian society forms its laws on biblical ones. Personally men do not have the body shape, skin texture, or feminine scent that makes procreation and sexual satisfaction a simultaneous possibility. I don't understand homosexuality as anything more than an offshoot of masturbation where a seeking of physical pleasure generates a trade.*

*Regardless of all the advances and the new morality of today, or whatever you want to call it, I still feel homosexuals are defective human beings, mostly brought about by themselves and rejection by society because of their own tendencies. I object to homosexual marriages, homosexual teachers, homosexual anything where a queer is allowed to publicly boast about his abnormality.*

*Homosexuality is a taboo because it's repulsive to most people. I feel sorry for queers as I feel sorry for sick people and I feel they should be encouraged to try to change. As long as they limit their sex to consenting adults they remain merely pathetic creatures. Homosexual marriage is a farce.*

> *Marriage is an institution of the family built around the family. Since men can't impregnate men or women impregnate women, then homosexuals do not have to marry. They can live together and play house if they like. Marriage they don't need. To let such homosexual couples raise children would be cruel to the poor kids. They would possibly not be queer but surely be ashamed of their parents, or at least the object of their peers' ridicule.*

> *I consider myself very broad-minded and liberated in MOST ways concerning sex, but I feel that our Creator made men with a penis and women with a vagina for a reason, and that's for intercourse, and male homosexuality in particular completely turns me off!!!*

> *While I've never been gay, and think to a degree it's unnatural and irreligious, I feel strongly about the rights of individuals. Each to his or her own.*

Indeed, some men had isolated homosexual experiences but found them distressing or had mixed feelings:

> *I half think I'm disgusting and disgraceful for doing it. Why do I crave men? Why don't I like my wife? I don't know. God help me.*

> *One of my pet peeves is people who say of gays, "Well, if you people want to choose to be like that . . ." I did not choose to be this way. Most of us did not choose to be this way. It's just the way we are. We did not choose to be gay any more than heterosexuals choose to be "straight." It's just the way we are by nature. Many of us have desired and wished and prayed to be changed, but as far as I can learn we cannot change or be changed either by psychology, psychiatry, or religion. Most people who thought they were changed by any of these means soon found that they were still gay. I would like to tell you one of my secular attempts at trying to make myself "straight," even though it did not succeed. I went to heterosexual porno movies and looked at naked women, and said to myself such things as "Look at that hot, tight, juicy pussy. Wow! I'd like to shove my hot, hard cock up there and fuck her good." I looked at the women and said these kinds of things to myself, but I have to admit I was lying to myself. When the naked men with their erections entered the pictures I was excited by them without any attempts to try to make myself think I was. As I have learned to accept myself, I have realized that being gay is not bad, is not sad, is not something to try to avoid or change. Our only reason, my only reason for wanting to change in the past has been because of society's disapproval, because I know/knew my friends would not approve of it or*

*accept it, or me. And because I had not accepted myself. I am finally learning to accept myself as and for who and what I am. I want to say, I am gay and I am proud. I'm almost there, I almost can.*

*Where I'm at now is I am more relaxed having oral sex done to me, but a penis still feels strange in my mouth. Where I'd like to be is: more relaxed in giving pleasure to other men. It's a self-appointed decision, and a part of this decision involves having more confidence in performing fellatio with other men.*

Strangely, in their teenage years many men do in fact touch each other and play sexual games together—something girls do not generally do as teenagers, although they have intense "best friends." Almost half of all men—a number that is increasing since Kinsey first tracked this behavior statistically—"mess around" with other boys in school.

One of the most startling findings of my research is the increase in the number of boys who, as teenagers, are having sexual experiences with other boys. How easily and naturally many boys share sexual activities with each other is truly surprising. For most boys, these activities seem to be remarkably free of guilt and conflict. In the 1940s Kinsey reported that 48 percent of the men in his sample either masturbated jointly or had sex with other boys as adolescents or in their early teens. In my own work for *The Hite Report on Men and Male Sexuality*, I found that 43 percent of the sample were engaging in this activity. In the late 1990s the figure in my sample increased to almost 60 percent. Does this change mean that the number of boys masturbating together is increasing, or are these percentages all in a range hovering around 50 percent—that on average, approximately 55 percent of boys have sexual interactions with other boys? What would this mean?

Girls, on the other hand, rarely experiment with sex together. Girls form intensely emotional and sometimes romantic friendships around the same age, in an atmosphere of strong feeling, but they do not look for greater physical contact. They create great intimacy verbally, in a way that boys almost never do, despite boys' greater physical intimacy.

What kind of sex do boys have together? It is common for boys to touch each other, masturbate the other boy, and sometimes perform fellatio together. A minority (19 percent) have experienced anal penetration or penetrated another boy. It is almost as if shared sexual activity is a secret reality for men, part of the bonding process.

### SEXUAL GAMES BETWEEN TEENAGE BOYS

Surprising findings about boys' relationships with members of their own sex emerge in my research.

One of the most startling findings of my research is the increase in the number of boys who, as teenagers and older children, are having sexual experiences with other boys. This number has increased substantially since Kinsey's research in the 1940s.

To hear how easily and naturally many boys share sexual activities with each other is truly surprising. Though some boys worry a little or more, these activities seem to be remarkably free of guilt and conflict. Indeed, most boys do not wonder whether they may be "gay"—they don't seem to worry much about anything; they simply enjoy the pleasure and camaraderie. The biggest worry is HIV.

The spread of pornography and explicit television programs has probably encouraged boys not to hide their sexual feelings and bodies from each other; is this change what is responsible for the increase in shared sexual activities?

However, many boys who feel that they are "homosexual" (as opposed to those who just feel that they are having sex with other boys for fun) still report feeling very isolated with regard to their sexual desires for other boys, especially if they live in small towns. Explained one respondent: "All through junior high and high school I was frightened. I was not aware of anyone else who was gay. I saw my sexual feelings as a barrier between me and everyone else, and felt completely alone with these feelings. I would hear the ordinary ugly innuendoes or jokes that every kid hears about gays. This deepened my isolation: I was frightened of having any of that scorn or hatred directed at me."

What is really surprising is the kind of sex boys are now having together. According to my 1970s data, this contact mostly consisted of joint masturbation, often without touching each other. Now it is much more common for boys to touch each other or masturbate the other boy, and 36 percent of boys also perform fellatio together; 19 percent have experienced anal penetration or penetrated another boy. Very few kiss.

Judging from these participants, it is almost as if shared sexual activity were a secret reality for men, part of the bonding process. Or perhaps it is a new way in which men, especially boys, open up to each other. Is a more "female" style of intimacy still "off limits" to men, while "sex" is not?

On the other hand, this increase in the incidence of boys loving boys could imply an impending denial of women, part of the current backlash against "women's rights." Is men's politeness to women a charade, a pose, in a hypocritical world where men know that they are closer to each other than they are to women? Is this revival of the completely male-dominated world of societies such as were standard in classical Greece or eighteenth century America?

## WHAT IS SEX BETWEEN MEN LIKE?

Is there a sequence or pattern of usual activities "performed" during sex between men, similar to that in sex between men and women? What are men's favorite activities during sex together?

Men together usually start with "foreplay" and end with orgasm, but patterns between men are much less rigid than patterns between men and women; most sex between men is further distinguished by the fact that both partners almost always reach orgasm. Here are some men's descriptions:

*Our sex consists of a lot of conversation; affectionate kissing, holding; body contact—a great deal of oral exchanges—deep tongue kissing— tongue in ears, on neck—all over the body—use of tongue, lips on penis—and hands all over the body—massaging—masturbating— lotion lubrication—on penis and hands—usually ending in anal sex— mutual or quite often 69.*

*If we both have an erection and we are rubbing our rods together, it's the same as masturbating. I like to slow wrestle with an abdomen and pelvis locked tightly together. If possible I'll rub his chest softly. Then it'll turn into a wrestling match that grows more vigorous as we reach climax.*

*In bed or on the floor or wherever I and the man I am making love to are at the time, I love feeling his body all over, front and back, head to toe, and at the same time he feels me (except I do not touch his cock during foreplay and he doesn't feel mine), I really enjoy hearing him breathe, his body flex, he perspires, my body does the same, I feel my balls begin to ache, we are kissing each other all the while. Foreplay differs from lover to lover, but when I can feel his joy and happiness because of what I am doing to him, this makes me happy. I have found older straight men like kissing, or if I am making love to a straight man and sucking him off, feeling his cock go from soft to hard is positively very exciting and rewarding. Then I might drink his cum down, afterward, his cock is drained, no longer throbbing, limp, my head is still between his legs, his cock in my mouth, I feel his stomach and he is breathing normally again. We are usually not in a hurry to get dressed. Gays stay all night, straights go home. We never wear clothes, we stay naked until he goes back home or I do.*

*In the gay world there's an unwritten code of tit for tat (you come, I come). Sometimes it is a relief for my partner to know it isn't essential for me to ejaculate, but unless I am very direct (which can feel a little awkward if you have not known them long) I will go into automatic pilot and orgasm. At those times it is more like masturbation with an audience for me, which I hate, because the potential for emotional connection is lost.*

*There is the utmost tenderness if we are emotionally bonded—all kinds of caresses, kisses all over the body, deep mouth kissing—kiss the lips, the nose, the eyelids, the forehead; be as tender as a butterfly. Of course, lying together nude is part of it—fellatio is very special; a lot of handling and caressing of the genitals, maybe mutual masturbation, some thrusting with the penis between his legs or against any part of his or my body, or thrusting during fellatio. Just fuse into one bonded relationship. After an hour or two of the above activities, we may wish to reach orgasm by either fellatio or penis-anal intercourse, or maybe finger fucking and fellatio simultaneously.*

*Close hugging and friction. If the mood is romantic (and I prefer that it is) dancing, petting, deep kissing, mutual fellatio, then "milking" during the ejaculation, that is, swallowing the semen, sometimes mutual masturbation, or reaching orgasm by body friction in a variety of positions— chest to chest, chest to back, penis wedged between thighs, or chest to side. Or my favorite, anal penetration.*

*If it's a very macho guy then he usually wants me to submit after some perfunctory petting. I refuse almost always. If the partner is a confirmed "catcher" then the signals become clear that he wants you to penetrate him. I do not always want intercourse. There are times when I would be more than satisfied by simple petting and sleeping together. I do sometimes fellate someone or sodomize someone because it is expected. Sometimes I sense their appetite and comply out of compassion.*

*Normally I like foreplay. I like to get sucked, I like to suck. Sometimes I shower with or without my partner (making sure they do) and then I love rimming a nice round, firm, hairy butt (analingus). My nipples are the most sensitive part of my body. I love grabbing and lightly slapping asses. My nipples are most important. But sometimes I like to just "grease it up, stick it in, and fuck to my heart's content."*

*I will tell you my favorite recent experience with someone I just met. The first night, I asked him to come home with me. When we walked into my living room, the first thing he did was strip to his birthday suit. I was a little surprised at the quickness of the action, but I followed suit and we sat down on the sofa with a drink. He had a nice body and I was ready, so I started to feel him on the leg. The minute I touched him—he was ready to trot. Went to the bedroom and in the privacy of darkness he really came to life. Rolled over on top of me and kissed me full-mouth. I thought he would suck my tongue out of my mouth. Then he sucked my breasts and went down on me. He wasn't very good but he tried some of everything. After a while, he worked back up to my face, and with a wet finger working into my asshole, he asked if I had ever had a piece of meat up there. I told him yes but if he wanted to do it, be gentle. He was and with me on my back—with the aid of a pillow—he really enjoyed it. After quite a while, he finally climaxed—with all of him in me and sucking my tongue out of me. I climaxed at the same time. It was such a close feeling. I shot up onto my chest and, holding me very close with both arms, he ran his tongue down to taste it. Sucked up some and brought it to my lips. We lay that way for a long time until I thought my legs were going to break.*

*There was a period when I was orgasmically dysfunctional. The dysfunction manifested itself for two years after I "came out" as a homosexual. The basic reason was guilt. I had a lover (he is still my lover now) and we did a great deal of reading on sexuality. And he was very patient in bed. Together we worked at freeing my hang-ups. I got to the point where I could masturbate in front of him. We began to enjoy mutual masturbation. We experimented with many positions and vicarious actings-out of fantasies. The dysfunction waned and I began to have oral orgasms with my lover.*

QUESTION:
What are your favorite things about sex with men?

*I love their nude bodies to be next to mine and my nude body next to theirs.*

*I enjoy holding and being held by a man most of all. Fellatio comes in for a close second, but I need the physical contact most.*

*I like my rod sucked.*

*My favorite is anal intercourse with a nice, firm, hairy butt.*

*I fuck my partner and he comes at the same time by masturbating himself. Or the reverse. I also like the "Princeton fuck" (the "collegiate fuck")—just rubbing together face to face to the ecstasy of orgasm, or jerking off together. I experience the warmth and closeness of my partner, while my own hand knows exactly what to do to my body.*

*I like to take his clothes off real slow and watch him get horny and hot.*

*The affections (hugs and kisses) are the best part.*

*My favorite is anal intercourse. It is most rewarding emotionally, although I feel strange admitting that—but after the act what I remember most vividly and savor long afterward is the union, the tenderness, the language that was established between us. Just being inside of a man makes us a unit and for that one moment of anal intercourse we are a complete "ONE" emotionally as well as physically. I love the feeling of his scrotum against mine. His manhood next to mine.*

A few men describe a preference for sadomasochistic sex with men:

*The older I get—I am thirty—the more I find that S&M allows for greater expression of personality than "normal" sex. When a man wants to dominate me it excites me. It makes me feel powerless but secure in his strength. Several times men have made me masturbate while I beg for sex with them. The cruising, the hunt, the relationships with strangers, satisfy my need for adventure. Sometimes I play the sexual master; sometimes I play the slave or any stage in between. By playing these roles I learn more about myself. I like to think of sex as an art. I have never had intercourse with a woman, and never performed cunnilingus. I think women's genitals are grotesque. Sadomasochism is appealing because it explores the frontiers, the hidden corners of personality. It teaches you to realize your own power and assertiveness. It frees you from socio-sexual restrictions. It can be, with me, an act of rejection of society. The S&M social group can be a sort of charm school in which masculine mannerisms are taught. I believe that mannerisms are learned from society. Many homosexuals learn to act "gay" or effeminate. They feel as though they are being free but I believe they are victims of their own stereotypes.*

*S&M is an emotional experience. As a slave I like the feeling of being in the hands of a more powerful individual. As a master I like the feeling of possessing someone and of teaching them. Physically I like experiencing unusual sensations like spanked bottoms. Hot wax allows one to explore degrees of pain in a fear-free situation. I also like humiliation, drinking and being covered with urine, and coprophilia. I don't know why, perhaps it is an aspect of infantilism. I've only been into it for a year and have not realized all my fantasies relating to it.*

QUESTION:
What are the disadvantages of sex with men?

*OK, it is truly enlightening to find out what other men are like intimately.*

*Disadvantages are social—it's highly dangerous to love another man for fear of social ostracism. I have found the safest affairs are with men who have something to lose if the affair is found out. That way the affair is secret, sacred, and safe.*

*Disadvantages: even today, and in this relatively enlightened society, we run the risk of losing our jobs, our housing, being fined, jailed, even killed for being gay. Advantages: no fear of pregnancy; heightened pleasure from its "illicit," "forbidden" aura; more flexible and enlightened attitudes towards fidelity, monogamy, and casual sex.*

*I would be very embarrassed if my family and most of my friends found out. Also many men are assholes and I want nothing to do with them, much less to share sex with them.*

*Disadvantages: specific health risks and problems which are not that big of a deal, if one has knowledge.*

*The only disadvantage of being gay is trying to convince non-gay people that you are a human being. Otherwise, I am very happy being gay. At the very best, a person can find a missing part of himself in a loving relationship with another man.*

*There is nothing I don't like about sex with men, but I am very tired of the gay men's subculture—it is so exclusively male. I spent my high school years and half of my college years mainly with boys/men (they were boys'/men's schools) and I still feel easy and close with men most of all, but now men's groups, men's subcultures, etc., do not interest me. I am much more interested in women and in mixed groups. Being with men only gives me the same feeling I have when I spend too much time just with white people or Americans. It is too confining.*

*You have to be able to cope with the negative or anti-gay attitudes of society, and the potentially traumatic problem of what to tell your parents. It can also be lonely. Intimate relationships tend to last only a short time, and many people have to be very careful on the job to keep their gayness a secret. If you're in a position to be able to accept your gayness and be open about it, the pressure is not too bad—but there is always that feeling of societal disapproval in the background.*

*The disadvantage is discrimination. It's something that every person should definitely experience at least once in their lives.*

How is sex with men different from sex with women?

*Men are more outgoing sexually. They want sex. Women will fight you off. Also men are better at "sucking" than women, and fucking a man is tighter than fucking a woman. I respond to it physically and emotionally in a way I cannot generate with a woman. My wife considered me a fantastic sex partner, but to me sex with her has been less satisfactory than masturbation.*

*Too many times when I have been with women, I found out that they were pretending to enjoy what I was doing, and afraid to do anything except just lie back and get screwed.*

*The tight fucks are great. Plus, you can both fuck and be fucked (something you can't do with a woman). Also, men are better off psychologically than women.*

*I've found my male partners less inhibited about caressing my body than women. I find more equality in sexual action.*

*Roles are shifted easily and thus there is more variety. Men are more vigorous and aggressive in sex than women, almost always more muscular and rougher in action. The chief attraction of males over women is having a cock.*

*Right now, most women I find boring. I feel better with men.*

*I don't like the heavy role-playing that always seems to result from male-female sex—when I, the male, wasn't dominant, it generally seemed that the female took over the dominant role. We had so much trouble being equals that we finally gave up. It's easier and more natural with another man.*

*Men don't give you the horseshit women do—I don't like the rat race women lead you on. You know you're going to fuck her, but you must go through a long ritual. If a man is willing—you get it right now.*

*With men it's honest. I like the honest level of the involvement.*

*I enjoy sex with men best because I can relax passively in the strength of someone else.*

*You don't have to worry about having to support her, or marry her.*

*With women, one must pretend to "love" or at least be strongly attracted before women will agree, and most still act as if in participating in sex they are doing a favor or at least giving more than they receive. Because of the need for entertaining them, even if only buying them drinks, sex with women costs much more. With men, except with very young ones, the treatment is as equals.*

*Society expects me to be dominant in my work, in social affairs, in my spirituality (vis-à-vis the Catholic ideology of male supremacy), and also in my home life including bed. That is too damn much dominancy. I need to be able to feel "catered to" emotionally at times too. Thus, I find a homosexual relationship much more rewarding in that I can have a healthy balance between dominance and submission in bed.*

*With a man the feeling of strength with strength is a fantastic feeling to me. Women are too soft and cannot give me the strength which I need. Being next to a man amplifies my own strength.*

## PERFORMANCE PRESSURES IN SEX BETWEEN MEN

*I hate to say it, but sometimes there is a big silent competition between who has the biggest cock, can shoot the most come, and stay hardest the longest, etc.*

*Sexual activity in the gay world is fraught with role playing, exaggerated postures, and too damn much emphasis on potency or "masculinity." Some of the rituals are unpleasant—the cruising routine in bars, for example, and heavy use of alcohol, marijuana, "uppers." Some of the bizarre interests are not too much fun either.*

*I think sex with a man can get to be a contest of wills—a question of who really is more powerful.*

*Sometimes I feel pressured by men to have an orgasm, especially in "quicky" situations with strangers. It's often almost a contest as to who can make the other come first.*

*Usually I am the one that makes the advances. I am unsatisfied if I have to make all the advances. It's as if your partner isn't interested. I like to be passive at least once in a while, to know they are interested in me and my body. But sometimes you could sit and wait and rot till it falls off if you wait for other people.*

*I don't like men who jump up after and have to leave right away, and don't show any affection.*

*I would like sex to have a greater emotional emphasis than most men are ready to give it.*

There is a need for many more subtle descriptive and personal terms in our vocabularies. What is a "homosexual" act? In one way, men are having sex with other men when they share pornography and discuss how they "have" sex with women or when they go to topless bars together. They are enjoying sex together and joining in a form of sexually related bonding. Is caring for another man "homosexual"? In some ways, as we have seen, it is considered even less manly to embrace or kiss a man than to have sex with him.

This attitude carries over into "normal" work and friendship relationships between men: Why can't men be close and affectionate? In fact, not only can men not touch each other and be close physically simply as friends,[10] but also in most cases they are not allowed to share real emotional intimacy. A large part of the problem is our language—or lack of it—and the ever-present fear of being labeled "homosexual." And yet many men seem to express a longing to relate to other men in a new way, differently, to become more open, close, and honest with each other.

## LOVE STORIES BETWEEN MEN

QUESTION:
Describe the time you fell most deeply in love. How did it feel? What happened?

*Being in love is the most all-encompassing, overwhelming experience of my life: I feel ecstatically happy when I'm with him, when we're doing something together, or simply spending the evening together at home. He means more to me than anyone or anything else in the world. I cried myself to sleep when at one point he said that he thought we were spending too much time together, and that we needed new experiences apart (including, potentially, other sexual things). I was desperately unhappy, both with him and when we were apart. I could barely stand seeing him be cold and unaffectionate with me. Although I agreed that we had become too isolated from other people, I didn't want our reaching out to new people to negatively affect our relationship. But we have more or less worked through this now, and the happiest period of my adult life has been the past year. Especially when we were away on holiday together, away from our work, doing new and exciting things together. Perhaps the closest I've ever felt to him was the last time I saw him, and we both cried on each other's shoulder about having to say even a temporary goodbye. Those tears were more expressive and real than any words could ever have been.*

*Does feeling deeply in love really need description? I felt that the most important thing in my life was the happiness of the person I loved. I subordinated my own feelings and interests to the objective of my love's happiness. I felt (no doubt irrationally) that had it been necessary I might well have sacrificed my very life for the preservation of my love. My whole existence for a couple of years was suffused with this all-important passion. What happened? The person I loved, who had reciprocated my feelings at first, grew less interested in me and by the end of three years of living together he was not any longer in love with me at all. It was a heartbreaking crisis for me, and the emotional agony and scars from that experience have left me permanently and clearly altered in my personality. I have never since had the same emotional capacity that I had before this experience. It is as though a part of my emotional capacity had been burned right out of my body or amputated. Eventually after many months I slowly resumed living. I have never, however, in the ten years since, been able to shed a single tear over anything. As I said, it is as if a part of my emotional capacity had been removed . . . cauterized away. I am basically a happy person. Only rarely do I feel a slight depression, but after that episode I think it must have been three years before I had a week when I could look at myself and say honestly, "I am happy this week."*

*The most deeply in love I have been was when I was nineteen, with someone I lived with for six years. There was a sexual attraction, but beyond this there was a sense of "comfortability," a tremendous joyful feeling of well-being. I don't like the gay term "lover"; to me that denotes something risque, spurious, without depth. This was a partnership, an equal sharing where we both used our talents to complement the other and shared the day-to-day responsibilities of living. There was no "he" or "she," simply two people who happened to be male and who happened to fully enjoy and respect each other. I do not recall that either of us felt any need to be jealous even when one or the other would seek a sexual encounter outside. We were honest about our relationships with others as well as each other. I believe that the honesty in our relationship gave to it a tremendous amount of security. I have never known such a sense of well-being or happiness since that time.*

*I have been deeply in love twice, both times with straight men who loved me also but could not totally express that feeling, sexually or otherwise. I have kept close contact with both and have continued to love them, one for seventeen years and the other for fourteen. The two times I was in love it hit me like an electric shock—like having a bolt of lightning hit me. I knew at that instant that this was going to be "the one." I was relatively speechless and fumbled for words. I became flustered. I was enormously aroused sexually although not aware of having an erection. The first time the fellow touched my hand (by circumstance, not intentionally), it was so intense it was almost painful.*

*I met my lover of two and a half years in a bar. I walked up to him and initiated conversation. There was immediately a strong attraction (physical). We returned to my apartment and had sex but it was more like making love. He was very considerate, and gentle in a way I had never really experienced before. After we had sex, we talked for a few hours, really candidly. I had to work the next morning and recall seeing him sleeping as I got dressed. He looked like a peaceful cherub. I knew this experience was a beginning, I knew it intuitively. We spent much time together, going to plays, movies, and art museums. I remember being turned on by his entering a room. Several times I couldn't tell whether I felt my penis or his. I missed him horribly when I was away. We became such good friends it permitted me to unlock much within myself and him. There was no question about the reciprocal nature of our relationship. There was a deterioration, however, when we took an apartment together. He became absorbed in his career and became distant, and very selfish about some things. I made all kinds of allowances and tried to talk things through. Still whenever things got rough for either of us we each supported the other strongly. When we began after two years to do fewer things together, I knew that my commitment was dying. So I decided not to move with him when he got a job offer in another city. He was surprised and hurt but made a fast recovery. I was upset, too. I still deeply love the guy. We visit each other at holidays, and have sex. But it is more out of a tribute to the past, I guess.*

## DO GAY MEN PREFER "PROMISCUITY"* OR LONG-TERM RELATIONSHIPS?

*I want a permanent relationship with someone who is "always there." The hardest thing in my life is ultimately being alone at night. I can have*

---

* Although it is common to hear that "now that there is the fear of AIDS/HIV infection, there is less promiscuity," this is not really accurate. Of course "promiscuity" is a perjorative word with negative connotations, a word which many men said they preferred not to use.

*great days and good times at work and in a variety of traditional ways, but it always ends in going home alone. I wish there were someone there to go to bed with me for the night; someone who cared and who was not there necessarily for sex.*

Some men preferred sexual freedom to a relationship, at least a monogamous relationship:

*I've had sex with over 2,000 men. I love to fuck and look at all men's penises. I'm what they call a whore. I love group sex and going to the baths. I would be bored with monogamy.*

*I am in love. However, I am not now in a steady relationship. To total the men that have wandered into my life would be foolish, but a conservative estimate would be 150 to 200. Monogamy doesn't work for me.*

*I don't like the idea of being tied down to one person all the time. Right now I feel that I have enough love and affection within me that I can share it with more than one person, but if I ever do go into a relationship I hope it will be for an extended period of time, because for me to give a good meaning behind my love I would have to concentrate on just one person. Right now I prefer having casual relationships, it gives me a chance to meet and like many different kinds of people and it's helping me decide the type of person I would like to settle down with.*

*My plans for the future are to stay single. I prefer to be free to do as I please without having to worry about the feelings of another person.*

Others were involved in, or preferred, long-term monogamous relationships:

*I have a steady male relationship. I do love him, but we don't talk about love. We enjoy each other's company and most of our talk centers around our careers. The relationship has been steady for one year. In my forty-four years I've only had sex with four men. I'm too busy to cruise and I don't feel safe in a multiple-relationship arrangement. The "gay" men I know are monogamous and are far from promiscuous. If there is any promiscuity, it's in younger men. I never make passes at teenage men. I never contemplate sex with my college students. I've only had sex with men who are professional and are generally colleagues. I really like most men I work with and feel very close to them, even emotionally close.*

*In my present life, homosexual promiscuity is a reality. It certainly was not so through most of my life until the age of sixty-nine. Even now I would greatly prefer emotional closeness with one person to casual sex.*

*My earliest sexual credo was the more the better—quantity without regard to quality. Over the years my attitudes toward myself as a sexual being have metamorphosed. Now at fifty, I prefer sex as an expression of deeper feelings rather than the simple act of getting my rocks off. I guess this is a sign of maturity, at least I hope it is!*

*Now I am "single" again for the last nine months. At first, after the relationship, I enjoyed being able to do exactly as I pleased, no longer finding it necessary to conceal any of my actions. I had two affairs (one lasting four weeks, the other two weeks). But I am very dissatisfied with what I have come to regard as insubstantial relationships. I wish more than I can convey to be involved in a strong commitment. Since there is no sanction for a gay bond, nothing societally that legitimates the commitment I crave, I feel somewhat at sea. I hope to find (and I am expending plenty of energy searching!) a meaningful relationship that incorporates both sexuality and deep friendship. What is depressing about gay life is that as much as you hope to avoid the banal stereotypes, they are almost inherent in the nature of this subculture. I mean, you may wish a life mate but it is a rarity among those I know. You also may dislike the prevalent emphasis in gay bar society on conspicuous sexual attractiveness, but you are forced to play the game—the bar routines— in order to meet people. It becomes a vicious cycle. I have found myself becoming more adept at bar communication but I attempt to mix sincerity with bar suaveness. My "success" (score) rate is high, but I do not pride myself in this, since my goal is a long-term relationship.*

Many gay men believe that a nonmonogamous but committed relationship is the ideal:

*I have a lover and we've been together for eight years. I occasionally have sex with other guys, but they are for sex only, usually, and there is little emotional entanglement. My lover does likewise. We have many gay friends, but they are comrades, confidants. Our love is not based on infatuation, but was something that took a period of years to build and nurture. There have been good times and bad times. Bad times (emotionally, financially, and sexually) have helped us grow and understand one another much better than if everything had been great always.*

*Age forty-one. Homosexual. Married thirteen years. Got married for children and respectability (1960!). I loved my wife in a way but always had to fantasize males while making love. I also had lots of sex with males outside. I wanted children and had two, adopted two more. I love my children very much. Now I'm living with one lover and have occasional sex on the side. The present relationship is the happiest and the closest. We never fight and are neither exclusive nor consider our relationship to be eternal. It is nice and cool in that we accept what we have as long as it lasts.*

*I like to be especially close to someone with a little casual sex on the side.*

*I prefer an open monogamous relationship, one in which we are primarily monogamous but realize that people do come and go that are attractive and friendly—those you might want to date for dinner or go out with.*

*I hunger for emotional and sexual closeness—don't know if I'm capable of casual sex without emotional closeness. But I think the term "promiscuous" is best applied to heterosexual relationships. For gays I would prefer to use the phrase "less sexually restricted."*

This style seems to be favored by most men in intense or long-term relationships with other men.

Yet men do not always want "freedom"; sometimes love can be more "consuming," or very romantic—as the following stories attest. One man tells the beautiful story of his feelings during his first romance:

*I was almost seventeen years old when I first fell deeply in love. The intensity and the depth of the feeling frightened and overwhelmed me. At the time I was working as a cashier in a large supermarket. I enjoyed the work and enjoyed the close contact with people, especially the employees. After work we often got together and went bowling or played pool, etc. I was especially attracted to one of the fellows and we double-dated. It was on one of these double dates that I started having sexual fantasies. While he was making love to a girl in the back seat, I thought of him while I was kissing my girl in the front seat and wondered what it would feel like to be made love to by him. After the date I asked him to spend the night at my house and he accepted. I knew that something was happening to me but I wasn't sure what. After he fell asleep I got up, put my clothes on, and went to a nearby church. I knelt there and prayed, begging God for guidance. I cried, dried my tears, and returned home to bed and the strangest, most enduring relationship of my life began. I was surprised when he responded to me*

*sexually and I discovered what his kisses were like. I was in a state of*
*shock at what had happened to me when I realized I was in love.*

*We both had feelings of guilt and fought the relationship. We stopped*
*double-dating and avoided each other like the plague. Once or twice I vis-*
*ited the places that he frequented and remained in the background*
*watching him. After a stint in the armed forces we got together one night.*
*The feelings were still there but I had developed some self-control and we*
*touched and kissed and that was it. After that we got together about twice*
*a month for several years, but didn't touch. I always remember the mag-*
*netism of his body chemistry in relation to mine.*

### THE POLITICS OF BEING GAY

During recent years, there has been a kind of right-wing shift in terms of attitude on the part of gay publics in the United States, the United Kingdom and elsewhere, as documented by statistics in those countries.

After New York City's Stonewall Riots and the "antiestablishment" period of early gay pride, centered on liberal politics, came a different atmosphere, many gays going out of their way to stress that they are a stable part of the society, that they form families with their partners (true), but with an underlying tone that this "legitimizes" them, because they are helping society uphold the traditional morality of the couple. Sexual "difference" was claimed to be a matter of biology rather than of "choice," and therefore there "was no reason" to punish gays by excluding them from society— an understandable point of view, though whether being gay is a biological matter or a "choice" is still a controversial question.

While such feelings and beliefs can certainly be authentic (why shouldn't gays be politically conservative?), they can also be part of a defensive reaction, people try- ing too hard to fit into the status quo or "traditional morality"—especially at this time in history when "alternative values" seem to be less and less acceptable to the overall society, when "family values" are considered by so many to be "the test of morality and maturity."

During the 1990s "biological determinism" became the fashion; its approach to the question, "What causes homosexuality?" led to the answer that "it's all in the genes, no one can help it, it's how you're born." This shored up a pro-family ideol- ogy, seeming to say about gay families: "They are not dissenters, just chromasoma- lly different."

Yet gays would be wrong to forget the downside of trying to fit in by conform- ing, thus playing exclusionary politics; it is an error to forget to keep an eye on soci- ety's need for diversity and freedom of choice in personal sexuality and way of life.

Many gays in the United States have now sued large organizations, including government military bodies, for discrimination. In the United States gay men began a movement for public acceptance when, in the late 1960s, they refused to be cowed in New York City and fought back in the famous Stonewall Riots. Tragically, the gay rights movement gained more gravitas with the appearance of the AIDS/HIV virus, which has killed so many, a number that is still increasing and a disease that poses a serious risk everywhere.

A current sign of the times: gays in public life are getting more powerful. In 2001 Paris elected its first gay mayor—yet that was never the issue of the election, nor is it often remarked by newspapers assessing his performance in office. This circumstance is quite remarkable, something no one would have thought could happen just a few years ago. Ten or fifteen years ago any politician who admitted that he was gay would have been dead politically! Now Berlin also has a gay mayor.

There were, of course, always gay men involved in public office and in corporations, but this fact was not public information (there have also always been some single men of "unknown sexual preference"). There were too, and are, many lesbian women in public office and in corporations, yet they too have been extremely quiet about their personal lives. (Being single is difficult for women in important public posts, whether gay or straight—the attitude is, "A woman should be married!")

Another famous gay man in politics is/was the mayor of New York, Edward Koch. Although the media knew of his sexual preference (and everyone knew he was "single"), at the time (the 1970s and 1980s) they did not write about his private life; this was several years before President Clinton's impeachment trial put "sex" on the map of public-figure profiling.

Let's not forget the most famous gay man of all, the political chieftain J. Edgar Hoover, head of the FBI in the United States for decades, spying on presidents, politicians, and film stars, in part to blackmail them into political conformity—yet he himself was secretly "married" to another man and enjoyed practicing what many would call "sexual perversions," such as dressing as a woman when having sex.

More gay people are involved politically today than ever before; what influence will this emergence have on the direction of politics in the future?

## ARE WOMEN STILL MARGINALIZED IN THE GAY WORLD?

Although today there is a strong movement of gay men that is visible in most Western countries, pushing for the right to love others of the same sex—in France, gay couples can register with the city government as a couple and gain inheritance and other rights that in the past were reserved for married (heterosexual) couples—lesbian women are still less visible.

Gay women are almost invisible on the streets in gay neighborhoods. One sees many more men together than female couples or single gay women, though statistically, around the world, there are as many gay women as gay men. Lesbian women are there, approximately 15 percent of the population, but much less visible. "Single heterosexual women" in their 20s and 30s may be slightly more visible, since the media has focused on them as a group, it would seem.

Beginning with the Stonewall Riots by gay men in New York, and continuing in the activist groups focusing on the AIDS/HIV virus epidemic, gay men have gone more public than have gay women. Inside most gay rights organizations there is an unfortunate tendency to put men at the top, women on the bottom as secretaries and helpers of men, not as leaders, just as in the "straight world" (in the overall "heterosexist" social structure).

Of course gay women may understandably feel less confident in public than do gay men, since women in general are more vulnerable to social aggression and exclusion; to identify oneself publicly as a gay woman can put a job in jeopardy.

Unless they "get away with it" because such "lesbian affairs" are seen as "girlhood flings," sexy and "harmless" sexual experimentation (often depicted in popular pornography as two women getting turned on with each other while they wait for a man), lesbian women rightly fear punishment for their sexual relationships with other women if they are "too outspoken" and visible. Thus lesbian women are less visible than are homosexual men.

Acceptance by society now is not yet the same for gay women as it is for gay men. Women are still marginalized: just as, statistically, there are few women at the top levels of government and other institutions (like corporations), compared to men, there are also fewer gay women in those positions, especially not women who are recognized as gay. Women at the top so far (the few that there are) are still almost always required to have a family too. Margaret Thatcher and Madeleine Albright were known as married women. The head of Unicef is not married, nor is Condoleeza Rice, the current secretary of state in President George W. Bush's cabinet in the United States, but they are unusual. For the most part women in public positions "have to be married" with children.

It is important for women to have the freedom to decide about their lives. If lesbian women feel that they have to hide their relationships and feelings, this situation is not good for the psyche, identity, and pride of women in general. Such a tendency, while understandable, is regrettable, depriving other women of all ages of the chance of seeing the possibilities that exist. After all, the sexual relationships of women together can be extremely beautiful.

Women own the world as men do! Women own the streets, and women own their own bodies! Let's see women together in the street holding hands and being together as they really are.

## THE FUTURE OF WOMEN

### WILL MORE WOMEN CHOOSE LESBIANISM?

A letter I received paints a vivid picture of the dilemma or crossroads women sometimes now feel in their friendships with each other:

*I am 40, married for 18 years with a daughter 14, living a normal married life with its highs and lows. Five years ago I met the mother of one of my daughter's friends at school, and we became friends. Our friendship has grown stronger ever since. Now I telephone her at least once a day and she is always in my thoughts, I have come to need her presence in my life. During the day, I worry that she might need something, I want to be there to help her, at least by being able to talk to her when she has some small problem. For example, I know she suffers a bit with her husband with whom her relationship is less than idyllic. I like her because she is refined, open and kind. I find great pleasure in talking with her. I like to have her near me and I want our friendship to continue.*

*Once before, several years ago, I had another good friend, but that friendship ended: out of respect for the customs of society, and to be a good wife as my family wanted me to be, I suppressed that friendship— before comments from my husband became too pointed, i.e., "You spend more time with her than at home!" (which was not true), and so on. This time I am not certain that the right thing for me to do is to put my family first, as I always have before. I don't want to mess up my life, but keeping up a semblance of "living a normal life" is not satisfying. In truth, I am happier with her than at home.*

*I don't know whether I should speak to her about my feelings, or let them fade and force myself to focus on my husband. If I let this relationship grow, if the feelings are so strong that I want to share everything with her, won't I have to renounce everything else? What would it be like if I let this friendship become the center of my life, can I still have a normal life? I don't want to give up everything, but I can't give her up either—well, I can't give up my feelings for her, with her I feel alive and happy and well. Yet if I continue in my present "normal" married life, I will be dishonest in some way. I am confused.*

The writer has a right to be confused, she is wading into uncharted territory. She is voicing an inner conflict that she feels in her loyalties, in her identity, wondering what is best for her (and the best use of her energies), and where her future lies.

Although the automatic interpretation of her letter might be: "Oh she's really gay and doesn't know it," I think what she is saying is more subtle and more complex than that and deserves to be heard and understood on its own (without this layer of supposition on our part).

Many women feel a preference for being with and talking to a best friend but do not go so far as to put their feelings into words or outline the dilemma and contradictions implied—though they feel them. Many women with such friendships accept, as women traditionally have done, that though they are happier with their friend, "it cannot be," they cannot spend more time with her because they have a duty to stay within the boundaries of traditional cultural patterns, and they need the physical contact they can have with a man. Yet women today question what purpose their traditional duty serves, increasingly concluding that their real duty is to their own honesty, strength, and happiness, believing that looking out for this aim will create more happiness than that provided by traditionally defined female duty—despite attacks trying to keep women in line, by calling "the modern woman" "selfish" for her consciousness of her own rights and desire for physical/psychological autonomy.

The question is: how close should a woman be with her best friend? Should a woman ever contemplate leaving her family and "normality" to begin a new life with a friend? What would such a life be like? Can daily life between two women with children be "normal"?

On an even deeper level, the unspoken question that is felt in many female friendships is: when the feelings reach a certain point, where should they go? Must a relationship grow in order to survive, or can it remain as it is without change and endure over time? Is it artificial to place a block or limitation on a relationship, does this action kill it? Perhaps women are closing off what could become the greatest relationships of their lives, denying themselves glorious and rewarding companionships in the second part or all of their lives.

If such a friendship grew up between a woman and a man, not between two women, these questions might not arise, since at a certain point both people would feel that living together was a logical expression of the growing feelings. However, since the friendship is between two women, the options are unclear (and also taboo). On the other hand, the opportunity to make something new is compelling; at this time in history women are taking themselves and their relationships with each other more seriously, thinking about them. In fact, women today have the chance, a unique opportunity, to redesign their relationships in totally new formats, expand the possible ways of having friendships. Their options are not simply to either be friends or be "gay"; there are various ways of living waiting to be discovered "in between" these two options.

Although most women have strong friendships with other women that can last for years, society has not fully acknowledged in a positive way or celebrated these relationships (as it does marriage, for example), indeed seeking to deemphasize and trivialize them—by means of such cliché remarks as, "Can you really trust another woman? Remember, watch out, a woman will knife another woman in the back whenever she gets a chance!" or, "Women are their own worst enemies!" and so on. Today women increasingly disregard such remarks, think for themselves, and size up their relationships on their own merits rather than experiencing them filtered through negative versions of "who women are." Of course not every relationship between women is positive (!)—why should it be, after all?—but most women enjoy close female friends.

What should the letter writer, a married mother in her forties, do at this crossroads inside herself, to determine the direction she wants to take her friendship with her best friend? Statistically she is not alone: surprisingly, in my most recent research there is a slight but noticeable increase in the number of married or divorced women in their forties and fifties who begin for the first time opting to live with another woman, a close friend, in lives they never imagined for themselves. These relationships are sometimes sexual, sometimes not—and can endure and provide a stable and lasting way of life, form a good basis for living as a family with children. (Think of the great popularity of the television series *Sabrina, the Teenage Witch*, seen around the world with its example of two women as the "mothers" of Sabrina; the three women—Sabrina and her two "mothers"—live happily together as a family unit.)

Designing new relationships with each other, whether or not they are sexual, taking these friendships seriously, is an emerging trend, one of the places where women are now planting their identity, establishing a new female flag and set of values.

## GAY MARRIAGE AND "FAMILY VALUES"

I am in favor of gay rights—women's and men's choices—I always have been. Each of my books documents many moving voices of those in gay relationships.

However, the current issue of "gay marriage" strikes me as more symbolic than central to gay rights. Of course gay relationships are just as good and valid as any other relationships (are or are not); if this is true, the logic goes, then why shouldn't gay couples have the same legal status and protection and rights that marriage bestows on other couples—even if these rights are overrated? Clearly, gay people should have as much right as anyone to be proud of their love and to show it, to have a celebration known as "marriage," surrounded with the symbolism and legal sanctions attached, a day of ceremony and public celebration, dressing up and inviting family and friends, promising "before God and all present" to love, honor, and cherish the other for a lifetime.

On the other hand, in the 1960s it was said that marriage as an institution should be done away with; many heterosexual couples did not formally marry, as a sign of rejection of the institution, a sign that they believed in individual rights and freedoms, which they saw being repressed/stifled within the institution. They continued to believe in love and long-term commitment and often designed their own ceremonies where promises were exchanged in front of invited friends. (Originally the 2001 French "Pax" was supposed to add the legal backing to such "alternative couples," but the laws as passed were watered down, so they did not fully serve the purpose.) In those years it was completely out of style to say that one was "married."

Now we have come full circle: to be married is the ideal again, not only in the West but almost everywhere in the world; "family values" are all the rage. Marriage has become truly trendy. For example in China (and Japan), the only question for the "bride" is whether to wear a white Western wedding dress or a traditional red kimono during the ceremony. In the West books are published and promoted telling women "how to get and marry your man"; some ask if women should return to withholding sex until marriage.

A cynic could comment that in today's world militarism, with its hierarchical chain of command, has also become trendy; military might with its hierarchies is back in vogue, while democratic demonstrations sending messages to governments in countries such as the United Kingdom are strangely unheeded (Prime Minister Tony Blair's Labour government took the country to war in Iraq, though clearly the majority of the population did not wish it). Is this sign of the times in some way equivalent to the current belief in "traditional family values"? Does the military chain-of-command system twin the man-dominates-the-family chain of command in the legal structure of the "traditional family," or (as put in more "politically correct" parlance), "Today we recognize the beauty of the female in the traditional, helping role, and the importance of the traditional family structure."

The current trendiness of marriage may be connected to a belief in hierarchy as the only "workable form of society." Some say that "democracy doesn't work, it is too sloppy, what you really need is to create order, so someone has to dominate, be the commander in chief." Corporations and armies follow this pattern, but democratic governments are supposed to be consensual, based on majority rule. For centuries heterosexual marriage meant a ritualized hierarchy: man as legal head of the family, woman as child producer and caring person, "helpmate," in theory "protected" by the man (though statistics on domestic violence demonstrate that "protection" can be a cover for exploitation). Although movements of the last fifty years have attempted to change the "balance of power" within marriage, legally the man is still "owner" of the children, also usually of "the wife"—though the days when a woman had no separate passport are gone. The family—especially the traditional family—remains a largely hierarchical institution, and marriage is the celebration and confirmation of that institution.

As marriage became unpopular in the 1960s and 1970s, it was widely believed that a better form of relationship (heterosexual or homosexual) could be developed outside of marriage, without the antiquated legal hierarchies of marriage that seemed, willy-nilly, to somehow exert their subtle influence and push people back into the old formula they were trying to transcend. Not every experiment was successful, but some were, some of the couples and relationships formed at that time and in that way still remain.

Gay couples today may, of course, claim that they are not hierarchical and that this is not the reason why they wish to marry, and they have a point. However, gay couples by definition are perfectly placed to develop new ways of living together that break ground, create lives that others can emulate. Many have done this, but they are underappreciated, seen only as "alternative" or "different" ("not quite as good as normal . . . but . . ."), and their contribution goes unrecognized.

The only institution that seems to exist that offers public recognition of long-term relationships is "marriage" (whether religious or civil); there has been no public spotlight on a new institution for celebrating publicly one's long-term relationship, though there should be. I would not like to ask gay couples to deny themselves rights, in order to stand for a principle, but should they? For gay couples to push to join an institution that for so long has been exploitative and problematic may reflect little more than the current trendiness of "family values." Attaining the right to marry is symbolically important, but in fact, marriage itself may be the opposite.

What do family values mean to nontraditional couples, gay or otherwise? "Family values" became a code phrase in the Western world during the 1980s and 1990s, continuing into the present, seemingly an unquestionable "eternal verity," the very basis of a solid society—but are "family values" really the primary basis of civilized society? Or are they tribal ("defend your blood relatives against outsiders")? Surely, extending our caring attitudes to the entire planet, making all races and peoples "our family members" should now be the ideal of global civilization. Old-style "traditional family values" were exclusionary (they created a them-against-us mentality), but the values we need now are inclusionary!

Of course "family values" have a positive meaning as well; to define "family values" is complex. Suffice it to say here, briefly, that the concept of "family values" is being used to pressure people today into being married and "fitting into their niche in society" (and to frighten them with being "left out"), while "individualism" is laughed out of court or ridiculed as "egotistical" (or, it is said, "you'll die old and alone"). Traditionally, however, family values meant that men had more privileges than women, women were divided into two categories, "the marrying kind, the good ones" (married mothers, especially by the age of thirty) and "the others" (sad and lonely losers, or "cheap prostitutes"). These "family values" categories are clearly related to an antiquated social order that discriminated against women, while at the same time alienating and confusing men, denying everyone full human status.

While I believe in long-term relationships and love, I have doubts about the goodness of what we loosely call "family values"; if these "values" mean enduring promises of love, sharing long years of life together, perhaps bringing up children, having a companion to live with until death (or to pass that important moment with, should one be so lucky as to be "the first to go" or die), also inheriting family possessions, homes, and businesses from each other, then these can be good things—but they can also create a kind of "me and my family first" mentality, a way of seeing the world with a closed mind.

In France, the Pax (as it is called) was passed into law approximately five years ago, offering those who live together for any reason (even "just friends") to be "paxed" by registering as a "couple" in the town hall; thus they gain the right to visit each other in the hospital "as family" and to inherit some things. However, the rights of the paxed partners are not as substantial as the rights married people share, although they could be if the laws were expanded. If the Pax were expanded and spread to the entire European Union community (both for heterosexual and homosexual couples), it might turn into a popular alternative to "marriage."

But marriage retains a kind of beauty, a mystique built up over centuries, deserved or not. People want to get married, they want to feel that their union and love is blessed by society. One cannot forget the images of absolute joy on the faces of those couples, lesbian and homosexual, taking their marriage vows and celebrating publicly after, sometimes, up to twenty-five years of living together, seen around the world on television sent from Boston in the United States during May of 2004. There is great appeal to the symbolism "before the world" of establishing the love-of-one's-life as a marriage partner.

I still fully believe in gay rights and think that anyone who would deny people the right to love others of the same sex is probably a bigot who should rethink. I also think that women's sexuality is frequently better expressed with other women than with men—certainly lesbian sexuality is more creative, does not follow a preordained formula, and women have more orgasms together than they do with men, they feel freer to express themselves, thus there is much that can be learned by everybody from what women invent together.

The question is: is getting married as a gay couple (female or male) really the bonus it is supposed to be? Clearly it makes gay people more visible and more "legitimate," and that is good. But it does seem a waste of good energy for gay couples to reinforce and support one of the major institutions of traditional society, when after all what they are seeking is to change that society. . . .

Yes, marriage should be legally possible, a choice between any two people, but I hope that many people—gay and nongay—will think twice or three or four times before embracing "the system."

NOTES

1  See the questionnaires in the Appendix, each of which addresses the issues discussed here.
2  Alfred Kinsey, *Sexual Behavior in the Human Female* (Boston: Scribner, 1948).
3  Ibid.
4  A good summary of the arguments can be found in Edward Brecher's *The Sex Researchers* (Boston: Little, Brown, 1969).
5  "Bisexuality: Some Sociological Observations," a paper presented at the Chicago Conference on Bisexual Behavior, October 6, 1973, Department of Sociology, University of Washington.
6  Ibid.
7  This information is in the appendices of the original *Hite Report*.
8  Kelly, Janis, "Sister Love: An Exploration of the Need for Homosexual Experience," *The Family Coordinator*, October 1972, pp. 473–75.
9  Carroll Smith-Rosenberg, *Disorderly Conduct* (New York: Alfred A. Knopf, 1985).
10  See also the documentation of boys' relationships (or nonrelationships) with their fathers in Parts 2 and 4 in *The Hite Report on the Family*.

# Part 6

# Sex, Human Rights, and Globalization
## (1996–2005)

*Building on the previous research-based excerpts in this book dating from 1976 to 2004, this section addresses the current political turmoil internationally. Focusing on how sexuality and gender identity impact our views of world politics—and in fact contribute to politics across the globe—it also suggests means by which the situation might be improved. What do the previous parts of this book imply for our larger political view of the world? Can we see some of the themes discussed sticking their heads out of recent global debates? Compiling essays written by Hite from 1996 to 2004, this section connects the material in the Hite Reports with international politics and the global situation generally.*

# Reevaluating Family Values and the Sexual Revolution
## Toward a New Vision of Sexuality

### WHERE ARE WE IN THE "MORALS REVOLUTION"?
### TRANSITION OR COLLAPSE?

Can we find a new way forward for our sexual morals, or do we feel that we must either "go with" the "sexual revolution" or "return to the tradition of family values"?

Another way to ask this question is: Is society now doing away with "moral structures" imposed for centuries on its behavior, without which people are nothing more than "amoral animals," or are we creating a higher moral standard amid the current confusion by integrating equality and democracy into sex and the family?

These issues have emerged dramatically in recent United States elections, as well as on the global political scene, in Middle Eastern and Afghan wars. The position of women in society, plus laws about female pregnancy/fertility/artificial insemination/abortion, have become central to today's political debates.

We frequently hear of "the collapse of the old moral order," which was supposedly as stable and eternal as the stars. Often the implication is that "the new woman" (even "the movement for women's equality") has caused hostility or a decadent situation. But does the change from a moral system in which the reproductive couple is seen as better, more moral and valuable, in favor of today's "new morality" automatically imply the "collapse of society"? Or is this a continuation of the demonization of female sexuality, in the tradition of blaming Eve-in-the-Garden for the "sins of mankind"?

In my view, we are in a process of reevaluation, renewal, transition to a new moral order: we are as moral as ever but in the process of rethinking who we are, reevaluating our direction—our sexual morality, the meaning of family, roles for women and men, and sexual identity.

Throughout history there have been various moral and sexual/reproductive orders unlike our own that were nevertheless stable and created "good citizens"—one need think only of ancient Greek or Roman civilizations. Thus the cry that "moral values are collapsing" is a little like Chicken Little crying that "the sky is falling"; what we need is change that builds on previous versions of family and morality, as well as human rights: we need progress, not fear of straying from the ways of the past.

The various essays in this section—most of them written during the past four years—discuss the ways in which change can come about to build a new sexual viewpoint.

We are on to something new: there has never yet been—that we know of—a moral order based on the full equality of women and men in society, nor a social order in which women had sexual autonomy and full rights over their own bodies and reproduction, as called for by the United Nations 1995 Declaration on the Rights of Women signed by 140 countries in Beijing, China. If we can manage to redefine sex in a way that opens up the energy and enthusiasm of women as well as men, we will have achieved something important. Currently the energy of half of humanity is being lost to the public good; this is a good reason for trying to rectify what has been a lapse in democracy for two centuries—a time during which democracy did not include women as full voting citizens. What will this new world look like? How far have we come in shaping it, and how can we stop the hijacking of "women's liberation" and women's sexuality by an old "sexual freedom" agenda?

We can construct a "third way" forward. We do not need to choose between either "traditional family values" (with rigid roles for men and women) or the pornographic views of the "sexual revolution." We can build on the best of both movements.

Remember, the "old order" did not reach its full moral potential if it did not include equality for women. In fact, it even enshrined inequality in law and custom, at the same time harnessing men into a reproductive straitjacket that they have resisted ever since.

Today, many people have ethical questions about their lives. Many men ask themselves how they could have more freedom, and they wonder how much time they should spend at work and at home; they are unsure whether they are "doing the right thing" concerning home and family. They also wonder whether they are having enough sex at home. Women, on the other hand, ask themselves if they are being honest in their sexual relations, and they wonder if they should follow traditional patterns, becoming relatively inactive sexually after they have children—yet something about this role troubles them. The same people, asking themselves such personal questions, have mixed feeling regarding the international political scene and its "conflict of cultures": What does it mean in the Middle East for women to wear a chador? Do women in "those parts of the world" need "saving," or do women/men there find more fulfillment in marriage than they do in the West?

This debate and turmoil means that we are in the midst of rethinking our moral values, trying to design the best way forward.

## FEMALE SEXUALITY

What is really new in the moral landscape that is trying to establish itself now is not only equality between women and men, but also a new sexual identity for women. Women's moral-sexual choices have become complex during the last thirty years—to have children or use birth control, to marry or "live together," to make love in a "romance-free" context or only when "in love," to be a single mother or not, and so on.

Increased divorce statistics and the popularity of counseling now—not to mention continuing statistics on domestic violence—demonstrate the problems in many "traditional happy families" (think of the television series *Desperate Housewives).* There was no "golden age of the family": the "happy family" image constructed in the1950's media was largely generated by post-World War II government policies in the United States, United Kingdom, and elsewhere, removing women from jobs in factories and elsewhere (held during the war), reopening those jobs to returning men. Thus the romantic picture that is drawn of "those days" should not be taken out of context to "prove" that couples in the 1950s (when divorce was rarely possible) were happier; after all, at that time domestic violence was hushed up, and some wives even received lobotomies or shock treatments to "quiet their complaints." Earlier in the century Freud had given his wife cocaine "to calm her," and today female Prozac (or other antidepressants) use is higher than male use.

The need for women's equality and a transformation of the institutions of marriage and family is clear; that transformation is now underway, amid great confusion as with any major change. The change is happening not only in the West but internationally.

We cannot transform "the family" or human rights without also transforming the definition of "sex" itself. Why? Because the core institution of sex forms the center of love and family relationships. It is necessary to transform this central institution in order to progress.

Women today are accused of being "less good mothers" than previously; this supposed decline is often blamed on the idea that "equality" had made women "selfish," or that "feminism is driving a wedge between men and women"—even though it is necessary to expose the problems (identify correctly a problem) before a solution can be created.[1] The goal of feminism is not to make women resent men, but to give men and women real information so that they can create a more equal world with better values, whatever that comes to mean. Though today's "family values" mindset declares a certain style of motherhood to be the sine qua non of civilized society, this has not always been historically true, even quite recently: in eighteenth century France, for example, children were regularly sent out to wet nurses until the age of three or four, away from their parents, until they were considered old enough to get along within the household; eighteenth century France was not uncivilized. Our view of "mothers" has come about during the last 200 years, when the idea of "childhood" was elevated and Mary, Mother of Jesus, became the focus of spiritual sanctity in Catholic theory.

The new moral landscape is an improvement on the old because it contains more egalitarian ideas of love and relationships, it no longer accepts as "moral" men's right to govern women (women today have passports, whereas they used to be included only in their husband's passport, for example), nor do men now take for granted the sexual or reproductive use of the female body. Why should we be afraid of change?

It is difficult today to imagine how the previous moral-social order could have been considered "just" and good when one group was automatically treated as second class to another, when women were expected to provide sexual services to men without question—yet people accepted the "justice" and "inevitability" of this moral order for centuries. Gradually society developed so that we no longer believe in slavery or serfdom; in the same way, we now realize that women should not be legally or physically owned by men, either. Divorce can be initiated by both women and men on equal grounds.

The changes now coming about inside men and women are fueling the rethinking of morality and ethics taking place in both public and private arenas. The atmosphere is a little like that at the end of apartheid rule in South Africa: many people no longer believe fully in the system as it was, thus creating a climate in which transition can occur.

## ARE WE GROPING TOWARD NEW GLOBAL VALUES ABOUT WOMEN?

The "war on terrorism" is a misnomer because it implies that eventually one can "win the war." In fact, what we are faced with is the long-term prospect of learning to negotiate with more dexterity than we ever have done before—unless, of course, we believe that "might makes right" and that therefore we can simply "lay down the law" whenever we wish, as we have the greatest military-economic might in the world. Most people believe that it is better to negotiate and evolve an international idea of fairness and peace—what we might call "mental globalization."

"The debate about women" is germaine to the process of "mental globalization" going on internationally now, as it involves the influential West's rethinking all its basic premises including the composition of "the family," one of its most basic premises. Obviously this includes the status of women and men within the family, how "work" will be defined, psychosexual identity, and so forth—the core relationship between a woman and a man within a family and democratization of the family. My research attempts to clarify some of the debates taking place concerning personal sexuality, the meaning of family, and personal expression—issues reflected cloudily in most media, despite the abundance of stories about them; think of such surface issues as clothing, "lifestyle," "sexiness," and the like.

These "private" matters are part of the current "mental globalization" or attempted international debate about "what is right" that is developing now, as we blithely state that women wearing chadors and scarves represent nothing more than "a different culture and religion"—yet women living in Europe during the Middle Ages also wore such scarves and continued to do so inside churches until quite recently, while men take their hats off. (What is it about women's heads that needs to be covered?)

Specifically, the process of many cultures groping toward a new "consensus" or new debate about "who women are" and "what women's rights are" is part of a general sotto-voce discussion that is taking place in the new "global village," our world, about what the position of women should be, what the "family" should be, and which ways of life are "good," and what is "evil."

What are our values going to be in the new "global village"—beyond the obvious fact that we all believe in "truth" and "justice"? In the global debate about values and justice, there are already various general principles accepted by all: honesty, dignity, and love, for example. Yet there is little consensus regarding the place of women in society: what should it be? Should a good woman be "at home," taking care of her children, a semisilent partner in a "good family"? Or should women be taking their place alongside men in managing corporations and businesses and in the professions? Can women be single and "good"? Is abortion acceptable, and if so, which type? Does "Western women's clothing" represent "women's oppression" or "women's liberation"?

Regionalism seems superficially to offer an alternative to this mental globalization or "standardization" of values and lifestyles—and as Jacques Chiraq pointed out, what we want is not a world that is unicultural but a world in which cultural diversity flourishes. (I do not believe women should have to pay the price for this, however; for example, for them to be denied education "to keep our flowers pure," as it has been put in Saudi Arabia.) Globalization, for better or worse, seems to be with us and upon us; modern technology is spreading ideas and beliefs rapidly, thus regionalism is not a real solution. The existence of global media makes it difficult for regions to stay out of the new "mental globalization." What one culture thinks of another is often faulty, of course, so the debate is flawed. For example, a large part of what some in the Arab world condemn, as expressed in "anti-American" demonstrations, are perceived ideas of "what life is like" in the West—that is, "women are too free," and "there is too much profanity and sexual promiscuity" everywhere, making life "vulgar." But I hope that globalization includes equality for women and doesn't hide behind such pretexts.

Unfortunately, some media's tendency to mix semi-pornographic images of "free women," "free sex," and "American military might," blurred into one picture, makes the general negative reaction from "other cultures" somewhat understandable. Of course, financial inequalities also beg for attention—that is, the difference between the standard of living in Western society and "the developing world." Some parts of

"Westernization" are good, such as seeing women as full human beings with more capacities than those of childbearing and childrearing; others may be less good, and we can learn from other cultures. Yet the issue of women's rights is most highly developed in the West, legally and socially.

Societies may find that implementing a new view of women in their own cultures has a different outcome than the "vulgarity" they so decry in "Americanism": after all, while the American "equal woman" will have an American style, the style of the Indonesian "equal woman" will be different, with an Indonesian composition, and so forth. There is no need to condemn women's rights just because the style in which "a free woman" is currently most visible is one that is detested by many.

As the United Nations Declaration on the Rights of Women makes clear, the basic issues for women around the world who are striving for autonomy ("their rights") involve having physical control over their own bodies, occurring in various ways in various cultures. This issue can be seen in terms of reproductive rights, freedom from cultural pressures for clitoredectomy and infibulation, as well as sexual rights to choose the way in which women (and men) express their individual psychosexual identity and feelings. And, of course, the rights to vote, own property, and have a bank account.

A sophisticated discussion of what is "right" and "good" could make the world into a more peaceful and harmonious place. This debate will become more and more pronounced as the century progresses.

## WOMEN'S RIGHTS IN IRAQ: THEIR FUTURE AND OUR OWN

A struggle is now going on in Iraq and elsewhere to evolve a new basic value system and a way of running society and government. Where will women wind up in all of this?

This struggle is also going on inside of women and men around the world. Many women—West and East—perceive that they should "take sides," either supporting their own "traditional society" or accepting "global Western secular values" and "new ways of living." Yet are these two options the real choices? This is a simplification of our worldview's two extremes.

We need to identify a "third way" or several "third ways" forward, new views of how to live—neither to return to a "traditional social order" nor to "leap forward into pornography and let-it-all-hang-out." (This is really only the reverse picture of the traditional morality.) There are some good values in both of these views, but one is an extreme version (even a caricature) of the other, not really a way forward. In my current research I find that many people are trying to evolve for themselves a third type of personal morality that combines the best of these views, looking for a way forward that is neither one extreme nor the other.

Although the current international struggle and debate is perceived to be between "true religion" or "tradition," and "Western secularism" (or even "democracy" or "sex, drugs & rock 'n' roll"), this is not really the choice.

What are the two competing value systems now on offer? Traditional countries present women in the home, taking care of children, or covered with a heavy veil when outside—at least these are the pictures the Western news media usually offer us of Islamic countries—while Western culture presents women's freedom to work in offices or wear skimpy miniskirts in nightclubs, to "go out." In both cultures, men are in charge of social institutions, from church to government to family (at least as presented in media). Pornography, now circling the globe via the Internet, seems to show a picture of "Western culture" in which women and men are equally sexually active, although the images shown do not reflect feminist ideas of equality: the seeming choice between "traditional family values" and "the pornographic commercialization of society" is reinforced.

Not only is such a choice not the case (hopefully, the West stands for human rights, but not in the commercially vulgar context that pornography implies), but also most people in my research do not behave in these ways in private. These two extremes, which seem to be "the choices," disguise the real crossroads we are facing now, which involves issues of human freedom and dignity.

The new choice is between an authoritarian view (often going under the name of religion or "tradition" or "family"), which places women in a subservient position to men/God-Allah/the family paradigm of "respectability," and thus diminishes men too, by permitting them to be no more than "dominators" (of nature, women, other men)—and a new way of being, controlling their own destinies, creating their own new personal set of ethics and values.

Most Western countries, of course, cannot claim to be models of perfection in presenting the "new ethical world" we are talking about—though one has to give the West credit for its idealistic goals, which many people are trying to bring into being. At least human rights and equality are stated goals.

By contrast, in some Middle Eastern and African countries, a woman (but not a man) could be killed legally for having sex outside of marriage, as in the famous 2003 case of a Nigerian woman who was condemned to death by stoning as soon as she had finished breastfeeding her baby. Will women in Iraq now be able to have freedom and equal rights? Will the condition of women be improved under the new government? Will these conditions be improved in Afghanistan? Or will some leaders' minds be clouded by the seeming choice between "righteous, traditional society values" and "porno culture," with women's rights taking the erroneous consequences?

I am wondering what will happen to women in Iraq and its surrounding countries, and here in the West, now that things are changing so drastically. The position Iraqi women carve out for themselves there will surely affect the position of women throughout the region and throughout the world. I hope for the best, I am thinking of them. There are a great amount of good ideas to build on, from all over the world. I know they can succeed!

# A NEW SEXUAL CULTURE TO GO WITH A NEW INTERNATIONAL POLITICS[2]

## "MAKE LOVE NOT WAR": IS THIS WHAT OUR POLITICS MEANS?

How is sex political, how is it linked to peace? This question is often heard, but what does it really mean? Surely it is not as simple as the wonderful slogan, "Make Love Not War"? Sex and politics are deeply connected, but how?

Unraveling the hidden rules behind what we are told is "the right way to have sex and pleasure" is key to understanding the construction of the entire social system; therefore understanding the ideology underlying sex will go a long way toward enabling individuals and society to become more egalitarian and less warlike, more peaceful. A new sexuality is part of an emerging new politics of planetary health, the environment, issues of "globalization" or "antiglobalization," and world peace.

This vision of sex is connected to a new international value system that is trying to emerge—a still hazy revised view of who we are as a species on the planet, what we are doing or should be doing with our lives. The central question of this new value system remains one of war and peace: why are there so many wars, is war an inevitable consequence of human nature? Could we be less warlike?

In its deepest sense, sexuality is connected to world peace—not because of a superficial notion that "sex" is "deep," but since sexuality is key in women's growing "equality" and activity in the world, central to the definition of "who a woman is"—and because sex is key to "who a man is," if a man rethinks his primary assumptions about sex, he will also revamp his ideas about himself and who he is as a man—society will be greatly affected.

No one should think that saying "sex is connected to world peace" means simply that "if people have more and better sex, they will be more satisfied, and therefore they will be less interested in war." While that is undoubtedly true, and while the slogan "Sex, Peace and Love" is good, the idea proposed here is something new: that through the physical movements of "the sex act," individuals learn lessons in gender behavior and psychology that shape their thinking and belief systems—gender is taught to children largely through sexual moral codes. If we critique "what sex is," as we are doing here, we can see ourselves (and "human life") as separate from this ideology, and therefore we can innovate a more positive future.

In the radical new analysis of male sexuality I present here,[3] I have written about boys at puberty ("Oedipus Revisited"). The construction of boys' sexual identity at puberty and earlier carries over into men's identity as adults: if boys are brought up to think that being "a man" means being sexually "big" and financially powerful, and the idea is pushed that "a real man" must be "cool and tough"—though "sensitive"—and that anyone who does not "show proper respect" should be "taught a lesson," then "the right reaction" for an adult man is an aggressive posture. The current belief in "sex drive" as "an inevitable hormonal mechanism" inside men props up this system, asserting that men are "by nature" aggressive and need to be dominant, that "dominance" and "command" are inherent to men's biology and hormonal make-up. In my thesis, the social commands to boys (software programming in the brain) are causing an exaggeratedly militaristic society; these commands can be changed once they are identified (as here), thus ending a major cause of today's wars, small and large. Beginning to deconstruct "male sexuality" is doing two things: creating more pleasure and space for individual men, and helping society develop a more peaceful global strategy.

Most people today are not only concerned about how they should feel about "sex" in their private lives, they are also agitated by heated debates about sex in the news—that is, public discussions of abortion/right-to-life, parity and equality, sexual harassment, "the veil" or chador (necessary for a woman to wear to express "modesty" and "humility"?) versus the "miniskirt," the sexual trafficking in women, and rape in war (as in Bosnia, Chechnya, and Rwanda), among others, such as President Clinton's "sex life." Most people fear that they have fantasies that are not "politically correct," and often they cannot "square" their personal sexual desires with what they believe to be ethical.

In the end, sex and social reality are connected. The definitions of both female and male sexuality are central to our culture's social structure. If one believes that female orgasm happens for most women with some form of clitoral stimulation, then this stance brings into question many of our most sacred beliefs about "the act," "who men are by their nature," and "who women are," whether we believe that both people should have orgasms during sex, whether we believe that we can fundamentally alter the pattern of what we call "sex" and what kind of intimate relationships we want, what kind of social values we construct.

The changes that come to mind need not be feared ("sex" can be "sexier" than it is). Revising this institution does not mean making it "politically correct"; we will be able to be more who we are, even if "incorrect," after this transformation than we were before.

## HUMAN RIGHTS, EQUALITY, AND SEX: WHAT WILL IT MEAN IF WOMEN TRANSFORM SEXUALITY?

Today an increasing number of women and men gladly accept that clitoral stimulation to orgasm is the basic means of female orgasm, and a pleasure. They believe that, adding this stimulation to the basic sexual script, two people can be quite happy together sexually. This stage is currently the most advanced.

Focusing on noncoital activities to orgasm will mean a major mental shift for most people. Though most women now agree that orgasm utilizing exterior or clitoral stimulation is "normal," some men's acceptance of this fact lags behind. According to my research in late1990s Europe, 71 percent of men today believe that they should know how to "perform" clitoral stimulation by hand so that a woman can orgasm in this way "if she can't come otherwise." However, 93 percent of women believe that it is "normal" for a woman to receive or use clitoral stimulation by hand to orgasm during a sexual relationship—whether or not they do so regularly. At the same time, 25 percent of men report that they usually perform clitoral or exterior stimulation of a woman, by hand or mouth, until she reaches orgasm, though 59 percent indicate that they only "stimulate her clitoris for a while" (not to orgasm). Only a small minority (11 percent) of women report that the men they meet (not regular partners) usually offer clitoral stimulation all the way to orgasm.

Most women state that, in their experience, men generally still expect that the woman will orgasm during "the act" and seem glad to believe that the woman has had an orgasm if she simply acts excited. However, things are improving, and more men are informed today than they were a decade earlier.

Another change: many more women now initiate sexual relations than did so in the past. Until quite recently women were taught that it was the exclusive right of the man to initiate romance, marriage, or sexual relations. Today most "younger women" feel that it is as much their right to initiate a sexual dialogue with a man, as it is a man's right to initiate this dialogue. Some men are pleased: "It's flattering, and why should I be the only one to risk rejection?" while others are more ambivalent, not liking feeling that they must be "ready to perform, get an erection, whenever she asks."

What has not changed is the basic definition of "sex"—the basic focus on coitus as "real sex," "the act." Society as we know it has provided only one mainstream institution into which all bodily lust and need-to-be-touched feeling must be poured—"sex." This, the pattern of activities we call "sex," was designed to promote reproductive activity. To this day we follow this basic scenario, though most people use birth control.

Today's woman, in an attempt to no longer be a "passive-receptive vehicle for the depositing of sperm," or teased and laughed at as "out of date," may graft her sexual needs onto this scenario ("the institution known as sex"), though it may not satisfy her deeper desires and needs, just as it has not fully satisfied most men's.

Though there are many people who would say that the way we define "sex" is "natural," because "biology" declares that "men want to penetrate women, and women want to be penetrated by men," and further, that the "resultant childbearing" means that affection and long-term caring are "natural" emotions that develop in "the correct sexual relationship," others are not so sure—for example, the orphans in Africa whose parents have died of AIDS, or the orphans in Southeast Asia whose parents died in the 2004 tsunami, "street children" in Brazil, and others. Are they to stop believing that their parents originally loved each other when they were conceived? Does "family values" make them feel that they are "lesser"?

Those who believe that the way we define sex—as basically revolving around penetration of the penis into the vagina—is "biologically obvious" and eternal (historically "always the way it was done") do not see the sexual changes that are happening for what they are: a search for a transformation of love and eroticism, beyond "equal orgasms."

Believing that the institution we know as "sex" is fixed and eternal—"how it always was" and "always will be"—leads quickly to a condemnation of same-sex love: Homosexual sexual desire must be declared "a perversion"—though historically it is clear that it is not; it is one of the ways people choose and have chosen to express their feelings for others. As homosexual and lesbian relationships do not follow standard patterns (there are no particular traditional patterns; each person must listen to the body of the other and invent her or his own way of relating), clearly heterosexual sex can become much more intuitive and inventive, it need not follow a pattern either. There does not have to be a "schedule of events" or map for people to follow, sex does not need to be scenario-led.

Though most people still believe (and most pornography still shows) the idea that "sex" is "coitus" while everything else is "trimming," today's widespread experimentation may be a sign that the reproductive pattern of sex is changing—although the standard interpretation is that "values are collapsing." To interpret games during sex as "dark" or "dangerous" shows the influence of the previous "moral order" on our thinking: we are frightened of change and imagine ourselves to be in dangerous territory, constructing situations to reflect this state. "Sex" is not antireligious, yet it has been labeled as such by some Easterners and Westerners—at least sex outside of marriage, when not intended for reproduction. Religion as we have known it has called anything other than standard reproductive sex (coitus) a "perversion," blocking new developments.

## UNDEFINING "SEX": A BASIC ISSUE OF HUMAN RIGHTS

Is the definition of sex ("fucking") instinctive, or is it a product of society? Can the definition of sex basically change, or is it a straightforward expression of our hormonal natures?

Sex, as the first Hite Report proposed, is a cultural rather than a biological institution—one formulated by church and state to suit reproductive needs. The institution as we know it—"foreplay" followed by "vaginal penetration" followed by "intercourse" and ending with male orgasm—is a product of a certain society and its psychological landscape. Being of historical and social origin, centered on the delineation of rights (of inheritance, property, and so on) consequent to reproduction, its definition can, of course, change. Indeed, it should change, since the basic definition as we have known it is sexist and discriminates against women, treating them as second-class beings. (He has orgasm, she knows how but doesn't.)

Seen in another way, sex between women and men is much more equal today than it was in the 1960s. Even in the 1970s many fewer women had orgasm with a partner than today, since "clitoral orgasm" (as it was then called) was not accepted because of the negative influence of psychological theories that decreed "vaginal orgasm" the only "real orgasm." (On the other hand, many women around the world today agree that sex as they know it with most men does not include much more than coitus.)

In brief, for the last 2,000 years, "sex"—the way we have institutionalized erotic feelings and the desire for physical intimacy with each other—has focused on a rigid reproductive scenario, always centered on intercourse, with "the main event" being coitus. Everything else was considered ancilliary, that is, "foreplay"—"trimming" or the "warm-up"—or "afterplay." Even today very little physical contact lasting more than one minute is condoned unless it is between lovers or "sex" is intended; friends can rarely walk down the street together holding hands, for example.

The reproductively focused definition of sex is now out of date, but it is still considered the "sine qua non" of "sex." Ironically, most women use birth control, and men increasingly use condoms.

The reproductively oriented definition of sex puts women in a second-class position, expecting women to help men with the stimulation they need for orgasm (coitus; not stopping in the middle and saying, "That was nice, now I'd like to do something else"), though the stimulation women need for orgasm was not included—unless a woman could manage to orgasm during coitus. Centuries of "scientific speculation" had shown that "the problem" of female orgasm during "the act" was ongoing; the clear solution is that the stimulation that brings most women to orgasm—that is, the stimulation women use on themselves during self-stimulation: exterior pubic stimulation or "clitoral stimulation"—should be made part of what "sex" is.

Sex in the traditional definition can be pleasurable, but it is also sexist; it teaches women that they are inferior and men that they are "different" and "more animal"—neither of which is true, but which has the effect of alienating both people, believing the other too different to be understood.

Sex should be redefined—or undefined. It should include "clitoral stimulation" to orgasm, of course, for women, but it should go further than that. The institution we know as "sex" (with its celebrated reproductive scenario) should be undefined (or deconstructed) to make sex an individual vocabulary of ways to touch another person. Our feelings are much more subtle and interesting than the body "vocabularies" currently available to express them.

## WOMEN REDEFINING SEX

Redefining sex to suit yourself . . . Women are making many changes in the ways they see and practice intimate physical relations—how they express and share their bodies— though working this out takes time.

Sexual freedom for women is not a clichéd version of the attitudes of the sexual revolution, turning tradition on its head for shock value and imagining that all that had been "repressed" now "good" and "worthwhile"—for example: "I am married, twenty-eight with three children, and currently in the middle of a Greek-Anglo affair, which began while my husband and I holidayed in Greece recently. I consider myself a liberated lady in tune with her own body."

Sexual freedom for women is closely related to economic independence. Intimidation, because of economic dependence—as seen also in sexual harassment at work—has meant that many women could not express themselves sexually and in other ways, nor take new steps; if a woman lives in fear, because of either economics or the psychology of inferiority, she will attend to the other person's needs and fear expressing her own, including her own sexual needs (perhaps especially during "sex"). Creating a new body language will not happen overnight.

Women are making changes now in the way they participate in sexual relations, the way they share their bodies, and they are hoping to make more changes. These changes will lead to longer lovemaking and more pleasure for both females and males.

Though currently women are pressured to act in sexually "male copycat ways," inside women there are new ideas of how they really want to behave and what they really want to do. Current stereotypes insist that if a woman initiates sexual activities long defined to be "sexual" by men, or acts counter to the past sexual stereotypes of women, then she is "liberated." In reality, being active in sex may have an entirely different meaning for women in the future.

The semipornographic images of women visible on so many advertising posters and in television commercials (often used by fundamentalists to point to "the decadence of the secular West," and women's "new selfishness" in this environment) do not represent "who women are sexually" but rather the use and selling of women's bodies by a double-standard tradition. It is no wonder, when female sexuality is equated with the images shown in many ads, that some women today recoil, deciding that "the old ways were best," imagining that women were more respected then, whether or not this is historically accurate.

In young adulthood the enormous pressure on women to "get married by thirty" and "have a baby by thirty-five" is usually claimed to be caused by the "biological clock," yet I propose that is caused not by biology but by society—in large part the pressure comes from women needing (subconsciously) to fit into the society's mythological icon of a "good woman" by being reproductive and appearing as part of a "traditional family," as a rite of passage; only this program will "legitimize" a woman's existence—according to the archetypes that form our psychological landscape at present.

Soon, I am certain, women will begin to demonstrate more and more fully the sexual feelings that are within them, leading sexual interaction in new directions.

## FAMILY VALUES: A REEXAMINATION OF THE SEXUAL REVOLUTION

Those who point out the positive sides of "sexual freedom" indicate the benefits for women (and men) of birth control, abortion, and self-expression. Those pointing out the negatives emphasize the exploitative nature of most pornography, the pressure to be "sexy" and young.

On the one hand the new power to control fertility, using in vitro fertilization and other fertility treatments, gives more and more women an increasing number of options vis-à-vis their ability to combine work and family. However, on the negative side the sexual revolution has pressured women to "act sexy" in a clichéd way, in a way that easily veers into the old clichés of women-as-sluts. It will probably take time for society to accept and see new kinds of sexual statements that women make, ways of being sexual that grow out of women's own thoughts and feelings, not ways that are foisted on them.

As one woman explains, "Where today's' female sexual freedom' goes off track is in thinking that' being overtly sexy' is the same as being sexually alive and a' new woman.' Neither is wearing black leather, whips and chains, or piercing your body somewhere weird automatically a sign of being able to take charge of your sexuality, though it can be a sign that someone is headed in that direction, trying."

Though women are told that they are "sexually free" (the birth control pill, no disapproval for sex without marriage), they often experience judgmental attitudes that condemn them—especially if they are over thirty—as "lewd" or "unfeminine" (Mary is pure, Eve is sinful; wives are good, mistresses are bad.) For example, the divisive arguments over "single mothers"—a hot political topic in many countries— shows that the double standard of morality is still alive, condemning women who have sex outside the nuclear family.

Many women responding in the original Hite Report in 1976 stated repeatedly that the sexual revolution did not represent them, that it was a male-oriented movement that demanded everything of them. It is not surprising that today, thirty years later, the "back to basics" movement toward "traditional family values" is preferred by so many women. It is a mistake to look back and think that women are betraying the movement of their own making; women still believe in feminism (equal rights for women—to vote, hold top jobs, have education, and so forth), but most women never believed in the sexual revolution in its true meaning. The fact that several democratizing movements arrived on the scene together in the 1960s—the civil rights movement, the women's movement, and the sexual freedom movement, not to mention the "hippie, peace, flower power" movement—caused confusion, many later simplistically lumping them all together.

However, women have continued moving forward sexually in another direction, according to my recent research. The soil of democracy has given voice to groups whose views are taken seriously. While today some in many countries proclaim that they do not believe in separation of church and state, the West, especially via the American and French Revolutions influenced by Thomas Paine, believes in religious tolerance under a benevolent and watchful nonreligiously aligned government, a government that represents all people of all views.

Today this tradition is under attack as "immoral" and "decadent," the change in the status of women being the usual target of such barbs. Attackers use images taken from pornography and media to symbolize "the new woman"—although most women are not represented by the "dominatrix" images of young, thin, sexually clad women that religious groups point accusing fingers at. What is it that such fundamentalist groups are protesting?

## A DEEP FEELING OF UNEASE

Women have been forced for centuries to perform the act of helping a male have orgasm inside the woman, even though today birth control devices or condoms are generally used. Generally women have had to shower or douche after sex, since the female body requires more elaborate cleaning methods than the penis, and because of the female genitalia's less obvious position inside the body rather than the male's external location. The vagina, being interior, requires more immersion than the penis, which can be washed more easily.

Though it is called "innate," "biological," "obvious"—the purpose of the "sex drive" is to ensure reproduction, it is said—is this really true? Or is what we know as "sex" a cultural ritual, the part that leads to sex (that is, coitus or "the act") glorified and exaggerated by a social order that wants to ensure male orgasm—a social order that has unashamedly defined men as those with the right to "run things?" After all, in the West until the twentieth century, only men could legally own property and have bank accounts. Women were thought of as those without souls, mostly defined in terms of the body—"Women are closer to the earth, women are the mothers of this world, those who give milk to the earth" and so forth, those who are subservient to men and bear children ("in pain and suffering," as the Old Testament may have decreed). Inheritance has been passed through men for centuries; patriarchy decrees that children belong to men, though in antiquity this was not true.

The sexual ritual, teaching men to be "on top," the "fuckers," and women to be "those who are fucked," has become banal as a result of the proliferation of pornography and endless mediatized discussions of "sexy things." This is not to say that people have become tired of having orgasms, they have not. However, they are tired of the sexual clichés that are all around them, seeming to represent sexuality in an ugly context. This vulgarity regarding sex seems somehow to be combined with a negativity toward female sexuality.

What many women and men are feeling in their gut is that sexuality is unequal. Thus, during the later twentieth and early twenty-first century, men increasingly wanted to "make her come too," to "be more sensitive" and to "have longer erections." Women felt increasingly pressured to have an orgasm at the same time the man did, or to fake orgasm. This attitude even went so far as the positing (on flimsy evidence) of something labeled the "g-spot" in the late 1970s—meaning a supposed spot inside the vagina that would lead to female orgasm during intercourse. Of course, statistically, most women did not regularly have orgasm from intercourse, most women had orgasm from more direct clitoral stimulation, but the idea that there was a spot inside the vagina "to make her come" meant that many men felt they did not have to learn new ways of having sex nor interact in new ways with women.

Today there is a feeling that the definition of sex itself somehow is to blame for the deep feeling of unease about the "immorality"—that is, inequality—of sex that people are experiencing.

## WHERE ARE WE GOING FROM HERE?

It is quite possible that many women, who have been force-fed a hyped-up diet of "sexy images" (purporting to represent them) by the media during the last ten to twenty years, are now reacting by becoming asexual or "politically conservative," wishing not to have sex with "those values." In other words, many people feel revulsion at images pushed on them that show what they are told are "sexy and desirable" people. Whereas women in the original Hite Report were engaged in discovering and creating new forms of sexual exchange for themselves in ways that were creative and individual, this emerging new identity was more or less drowned by the flood of pornographic or semipornographic material that poured out purporting to represent "the new female sexuality" and "what is really sexy" soon thereafter.

In reality, for women to be more themselves during sexual activity will mean something that is still being developed—not, as is often portrayed, clichés like "Now women are dominatrixes, women can be on top like men used to be," or "the new woman" is good at fellatio and "not afraid to do it." It will mean a mutual exploration by sensitive and intelligent partners who want to create something new together.

## IN PRAISE OF SECULARISM

"Secularism" is not an amoral philosophy, and we do not need to apologize for it. We can be proud of it. It is a development that took Western culture over two centuries to create, combining the ethics of religious tradition with its own new theories of democracy and equality. These "secular" values of equality and democracy represent the progression of humanity from a hierarchical, feudal society to a system in which individuals are respected. This is a deeply spiritual evolution. In fact, secularism is the most spiritual force in the world today.

We should not confuse the progressive parts of our tradition with the excesses of what we call "the sexual revolution," nor imagine that "the women's movement" has created or is responsible for the sexual revolution. In fact, the reputation of the sexual revolution was wrongly enobled and glorified by coming at the same time as the antiwar movement, the black civil rights movement, and feminism. At times the achievements of these movements are confused with the sexual revolution.

To be true to our own values and spirit, we in the West should defend the rights of women everywhere against religious extremism. This is a "secular" viewpoint, since religious traditions in various cultures have or have had as one of their aims the continuation of women in a second-class position, one in which their sexuality and reproductive capacity is ruled by religious dictates (such as that a woman must cover herself with a scarf or a chador, but not men; or that a woman is unclean during menstruation and must bathe herself in certain ritual ways, including prayers, before she is "fit for her husband," and the like). Secularism accepts a philosophy of equality, giving women and men space in which to work out what this new philosophy will mean in their lives.

The religious and political battle going on now in many parts of the world is not really about "ethnic minorities" (though it is that as well), but more profoundly about a split between two possible views: One is the system of the old woman-suppressing patriarchy, in which men are viewed as warriors and crusaders who need, "by nature," to conquer others; the other is that of "individual human rights," a world in which thinking for oneself and allowing, even encouraging, a diversity of beliefs, opinions, and equally shared peaceful views of others is the goal. This latter is generally called democracy.

## HAS WOMEN'S LIBERATION BEEN DERAILED/HIJACKED BY THE SEXUAL FREEDOM MOVEMENT?

For much of the last two hundred years, women have made great progress; on the whole they have been on an upward movement toward attaining "equal rights for women in democracy."

Originally left out of the constitutions of both France and the United States, at their inception, women gradually inched their way into having voting, legal, and financial rights and now are trying for equal power in government and business.

Yet, was this "equal rights" agenda derailed during the late twentieth century by the "sexy woman" statistic seen often in newspapers and "women's magazines"?

Women began to hear, especially from certain "women's magazines" in the early 1970s, that they were now "sexually free" and had nothing to fear. They could search for their orgasms (I shudder to remember how my own work was exploited by some media in this way) and "behave freely" as "men have always done"—that is, "what's good for the goose is good for the gander," and so on, using similar simplistic clichés.

At the same time women were pressured to be "young and hip," "sexy" in the way the magazines dictated—young, "pretty," dressed in the latest seminude or body-revealing fashions, with bare legs and short skirts, long hair with a baby-doll look, and so on. On some young women, this look was sometimes attractive, but all women were pressured to have it (not to have it meant that one was "out of the game" and "undesirable"), so that eventually an anorexia epidemic shook the West, and reproduction fell to almost a negative number. How could you stay young and thin and "beautiful" if you were "fat" and pregnant, your skin stretched, or you became a "mother," "one of THEM"? Instead of being able to be proud of our full hips that create new life in the womb, we were shamed into dieting until we appeared to have the skinnier hips of boys.

Under pressure from men and advertising, women saw that "older women" were made fun of and/or fired from their jobs or not rehired ("too old"),* and they reacted by trying to remain young and thin and "beautiful" for as long as possible. Understandable.

Many women today are leading double lives. In their minds they are fighting every day a war between one side of themselves that says, "You are a rational full adult human citizen," and the other that says, "Better to play the part of being a simple girl, don't seem to know too much, don't get fat, or men won't like you!" Many feel like hypocrites or at least have a confused sense of their own identities, and often they cannot express themselves well in groups that include men. In the name of "sex" and "freedom," women are being contorted even further today, pressured into feeling that they must be sexy until they die, remain sexy during and past menopause even if they don't feel like it, remain sexy when they are not in love (at any age), that they are wrong if they choose celibacy for a period, and so on.

Most of all, women are told that they are "achieving liberation" when they have sex often and behave in a sexy way. Yet this may not be true, because the two are not the same. This is how women have been cheated, temporarily, of their progress and momentum, by being told that they must be "sexy" in the traditional scenario and resolve any remaining doubts they have about the "goodness" of sex, lest they be considered "old-fashioned" and dull.

Even if there has been a temporary setback—that is, the "free sex" movement of today looks a lot like the 1960's "sexual liberation" movement that exploited women in the name of "freedom"—if history is a teacher, then the 1960s soon becomes the 1970s with its full-blown women's movement agitating for more equal rights than before and condemning the time-worn attitudes of "sex" toward women. Will we see this movement erupt again today? Or is it perhaps erupting under the rubric of "family values"?

### THE SEXUAL REVOLUTION AND THE DOUBLE STANDARD: SHOULD WE RETURN TO "FAMILY VALUES"?

Women who participated in my 1976 research had quite mixed feelings about "sexual freedom" and the demands it places on them.

> *I think the sexual revolution is very male-oriented and anti-woman. The idea is that men are telling women they're free to fuck around with whomever they want. But the catch is that the double standard is still*

---

* I remember when my friends waged a successful campaign to force airline companies not to fire women when they turned thirty, though they had never fired men at thirty. Midge Kovacs, head of the National Organization for Women's "Image of Women in the Media" committee at the New York City chapter for several years, deserves much of the credit for this success.

*employed. A man who has many lovers is "sowing his oats"; a woman who has many lovers is a "prostitute" or "nymphomaniac."*

*Usually after they know they "have" me, I get the feeling I am a piece of ass. I feel their hostility and their contempt. The double standard is alive and well.*

*Although I live at a college campus, which is considered nationwide as a place of avant-garde sexual and intellectual ideas, it is not. Men here still disrespect women who have sex with those they're not "in love with," and if a woman cares about her esteem, it is only safe to have sex with either a male who cares about her so he won't make her feel bad and talk about her to other men so they disrespect her—or else with a person no one finds out about (like flings at ski resorts or vacations, etc.). One male, considered a leading radical here, was talking to a supposed female friend of his day before Halloween. They were invited to a costume party and she, having trouble deciding what to wear, asked him, "What do you think I should go as?" Very cruelly, he replied, "Why don't you go as a virgin? I'm sure nobody will recognize you!"*

It sounds as if women were saying that when they did try to be open and to share with men, having sex in a free way, in all too many cases they wound up being disrespected and hurt, because the double standard is still operating (it's okay if a man "plays around" but it gives a girl a bad reputation if she does).

Most women who answered my questionnaires were brought up to be "good girls," including those who were still living at home. Girls are still being admonished to hide menstruation and discouraged from being proud of their reproductive cycles, as well as restrained from exploring and discovering their own sexuality—called "bad girls" or "rebellious" when they try. Today at puberty girls are given information about their reproductive organs and menstruation but rarely told about the clitoris! So we still have some way to go . . .

## SHOULD SEX BE CONNECTED TO EMOTIONS? WHERE DOES LOVE COME INTO IT?

Some of the sexual-revolution ideology states that it is old-fashioned to want to connect sex with feelings—this means that you aren't "hip." Not only marriage but also monogamy and love or even tender feelings are often considered to be something only "neurotic" women want—yet why so? The idea is that "people should spontaneously have sex and not worry, just behave freely and have sex, no strings, anytime with anybody, for pure physical pleasure."

But almost no woman in this study wanted that kind of sexual relationship; not only did women find it boring, but also it made them feel "cheap," and frequently they worried about the man's opinion of them "later." Bottom line: overwhelmingly, women want sex with feeling.

To be told that we should have a regular "appetite" for intercourse does not coincide with how most women feel: periods of greater interest in sex with a partner, for most women, fluctuate according to attraction to a certain individual and (to a lesser extent) according to the menstrual cycle. Most women emphasize that the appetite for sex with another person becomes really intense only in relation to desire for a specific person, although, of course, they could enjoy sex at any time. What causes the awakening of this intense desire or love for another specific person is very personal and mysterious, as this woman explains:

> *Leaving out love and even commitment for the moment, good sex has to be more than anatomy or "psyching" yourself into it. It has to involve a certain amount of chemistry between two people. After a singularly disastrous experience trying to make a sexual relationship work when there was no attraction (just affection), I don't want to try to add sex to my friendships unless I feel attraction too. I don't understand it, but there certainly is such a thing as sexual attraction which can't be forced into existence.*

## THE RIGHT NOT TO HAVE "SEX": IS SEX NECESSARY FOR HEALTH?

Since the sexual revolution, with its tenet that sex is no longer "serious" (you don't have to fear pregnancy, and marriage is optional), it seems that women themselves are taken less seriously by some men in dating situations. Since marriage or commitment is no longer a requirement, it has become "hip" to have a lot of "sex" (intercourse). Women are often told that the sex "drive" must be regularly expressed to maintain "healthy functioning."

Yet many women in my research resent what they feel is commercialization and vulgarization of their sexuality—"beds on the sidewalks and pills in the vending machines," is how one describes the feeling she gets. Another reports:

> *We are taught that every little twinge is a big sex urge and we must attend to it or we'll be an old maid. I'm getting sick to death of sexuality—everywhere sex sex sex! So what? Sex is not the end all and be all of life. It's very nice but it's not everything!*

Or:

> *I wish there wouldn't be as much of a "hype" about sex as there is now. I hate the media's exploitation of sex and women. I would hope that*

*women wouldn't be looked upon as things to look nice and to have sex with. For the most part, women are judged by their potential sexual worth. I would like sex to become more personal. In a way, I'd almost like to have back the hush-hush good old days when you just didn't talk about sex. It would not be hidden because it was dirty, but because it was a sweet, private thing.*

Unfortunately the idea that sex is necessary for health had become big business even by 1975. Magazines, books, television ads using sex (or the happy couple) to sell their products, some psychiatrists, counselors, sex clinics, films, and massage parlors all continue to have a vested interest in the idea. We are constantly being reminded of sex in one way or another and subtly coerced into doing it: "Why aren't you doing it? Everybody else is. Get on the bandwagon! You're missing all the fun if you don't!—And you're probably neurotic and mentally unhealthy." Many women in my study felt defensive about the fact that they did not want to have sex more often:

*I think our culture has made sex over-important. Everyone thinks that everyone else is having a great time fucking all the time and so we all compete against the American myth. Given this, I think that sex in my life has assumed a correct proportion, that is, an expression of love between us; yet, I still feel hung up about the myth sometimes—maybe having sex is less important to me than to others.*

*The thing I enjoy most is making love with people I have that "special" feeling with—this is when it's most satisfying totally, even if it never gets down to real sex—it's still beautiful just holding them and feeling warmth and love with them.*

Of course some women prefer relationships to be based more on friendship than on passion. But they still indicated clearly that their desire for sex with another person is usually based more on feelings (erotic or romantic) for another person, rather than on a purely mechanical need for "release."

In fact, there is nothing unusual about spending various periods of one's life without sex:

*I am currently celibate. I enjoy it but the society makes it hard to be partnerless sometimes. There are activities I avoid because they will be "couply." People often think there's something wrong with you if you're not part of a couple, but being independent is worth it.*

*Periods of celibacy can be useful for reevaluating your life and rediscovering your sexuality—the fallow period before new things can grow. I did it for five years on and off once. By not having to please anyone else, I was able to get really deeply in touch with myself, and develop my understanding of the world—whereas before, always having boyfriends had kept me so narrowly focused on them that I hadn't had time to think about my relationship to the larger scheme of things. I found that giving up physical sex was a small price to pay.*

However, other women felt cut off and isolated during periods of celibacy, since sex is almost the only activity in which our society allows us to be physically close to another human being—since all forms of physical contact are channeled into heterosexual intercourse:

*When I go without sex for a while, I begin to crave affection and reaffirmation. I feel closed off from others, and begin to notice an intense need for affection, warmth, and any form of contact with another human being.*

*It doesn't seem to bother me physically, but emotionally I tense up. I miss body contact and find it extremely frustrating. There is a special kind of loneliness in being one in a culture that seems to think in terms of pairs.*

*I miss feeling wanted and needed, and the body warmth when I wake up. I usually start feeling unattractive and undesirable too—mentally depressed, bored, low-energy. I lose my sense of humor.*

Physical contact, "flesh to flesh, warm and tight," is tremendously important, and sex is almost the only way to get it in our culture after we are grown up. As one woman explains:

*If I am deeply depressed, cold, lonely, even with a stranger sex could be regeneration to me. The closeness gives me a sense that I am not alone, and that life is not all rough edges. It makes me feel loved and special.*

Another reports that what she likes best about sex is:

*The feeling of crazy friendliness it gives, sometimes falsely, plus the reassurance, however momentary, of being held. The closeness, intimacy, honesty—after that you feel alive and happy in a way you never do at any other time.*

## WHAT WAS THE ULTIMATE SIGNIFICANCE OF THE "SEXUAL REVOLUTION" OF THE 1960s?

Although sexuality is very important, it is questionable whether it is important in and of itself, apart from its meaning in life as a whole. The increasing emphasis on sex and personal relations as the basic source of happiness and fulfillment is connected to what may be a lessening chance of finding fulfillment through work. In the first place most people do not have the luxury of being able to choose work that they would like to do; for most people it is a question of finding some way to support themselves as quickly and as best they can, from the limited options available. Now, added to this, most jobs have become very repetitive, impersonal, and boring, so that most people today cannot hope to find any real personal fulfillment through actual work they do.

As one woman puts it, "Sex is clearly used as a universal panacea, to keep the masses quiet and stop them from realizing the emptiness, meaninglessness, and alienation of their working lives." It is interesting in this context to note that the sexual revolution came at a time when social and political unrest in the United States was a problem. Sexuality and sexual relationships can be surrogates for (or obscure our need for) a more satisfying relationship with the larger world. Meanwhile the commercialization and trivialization of sex advances further and further into our private lives and obscures its deeper personal meaning for us. In fact, we haven't had a sexual revolution yet, but we need one.

## BEAUTY AND WOMEN: RED LIPSTICK AS A SYMBOL OF THE FEMALE BODY

Women have the right to sexual appearance; make-up is not sinful. Two female friends lived together as a couple for six years. Both are beautiful, one likes to "dress up" and wear red lipstick, has long black hair, and wears clothes that fit her figure. Once she went to a lesbian meeting and came back complaining, "No one would even speak to me! They acted really suspicious. I was the only one wearing lipstick in the whole place! I looked like a 'girlie' to them, I guess—my skirt was short, too. Talk about politically correct, I mean they were all wearing more or less the same thing— either denim jeans and jackets or black leather pants and jackets, their hair short and no make-up. I was really out of place."

The fashion for refusing to wear the traditional types of feminine clothing, use make-up, or wear one's hair in a way that would seem to be an adornment goes back to the twentieth century protest against the ways women had been forced to be "sex objects" for men: "the prettiest girl gets the richest boy," and so on. Before women were allowed to have university educations or good-paying jobs (we're still working on this goal), they had to enter what was known as "the marriage market." They had to barter their appearance and "charm" to "get a husband," then later to "provide him with children."

In this context, use of the traditional adornments of "the female"—lipstick, powder, rouge, earrings, long hair, brightly colored sensuous clothing—became anathema, since it symbolized the craven situation of women "before." Women stopped wearing beautiful clothes and make-up because they didn't want anyone to think that they were "dolling themselves up for men." They wanted to show solidarity with women, not "compete with women for men." This new antitraditional dress code for women also included not shaving one's legs or other body areas. If women were not ashamed of their bodies, the thinking went, why spend an inordinate amount of time taking care of them? Why heed the advertising of cosmetic firms that wanted to make women feel insecure—about their skin, about the size dress they were wearing, about their hair (is it shiny enough?), and so on. The new woman would not bow down to these cosmetic companies and would not conform to traditional feminine stereotypes. She would be strong, whereas the traditional image of "female" had been of a weak creature.

While many of these changes are good—and certainly there was a point to asserting the rights of women by using the symbolism of clothing, making a statement by wearing a pants suit to work, refusing to look "feminine" as expected—today what began as a political statement has turned into a conformist mentality. There is too much pressure on women to "show their allegiances" through what they wear, too much of a "rush to judgement" by those on both "sides" who "decide who a person is" simply by observing her clothing and body language. Many people who are not lesbian point to other women and declare authoritatively, "There's one." Many lesbian women, especially in groups such as the one described above, tend to freeze out any woman who is not dressed in the "uniform."

Perhaps this situation is changing. I received a letter from a teenage girl in the south of Spain who reports that she is lesbian and likes dressing up but so far hasn't encountered any problem about this:

> I am nineteen, studying journalism in school. Although I don't look like it, either in the way I dress or in my physical appearance, I am a lesbian—a lesbian who lives a normal life, a pretty lesbian (so I'm told), very feminine. Well, I'm tired of hearing idiotic remarks about my inclination and desires.

All of this begs the question: What is beauty? Is it a concept that is infected with the values of the social order, so that women cannot simply say, "Each woman should choose to dress in her own way"? If "beauty" or "physical perfection" has been prized by men looking for wives ("good reproductive material"), then is there really any such thing as an independent standard of beauty? Why is the idea of "beauty" so emphasized for women, in the first place? The answer is: because the body—beautiful or not—was all that women had in "the old days" to use to find a husband and home. In the past, of course, ideals of female beauty changed: women such as Marilyn Monroe and Sophia Loren, famous film stars of the 1950s, were much heavier than women today are supposed to be. Today's beauty ideal has become so thin that the European Union put out a health warning, asking magazines to stop pushing the ideal of "thinness," since so many young women all over Europe were becoming anorexic.

Twenty thousand years ago, the famous Venus of Willendorf statue depicted a very round, possibly pregnant, woman as the icon of "the female"; for decades since the discovery of this statue, male archaeologists could not imagine that she represented a woman-headed social order (one that saw the female body's ability to give birth as miraculous), and instead "interpreted" her existence as being that of an early sex-object toy! Their only quizzical comment was that men in that ancient past must have preferred fat women . . .

Is it legitimate for us as women—whether lesbian or heterosexually oriented—to "reclaim" the symbols of female beauty, such as lipstick? To wear clothing that does not hide our body's shapes? Or are our politics more consistent if we do not try to "be beautiful" or "stand out" from others by being "attractive"? Does trying to be "beautiful" mean that we are placing ourselves in competition with other women, subtly flirting with men? If we try to be "attractive," does this effort mean that we are not in solidarity with "people everywhere who are living with very little, with few resources"—that is, "You shouldn't spend money on frivolous things like bracelets and scarves, you are spoiled! People in developing countries don't have time for such nonsensical things, they focus on more important matters, such as getting food to eat and taking care of children."

A museum in Tehran exhibited Western women's clothing, including the miniskirt, to demonstrate to Iranian women how privileged they were to live in a country where the government wisely expected them to wear the chador—so they wouldn't be exploited "like those Western women—it's terrible how they have to live." Western white women have become the international symbol of the "living in luxury, spoiled identity" of the Western world.

Can women reclaim for themselves any of the traditional feminine style, such as long hair and lipstick, or will these symbols prove to be too strong, still sending out their perfume spelling craven submission, betrayal of other women, and insecurity?

## TOWARD A NEW SEXUAL CULTURE: LINKING SEX AND POLITICS

Sex can become the personal expression of a wide-ranging sensual vocabulary that individuals want to use—not overlooking either women's or men's rights. Sex has been a grossly sexist institution oppressive to women and to men.[4] Revising the reproductive scenario, expanding it to become a wider, more erotic experience, will enable people to feel much closer, and this change in turn will enable them to see how understanding and communication will work in international politics; domination of one by the other does not lead to long-term stability, though it can do so for a period; equal partnership, on the other hand, is much more lasting and productive.

Reinventing sexuality means going back to basics: What do women want? What do men want—is it the clichés of "male desire" we see in pornographic magazines? Who would want "sex" without the overall head-to-toe physical contact it involves? This is one example of the undervalued-by-lack-of-vocabulary parts of erotic contact.

Though some would think, "if only men would understand the female orgasm, sex would be fine," much more is involved in today's changes than that—worthy as that may be! Yet it is a first step in making both orgasm for men and orgasm for women equally important steps in sex. However, most women want a more profound change.

First, many women want to take a profoundly new direction, not by being "dominatrixes" but by focusing on discovering what pleases them and involving men in these activities, rather than giving over autonomy, "playing the part" expected, being enslaved by the ideology with its "old dance steps," the choice being either "passivity" or "dominance." Women may at these times try activities that men do not recognize as "erotic," but they ought to try anyway, and stay tuned. . . . Men might do the same thing, if they began to try to reinvent sexuality based on their own bodies' voice.

Sexually, in my research, most women still feel that they have not yet fully flexed their muscles, tried their wings, that there is still some distance between their sexual "abilities" and the context or institution they are being asked to fit them into. It is almost as if women have been taking a "breather," resting, before continuing on to develop the meaning of their inner selves in new directions. (Is this true for men, too?) In politics, similarly, women no longer feel that they should "wait for someone to ask for their ideas," since "probably no one will ask"; they themselves decide to carry out their visions on their own.

Doesn't this direction imply that there would be a battle of the sexes, that women would no longer be happy pleasing men? No, because the construction of women and men in opposition to each other is part of the extreme separation and fetishism regarding gender difference that has been part of the culture for so long.

## NO MORE "BATTLE OF THE SEXES"

Wouldn't the battle between the sexes always exist, wouldn't the fight keep going, even with improvements in sexual understanding?

Although the battle of the sexes is referred to almost everywhere as if it were "a funny but inevitable, enduring part of life," not a socially created situation reflecting the outdated power inequalities between men and women in the general society (which will disappear), what we are living with is a highly exaggerated version of "the differences." Now that the socially endorsed power disparity has been challenged and is perhaps beginning to disappear, no doubt the phrase "battle of the sexes" will gradually fade from use. After all, according to my theory, it is arbitrarily created, not permanent. The battle of the sexes, or gender power struggle, is artificial, imposed on people by a social system that makes the two enemies.

This social system as we have known it fetishizes "gender"—whether you are female or male—making these the two most basic categories of existence. (Aren't you asked on every banking and insurance form to state if you are male or female?) Though in the United States during the 1970s, feminists fought to make this question illegal, arguing that it usually worked against women by discriminating against them as a result of clichés in the minds of reviewers, among other causes, these questions are still routinely asked on many international institutions' applications. Yet it is possible to envision a society in which gender is not the basic focus, nor are the "two sexes" trained to go in different directions with their needs and desires, how they see the world.

The way sex has been and is being defined makes men—who are more laden with power, thus "guilty" and "arrogant" vis-à-vis women and psychologically alienated from themselves—and women simultaneously long for and fear each other. Just think how many men fear "performance pressures"—as seen, for example, in the popularity of such drugs as Viagra and Cialis, which shows that men still believe in the talisman of a "hard penis" as their ticket to intimacy and "good performance." How many women fear that they do not have orgasm "the right way," that they cannot orgasm during "the act" or "are not pretty enough/thin enough"? These worries need not exist, were it not for a definition of sex that sets men and women against each other. A simple acceptance of the scientific fact of the wonderfully easy and pleasurable way that women have orgasm can set both men and women free from these performance worries—and their fear of the other. Of course this change should be accompanied by a simultaneous economic improvement, so that men and women are no longer economic enemies; at present, women in the West earn approximately 20–30 percent less than men in similar employment, while women worldwide are the world's poorest, least educated group.

There is no real opposition between a human being who is male and a human being who is female. The social system, denying "female human beings" their rights in terms of voting or even owning property or having their own money—and the religious system, for centuries declaring that women had no souls, murdering women by burning them at the stake, "justified" by a desire to "purify" society—have set men and women against each other. Most men have bought into this system, believing that they were given higher status and more rights and privileges.

If society creates "human nature," as proposed in my theories (and those of Jean Jacques Rousseau, Voltaire, Thomas Paine, and others[5]), then the positive news here is that we can change it by our actions. If we analyze "sexual nature," we are investigating the major underpinning of what is called "human nature" and its meaning. The body, important and wonderful as it is, is only part of who we are sexually;

much of how we decide to use our bodies in sexuality comes directly from the culture—a culture that we create every day—as well as from our individual makeup. Some believe that "human nature" is fixed, unchangeable, but this is not true; human history and culture go back 40,000 years; our version of "human nature" is only approximately 3,000 years old.

This work hopes to help transform the age-old face-off in the heart of the relationship between the genders: sex.

## PURITY AND IMPURITY EAST AND WEST: IS SEX "DIRTY"?

Ever since the Garden of Eden (featured in both Islamic and Christian scripture), sex has been seen as "shameful," not "holy"—having to do with the "lowly life of the body," not "things spiritual" (better).

As sex is seen as the opposite of things "holy," Catholic priests are expected to be celibate, even though Jewish rabbis may be married and have sex for reproduction; in various other religions, such as Islam or some sects of Buddhism, only men are allowed to be priests, as men are considered more noble and of "higher mind." Gender is a focus. Of course homosexuality is forbidden and masturbation is questionable.

How did the association of sex with the "unspiritual" come about, the association with "dirtiness" and "impurity"? Some see it as "obvious": the body is "animal," the spirit is separate. A related theory is that the proximity of the genitals to defecation (as well as urination) means that this is an inevitable connection—that is, "dirt" and sex.

In my view, the reason is historical: there was an earlier elevation of the idea of sexuality, and especially female sexuality, as positive (because it led to rebirth); when the new monotheistic hierarchical religions came along, they needed to overturn the previous viewpoint. Others feel that men have always envied the female reproductive capacity, and that this is what has caused men's desire to dominate women.

Yet another theory has it that the idea of sexual impurity emerged during the developmental stages of the two religions around the sixth century BC by way of a dualist philosophy about "body" and "soul" that existed in classical Greece. "Sex" was not seen as "dirty" before that time in most of the ancient world, as it was not so considered in the Bible's Old Testament (excluding homosexuality and masturbation); thus rabbis may marry. In this view each person is divided into two separate parts— "bodily sexual-animal drives" and "higher, purer thoughts, soul and spirit"—and these are an inevitable part of "human nature" or "biology" (our "explanation" when we do not understand something). This philosophy became entwined with the developing Christian and Islamic religions during early times. Perhaps it fit in well with the new system of father right.

Today the "purity/impurity" theme has come to pervade our sexual morality;

there is almost no morality without purity. This dualistic system merged with gender division (or was part of it from the beginning, since it was Eve the female, not Adam the man, who "caused the fall of mankind"): the female, such as Eve in the Garden, came to represent the "culpability" of humanity. Thus, in the double standard of morality that continues to this day, men are seen as representing "mind and spirit," while women represent "body/food and sexuality"; this cliché is endlessly reflected in paintings, philosophical writings, novels, and other cultural artifacts. In the dichotomy separating "the body" from "the mind," men are traditionally given higher status than women; for example, in fundamentalist Islam, men have the right to several wives if they are well-off, and the right to divorce by simply clapping their hands, whereas women have no such rights. The sexual double standard further divides women into two categories: mothers and sexy seductresses ("good women" and "bad women"), the "pure" and the "impure."

The bottom line is that female sexuality is considered most impure.

Although some have attempted to conclude that since both Islamic and Christian society place men at the head of family and government, while women hold inferior legal and social status, this arrangement is inevitable and therefore not unjust, but of course it is indeed unjust. Such arguments are illogical, and many other causes are possible; for example, since both Islam and Judeo-Christianity grew out of the same historical tradition developing in the same region, the Middle East, it may be that these developments have a simple historical genesis in which one group fought with and overcame another group. It is therefore not surprising that what are now two world religions share similar views of sex and women's and men's place in society. As these religions represent only 3,000–5,000 years of 40,000 years of human culture, it will be important in the future to learn how society was organized in the preceding eras of hunter-gatherers and others.

Will the world's major religions now move forward to revise their ethical views of women's sexuality and equality, or will they hide their heads in the sand, proclaiming a "return to tradition" virtuous (and all other views nonvirtuous)? Questions of morality need moral leadership; do we have such leadership today? Admittedly the issues are complicated, yet following laws created centuries ago (and translated many times over) to the letter is not a way of addressing current moral concerns but a lazy way of avoiding taking ethical decisions that urgently need to be made. The world is in turmoil over the issue of women's place in society, whether in Islamic traditional societies (in part the Iraq and Afghanistan wars were about this issue) or in the West.

Applying an ethical sense to current world questions such as "family values" or the position of women/abortion rights—and the definition of sex underlying all these issues—is very much needed. Thus the current research and debate hopes to provide some basis for reevaluation.

## ARE WESTERN SEXUAL STANDARDS "DECADENT"?

A charge often heard is that secular Western society is suffering a morals collapse. ("Secular" means a nonreligious state—that is, democracies that include the separation of church and state.) The supposed evidence that is usually provided for this charge is the prevalence of pornography and of media/advertising images of "sexy," scantily clad or consumeristic women, as well as pornographic depictions of sex. Are such symbols justifiable as representing "the problem with the West," if there is one? While many people may agree that too many images of vulgar sex surround us, this does not mean that Western society has become decadent and immoral.

The West today has come to be seen as the home of "liberalism," "secularism," "feminism," "women's rights," tolerance of personal "life styles" and sexual diversity— all of which the West can be proud of. They are part of the tradition of secular democracy that has made the United States such a strong country. However, fundamentalists from the Middle East as well as the West complain that Western society is "too free," accusing it of being amoral and decadent. In both Japan and Saudi Arabia, for example, some say that "Western influences make us lose the graceful beauty of the traditional Japanese/Saudi woman." Thus most fundamentalists focus on the position of women in their accusations, in fact insisting that women return "to how they were before." The demand to return to "family values" is, in effect, a demand that women return to their former role.

Are fundamentalists correct in their view of sexuality—that women should be mothers in the home, that men are immoral unless they are married fathers—or is the liberal secular West going in the right direction, with openness and sexual freedom, choice of partners equally for women as for men? Is "openness" about "female sexuality" an advance, or is it a coarsening of women, making "all women too available"? (As some women in the 1976 Hite Report responded, "Now I am expected to say yes to sex with every man who asks, it's worse than before when I was the property of only one man.")

## IS THE WESTERN "SEXUAL REVOLUTION" AN ADVANCE OR A DECLINE?

Though we frequently hear of "the collapse of the old moral order" as if it were a "catastrophe," "a decline of civilization," this view is inaccurate grandstanding. Yes, this is a period of chaos and change, but it is moving toward an improvement in the moral code, as people try to digest the meaning of women's equality within major institutions such as sex and morality—private life, home and family. How could we lament the end of the old moral order when it was based on such inequality, putting women in a perilous, secondary position? Over three centuries in the Middle Ages, millions of women were murdered as "witches" in the name of religion and tradition. A change from a moral system in which only the reproductive couple (man as head of the family) was considered good, in favor of a new, more complex morality that values "single parents" as much as the two-parent family—or, for that matter, any individual—is not accurately reflected by the images being used to discredit these changes: pornographic or consumeristic images of women "demanding power." These images are used to manipulate people's views, make them feel guilty, or fear the changes. Restoring female sexuality to its "proper place" in the symbols of humanity is important in this redesign of culture to make a more just society.

One of the central concepts of sex in both Islam and Christianity is that of purity. Beginning with the Garden of Eden, humanity was punished by God/Allah for sexual knowledge caused by Eve's curiosity; after Eve ate the forbidden fruit, Adam and Eve were "shamed" and had to cover their genitals with leaves and leave the Garden, thus depicting the idea of sexual impurity.

Perhaps because of this early story quoted by both religions, ideas equating sex and impurity are similar in fundamentalist branches of both Eastern and Western religious traditions; this similarity does not prove that "there is a natural connection between sex and impurity;" rather, it shows that both religions have a common historical root, one that shares the Garden of Eden myth and "fall from grace," among others. Both religions share the belief that only men (not women) should be priests, that female sexuality and the female body are somehow less "pure" than the male body: for a number of centuries, the Catholic Church denied that women had souls.

Now the West has in part changed its view of sex—think of religious tolerance, gay rights, and women's equality—causing some fundamentalists to label the West "decadent"; this book argues that the fact is just the opposite, that the pornographic images of "perversity" being pointed to by such religious groups represent their own system "acting out," not the new moral system that is trying to come into being. My latest research shows that people are personally struggling with complex moral issues, in private as well as in their voting decisions involving international global events. Most believe that women's equality is worth struggling for yet find that integrating it into their personal sexual life is not so easy.

The central point at which the moral issue of equality must be addressed is in the very act of "sex." How should it be redesigned, now that it is clear that most women can have orgasm easily but not usually via coitus, the way that men do? How should it be redesigned, beyond orgasm, if men find the "performance" involved boring and stressful? Even though this is a personal issue, people's choices—and their communication of their choices to others—will change the complexion of the overall society.

Will societies in Africa that now permit clitoredectomy and infibulation come to realize that these customs deny women and girls the right to autonomy over their own bodies, and will these societies change their views? Will Islamic countries, such as Saudi Arabia, evolve to become more "liberal/tolerant" in their valuation of women's rights and cease penalizing women for expressing a nonconformist sexuality? Issues of clitoredectomy, sex trafficking and sex tourism, abortion rights, and free choice of jobs for women—all are linked: sexual and physical autonomy are important for women, as the United Nations Declaration on the Rights of Women (Beijing 1995) announced. While we may agree that making this truth a reality will have more effects than imagined, we find ourselves trying to work out our belief system today—mostly as individuals, without what could be valuable spiritual guidance from "church officials." However, this is a great opportunity for us to renew our society and its democratic inheritance.

Today men, not only women, have ethical questions about their lives—for example, men often wonder how much time they should spend at work and at home, whether they are dividing their time correctly, questioning themselves about their priorities and commitments. This self-questioning about these and other questions, on the part of men and women, is causing an evolution in human understanding about the nature of sex and personal identity. We are all involved in this rethinking, even people "halfway across the world" feel confused and personally conflicted, desiring to be "pure" and yet feeling excited when viewing "Western pornography." This new self-consciousness is part of the global search for a new sexual value system.

What we are witnessing, and ourselves creating via our personal questions, is a transformation to a new moral and ethical system, one more diverse and individually honest than the previous rigid "good traditional family" value system, which excluded so many people. In the past, the "traditional family"—with a "proper father" and "proper mother"—forced many people who did not happen to "love the right person" to nevertheless build appearances of such a family, falsifying their feelings or forcing themselves in any way possible to fit into the system, lest society categorize them as "immoral," "immature," or "psychologically disturbed." Today we are trying to build a moral code that goes beyond that.

The very reason many in the West find Islamic accusations of "Western moral decay" so irritating is because they believe they are true, since Western religious tradition is so similar to Islamic tradition. The medieval Christian view of sex (declaring that women had no souls) and the current extremist Islamic view of sex and women have much in common.

Western moral progress is fragile as yet, and many people are not quite sure they have made the right choices, since they are still frequently wracked with doubt and torn within themselves, engaged in "soul-searching."

In my research I find that many people (male and female) are of two minds: on the one hand they believe that true morality means that they should behave honestly and in a way that reflects their inner identity (you should live with the person you love and not hide that affection, no matter how this might upset anyone else or society's view of you); on the other hand, there is a strong call to "be respectable" and follow the tried and true paths society has prescribed (stay married if you are married, this is your duty and may turn out to be prudent). Yet more and more people in the West today are applying personal ethics to situations that used to be governed by religious edicts and norms (such as birth control); today many people perceive that morality is a personal responsibility and choice. Supporting my research, population statistics for the last ten years in major Western countries have been showing that 50 percent of the populations of major Western cities are officially classified as "single"; this statistic indicates, not the "collapse" of society but, more probably, an attempt at its renewal by millions of individuals who try to make honest choices rather than staying married at all costs.

Why has the West changed its view of women, evolved a view leading to "equal rights" or "sexual equality," whereas many Islamic societies have not? In the West, women's rights (and experiments in sexual expression) have become more accepted during the last one hundred years; is this an inevitable future trend for Islamic fundamentalist societies too? Or was this "human rights" and "equality" idea unique to the West, part of the democratic tradition?

Female equality inevitably brings up issues of sexuality, since the society has been based on the rigid structuring of female sexuality—and indeed male sexuality—channeling their erotic feelings into reproductive scenarios.

Many fundamentalists, Islamic and Western, see the last hundred years in the West as a wrong turn in terms of women's role in society and family, also believing homosexuality is a sin or a "mental disorder."

Sexual equality is a concept that is changing from the inside the ways "sex" and human relations are defined. Some say that the changes of the "new sexuality" demonstrate the collapse of the old moral order, a decline in values, but others insist that that "sexual freedom" is necessary in order to have political freedom. This book contends that neither answer is going to lead to a positive solution but that the solution is being sought by millions of individuals everywhere, a "third way" forward, based on neither "traditional family values" nor "the sexual revolution."

Clearly equality and self-determination for women, among the most important issues of our time, are having a major influence, in large part creating these changes. Part of this process means revising our idea of "who men are," including sexually[6]; this will reduce the number of wars that are carried on internationally as our value system transforms.

## ARE "SEXUALLY LIBERATED WOMEN" IN THE WEST CAUSING "THE DECLINE OF MORALS"?

To say that Western women and Western sexuality are "decadent" is a superficial view, merely reversing the stereotypes of "female sexuality" from passive to active ("woman on top") does not change the basic presumption of the acts to be performed—they have already been defined. Truly authentic sexual expression for women will come with economic and legal autonomy and independence. Now that many women make their own money, their change in status is causing a huge moral shift for the better, although during the transition it may not seem so.

In part the current fundamentalist reaction against "women's rights" or "women's sexual freedom" may not really be against women's rights but against the vulgarity sometimes used to depict "free women" and "women's rights"—which grow out of the ideology just defined— that is, that sex is "dirty" and, especially, female sexuality is "bad." Unfortunately such images influence many people to believe that women's freedom and equality are vulgar, that female "sexual liberation" means women becoming unpleasant "dominatrixes" or "too aggressive at work"; some can only envision "equality" between women and men as women becoming as "ballsy," "insensitive," and "power-driven" as men are stereotypically portrayed to be. In other words, the old culture that saw women as nicely in their place is playing tricks on our minds, portraying all "this new sex" and "the new gender behaviors" as ugly, bizarre, and immoral. How often have you seen, for example, the citing of ads for penis-shaped dildos, penis enlargement devices, and sex toys like whips and chains, as evidence of "widespread perversions"? A serious examination of the facts, as in my ongoing research,* shows something different.

Sex and human rights are part of a larger debate about Western values, seen also in the international debate about the war with Iraq; fundamentalists cry that the "collapse of civilization" will occur if values relating to women and "the home" are not continued without modification. Despite such cries of gloom and doom, however, a new global "secular society" is developing—perhaps "more moral" than any ever seen. Of course, since we are still in the midst of these developments, it is difficult to know the outcome. However, the debate is part of an international debate about what the spiritual New World Order should be; although lip service is paid to "individual cultures" being "unique," in fact today's technological innovations, such as the Internet, films, and television, mean that we increasingly inhabit a global village with what will probably become a global set of values. Thus the debate is about equality, human rights and women's place in society—difficult concepts to integrate into "sex" and eroticism.

Some of the changes of the last thirty years in the West may have gone in the wrong direction, while others were good. The 1960's sexual revolution made several mistakes, while it also made advances. It decreed that women were no longer required to remain virgins until marriage: sex was declared to be healthy, necessary, and good, repression of sexual feelings a cause of grave problems or a sign of "blocked thinking." Whereas in the 1950s, "a girl's reputation was ruined if she was found to be having sex before marriage" ("damaged goods"), in the l960s the reverse pressure was applied to women: "You're hung up if you don't have sex regularly and enjoy it." The birth control pill for women enabled much more sex to take place without worry than previously, yet "the pill" was a mixed blessing: with it, women

---

* For example, today most people no longer consider specific sexual acts, such as oral sex, whether fellatio or cunnilingus, sinful; the focus of morality has shifted to the sphere of relationships. The new center of moral focus is on issues such as violent pornography, child molestation, rape, domestic violence, and sexual harassment.

achieved more control over their own reproduction but also came under greater pressure "to have sex at the drop of a hat." In fact, now that many women make their own money, much is made of the sexual independence Western women enjoy.

The changes brought about by the "sexual revolution" and the birth control pill have had positive and negative sides. The positive side was more often contributed by the feminist movement—the claiming of women's right to birth control, orgasm, abortion as a choice and self-expression. On the negative side, the sexual revolution seemed to mean that whereas in the past a woman was owned by one man, now she was owned by all men, as she should "take the pill" and "be available for sex if a man asked her." The sexual revolution also led to the proliferation of pornography, with dehumanizing and dangerous caricatures of male and female sexuality, an increase in sexual violence to women and even murders (especially of young women who fit the images in pornography of "vulnerable young women"), and pressure on men to "desire every woman under forty," exhibit an erection as often as possible, and so on.

There is now a movement in opposition to these changes, known as the "pro-family values" movement, claiming that the sexual revolution destroyed moral values and led to a decline in moral "goodness," even to the sexual molestation of children. Unfortunately the "family values" movement defends "morality" by trying to reinstall the double standard of morality regarding women—surely an anachronism, judging women badly and harshly if they are "too sexual."

While fundamentalist religious critics are correct in that the "sexual revolution" did not always go in the right direction, the goals of women's rights and equality—now lumped together and called "the sexual revolution"—were and are good: to create equality in the basic physical relationship between female and male, to make private life equal, with greater justice.

The final question, then, is how best to go forward: return to "family values" or embrace the "sexual revolution"? In my view a third way forward needs to be identified—an imaginative way to integrate women's and men's sexuality and equality with overall identity, in the process changing how one thinks of others, plus of course allowing those of the same sex to love each other without shame. Images of "swinging hip sexy women" do not represent this ongoing long-term change, nor do images of "gay men with whips and chains and leather," nor today's women's magazines that shout, "Be a sexy woman!" leaving many women feeling doubtful that they want to be sexy in the way the magazines intend. However, despite the confusing clichés of "the free woman," women in many parts of the world are slowly but surely now making small but radical changes in their daily sexual self-expression—changes that have nothing to do with commercial images, but are very private and personal movements. They believe they can combine being "graceful" and nonaggressive ("old style femininity") with nontraditional sexual acts. They are creating their own process of sexual evolution, experimenting with new forms of sexual self-expression.

Is secularism "decadent" and "immoral"? No, Western secularism is becoming more moral, trying to integrate ideas of justice and equality into sex and society—imperfectly, so far. Although Western sexual morality may have taken a few wrong turns over past decades, this is not remarkable when a society is emerging from centuries of an unequal social order, a social/sexual order that used to be based on "female submission." In fact, overall society has been going in a positive direction. The excesses of the present and the attitudes and images now fashionable (as in "trendy" pornography) are obviously parts of a transition out of a long, numb slumber.

The new morality—aiming at equality and human rights, even when it has not yet reached the target or has even gone off in a mistaken direction—can lead to a more stable and happy society than either a simplistic return to basics or an unmodified acceptance of the sexual revolution.

Based on my research, I believe that many people are now privately and quietly constructing another way of life inside their relationships, a way of sexuality that is not like the past but also not like the images of "let it all hang out." What is new in "the moral landscape" that is trying to establish itself is not only equality between women and men, but also a new sexual identity for both.

The new moral acceptance of "equality" as applied to sexuality is leading to changes in thinking within men and women about their personal sexuality—as well as the focus on public issues such as "birth control," "monogamy," "adultery," and "the female body" (should women wear the chador?); the question in private is, "What should our relationship be like?" As at the end of apartheid rule in South Africa, we may be at the end of one rather rigid version of morality and at the beginning of the democratization of morals: many people no longer believe fully in the system as it was, only accepting parts of it, thus creating a climate open to change.

In my view what is being constructed is more moral, if that term should be used, than in the past. People today no longer feel that it is right to simply conform, no matter what they feel, to "family" stereotypes; they want the world to recognize their love for another, whoever that person may be; they no longer want to seek approval from society by simply conforming to social expectations, since they often feel that by so doing, they are being immoral and not honest.

In summary, secularism is not "decadent" because it has "sexy free women" (who should be more "modest," so there would not be the vulgar images seen everywhere). There is a confusion in the public mind between women's liberation and images of "sex, sex, sex" that depict women as "free, hip, and sexy." These images hark back to earlier views of women and soon will go out of style; we are now in a transitional stage moving toward a new kind of social organization, although it may take several generations to see this clearly. Fundamentalist Islam and fundamentalist Christianity need to review the meaning of morality and thus the relationship between women and men. Religion stands for moral justice, yet inequality is a form of injustice that must be rectified.

Fundamentalist Islamic societies and fundamentalist Western societies should move forward in terms of women's rights, take a new look at their views of sex, women, and the definition of "men"—acknowledge that a revised sexual moral code is necessary. Religion should offer leadership in the area of morality, not hold us back; equality is obviously part of what most of us believe today to be ethics, we no longer believe that slavery is "right," even if it existed in biblical times. Therefore religious doctrine now should be updated in the matters of "equality" and "human rights" to create a rebirth of religious respect.

Attempts at equality between the sexes inevitably lead to the redefinition of sex, since sex is the pivotal point of the relationship between male and female. A fundamental rethinking of women's position in society inevitably involves a fundamental change in sexuality.

## LOVE AND FAMILY VALUES PAST AND FUTURE

### SOCIETY BEFORE THE GREEKS

How often have you heard it said, "It's human nature, it's biology, you can't change it!" I'm afraid this argument is lazy rationalization of the status quo. Our design for living is a combination of the physical and mental; society's influence is quite pronounced.

We urgently need to redesign the way we are living, including our ideas of family, sex, and work—the basics—and this in turn will create new global political ideas. At the moment, the world is "topsy-turvy," we find ourselves involved in a large-scale "war against terror" and can't seem to find a way out. Understanding prehistoric ways of life can give us a broader canvas for thinking, and free us from the confines of what we are told is "realistic and possible." Understanding "who we originally were," we can better design our course of action, review what love means to us.

How have we become so myopic that we lack vision to see a way forward out of the current global conflict? Are we "missing the forest for the trees"? We rationalize "the way things are" as "inevitable human nature" or "biology," probably so that we won't have to change, selecting those parts of "science" that support us. A knowledge of pre-history offers a good counterbalance to this myopia, a bigger picture of the universe and of what is possible. (The term "prehistory" refers to milennia of highly complex cultures that did not use written records; many people consider such societies "lesser," but it is precisely the fact that they used other means of communication than writing that makes them so interesting.)

One example of how wedded we are to specific views we consider unquestionable—values we consider "obvious"—is terming "the night" a less realistic time than the day. Possibly humans once lived in the night during centuries when the lunar calendar was favored over the solar or Gregorian calendar; we still have night vision in our eyes. It is also possible that it was not simply "our biological identities" that created the transition to sun-calendar culture, but an ideology and lifestyle (farming) that caused the changeover. Some scholars believe that the change from a moon calendar to a sun calendar (with accompanying social reorganization) represented a new social order that was imposing itself. While the earlier lunar calendar had been handy for women mapping their menstrual cycles (which are linked to lunar cycles), thus avoiding/encouraging pregnancy, since women timed their "fertile periods" via the lunar calendar, this was no longer possible with the sun calendar. With the change to the solar calendar, women lost status, and female deities were demoted in rank (in the pantheon of goddesses and gods),* later struck off the list of "creators."†

The discovery of fire was one of the earliest basic inventions of humankind. As fire was necessary for cooking, this was probably linked to the changeover from the lunar to the solar world-view (happening at the same time as the change from gathering-hunting to farming and the growth of cities). Many archaeologists believe that the beginning of farming and agriculture—when several types of grasses were blended together to create "wheat" and bread was invented —coincided with the formation of cities. Before the rise of agriculture social organization seems to have been quite different, including a profoundly different view of the universe, one that we might not recognize; it is even possible that "human nature" in prehistory was not warlike, since Catal Huyuk, an early town excavated in Turkey, had no walls for defense.

For over twelve centuries archaeological remains indicate that a single culture extended from the Black Sea in Russia to the Lassaoux caves in France and the

---

* Although earlier societies hailed Athena the goddess as "leader," later societies demoted female goddesses or eventually deleted them altogether from their pantheon of deities. For example, Athena was originally chief of all the gods, then she was demoted: whereas originally she had been "simply herself," in later myths she was described as being "daughter of Zeus, born out of his head"; today she is only a word or invisible. Similarly in archaic Egypt, whereas a statue of Isis once stood over the waters of the delta of the Nile and Tigris and Euphrates Rivers (often called "the cradle of civilization"), Isis being the central deity of society in that place at that time, later she was demoted and termed nothing more than a "fertility goddess," connected with water and the like; venerating her was declared "blasphemous," and she was spoken of as a sexual or breast-feeding mother-goddess. It is worth pointing out that societies of the time based on the pantheon view seem to have been at least as moral as societies today.

† In the sixth century BC, much of the mythology and ideology of ancient Greece was reshaped by famous playwrights, as the new social order was still being put in place and digested. Sophocles, the playwright, for example, rewrote the myth of Oedipus, attempting to make a statement showing the "wrongness" of Oedipus the boy wishing to have sex with/love/marry his mother—Sophocles implies this love was "wrong," not because she was older, but because she "belonged to" his father, and probably a son should not go against his father or another man because of a woman—this version of Oedipus went along with a new ideological view being shaped at that time of father right (men on top); the matrilineal social order with its pantheon of powerful female and male goddesses and gods was not long past in historical memory and still needed to be overcome "in the gut" or psyche, even though the new social order had been successfully imposed (we don't know how, this has been lost to our history). Also in those early centuries, a movement toward monotheism headed by a male god became pronounced, whereas previously societies in the Middle East had believed in multi-deitied pantheons, which still survive in Hinduism in Southern India. A multi-deitied pantheon creates a psychology that is more accepting of diversity.

southern part of Austria. What we know about this culture demonstrates a matri-lineal gatherer-hunter way of life, but beyond that we know very little. "Writing" had not been discovered; the writing that preceeds Linear B on Crete at the end of this period, Linear A, is still untranslated. (John Chadwick, who attempted to decipher Linear A, after several years believed he had failed "because it [what he could deci-pher] seems to be nothing but a list of names of women and their daughters"—I hope readers understand how ironic his conclusion was, since in those earlier civiliza-tions, when descent went through the female line, keeping a list of the names of mothers and daughters would have had a great deal of purpose; so perhaps his "fail-ure" was in fact a success that he failed to recognize, simply because he didn't find what he had been expecting.)

If the earliest known societies were quite possibly societies in which children were cared for and "owned" by the group, not the mother or the parents, then these were societies in which the family was structured quite differently—and flourished/reproduced—this structure tells us quite a bit about our own possibilities. It offers a brilliant contrast with our own belief that only the basic biological family will create stability and growth and opens our minds to seeing new ways of social organ-ization; it does not, of course, mean that our only choice is to copy those ancient forms of social organization! It simply means that if things were once so different, then we can imagine whatever we want that could work, we are not limited, as many claim today, by the necessity of setting up "the biological family," without which civilization will collapse. (Many children in Africa whose parents have died of AIDS and children in Brazil who live in the street will be happy to hear that their forms of family can be just as good for them as the biological family may or may not be for others.) Margaret Mead was possibly trying to provide us with the same kind of contrast when she, an anthropologist, documented an alternative social order that she found still flourishing in mid-twentieth century Polynesia. Contrasting soci-eties offer us the chance to gain a more objective view of our idea of "the family."

What do we mean by "family values," "love," and "proper upbringing of chil-dren"? The goal of families is to raise children with positive values. It is clear that in many early times children were raised as a group by all the adults, not by "one mother and father" as depicted in the Catholic "holy family" or the "biological fam-ily" that today we assume is "best." Perhaps father lineage was not standard practice in the earliest societies, which were matrilinial, because men were rarely certain that it was their intercourse with a woman that led to her pregnancy (male ownership of women via marriage was not yet instituted); thus fatherhood was less clearly a con-cept than was motherhood (it was easy to see which woman gave birth to a child). Or maybe there was another reason.

"The family" was not always the trilogy family we have grown up believing to be "the normal family"; in fact, when the "single-mother family" was the norm, society flourished. In the 1970s, scholars debated whether the historical changeover from mother right (female-descended societies) to patriarchy/father right (male-descended societies) was caused "naturally" by "the growth of cities and social organization," with their homebase thinking, or whether the change was caused by a series of physical battles between societies with different social structures/"religions." As concrete evidence of such physical battles, we can today see (among others) the stone depictions of "female Amazons fighting foreign male invaders" carved on the famous friezes now in Berlin's Pergamon Museum. The archaeologist Marija Gimbutas developed this subject in some detail before her death in 1994.

Though the 1970s scholars never reached a consensus on the nature of the earliest families—the question was left open[7]—the change in approved family structure seemed to take place around the same time when the lunar calendar was dropped and cities became important. This early social organization is a puzzle that is still being investigated.

Today the shapes of families are changing yet again. We need to realize how culture-bound it is to label "single mother families" as "less good" than "the traditional mother-father family." We should be glad that reproduction is taking place and open our minds to new forms of love and family. Many people want to rebalance our way of living with nature and other cultures. While we wish to retain the ideas of loving and caring for others found in "family values," we do not wish to create people who selfishly protect "their families" while children in Africa starve; we want to expand the idea of family. "Family values" is a private-property version of loving others, whereas "family love" should be extended to others all over the planet.

Our view of what is the "obvious order of things" is much more flexible than we generally believe. "Human nature" is plastic, and we can improve society and ourselves by seeing more clearly "where we come from," "what is natural," and what love and "family values" are all about.

## PERSONAL POLITICS: HOW PERSONAL THOUGHTS ABOUT SEX ARE CONNECTED TO INTERNATIONAL POLITICS

Private and personal decisions about sex are related to larger political debates going on today, such as the position of women in the Middle East, the meaning of family, as well as love and sex in Asia (think of sex trafficking of children), the Middle East (think of women wearing the chador), and the West (think of the scandals related to pedophile rings), and many other issues.

As mentioned previously, most people today are concerned with the heated debates about sex in the news: public discussions of abortion, equality, sexual harassment, "the veil"/ "the chador"/"the secular minijupe," the sexual trafficking in women, the rapes in war zones (as, for example, in Bosnia, Chechnya, and Rwanda), even "President Clinton's sex life." Undoubtedly their views of these matters influenced their voting patterns in recent elections in Western democracies.

They are also concerned with how they should feel about "sex" in their private lives; they wonder if the sex they are sharing with another/others is "complete" or "who they really are/want to be." Is life "passing them by" without their really having the great experiences they hope to have?

Black-and-white choices seem to be on offer, yet most people find that some of the "traditional family morality" and some of the "new morality" (right to divorce, non-penalty for masturbation, and the like) are good. Thus they live their lives with a mixture of values. However, in the international sphere the choice is more cut-and-dried, it does not so far seem to allow for variation. Will it in the future? Or will we reach moral/sexual consensus that is translated into our value system before too long?

Though women are told that they are "sexually free" (the birth-control pill, no disapproval for sex without marriage), today they often still experience judgmental attitudes that hark back to the mythological images (Mary is pure, Eve is sinful). For example, the issue of "single mothers" is a hot political topic in many countries, showing that the double standard of morality is still alive, condemning women who have sex outside the nuclear family even in these days of reproductive need.

To be quite clear, think about this: if women know perfectly well how to reach orgasm when they stimulate themselves, yet most women do not have orgasms during "the normal sex act," what does this tell us about equality? It tells us that sex is an outdated institution that is reinforcing inequality in that it centers on the stimulation most men need to reach orgasm, glorifying that, and does not include (or calls "special stimulation") the stimulation most women need. We need to change this, create a new kind of sex.

## SEX AND WORLD PEACE

Understanding the sexual ideology can indeed be "a road to peace." How? We cannot simplistically smile and say, "If everyone would just make love, forget about war, the world would be a happier place!"—though that may be true. In fact, the definition of female sexuality contains all the elements central to our sociocultural structure; to analyze female and male sexuality takes us—as seen in this book—on a long examination of the underlying social ideology.

If most women reach orgasm via a form of clitoral stimulation and not "vaginal penetration," this circumstance brings into question a number of our most "sacred" central beliefs about "what sex is" and "the act," also "who men are by nature." In its most profound sense sex is linked to "world peace" because striving for a new understanding of how to conduct our private lives and our sexual lives is part of a general striving to formulate a new international system of values and relationships.

What is being proposed here is a rethinking of the meaning of sexuality, including a new analysis of women's and men's sexual rights. Can we change "human nature" by reprogramming ourselves about sex?

## FEMINISM, FEMALE SEXUALITY, AND WORLD TERRORISM

For most people the recent attack on the United States and the wars in Afghanistan, Iraq, and elsewhere in the Middle East mean that the concerns of "the women's movement"—"equality and all that," sexual rights—are pushed far into the background of the international political stage.

The reality, however, is just the reverse: the issues of women and women's "place" in society, the meaning of female sexuality and the female body, underly this conflict on the global political stage. In fact, female sexuality and its place in the social order is one of the fundamental issues underlying current world political clashes.

Current extremist or "terrorist" movements—Islamic, Western, and otherwise—can be seen as in large part a protest against the growing power of women, a condition variously referred to as "the collapse of the family" and "Western secularism."

Of course poverty and issues of "rich versus poor," exclusion/inclusion, as well as "religious values" play crucial parts in this developing situation. However, to see how "feminism" and the current conflicts are linked, one has only to look at the part played by the oppression of women in Afghanistan (denying them education, jobs, and the like) in the current global reshuffling of power; people now doubt that the treatment of women in Saudi Arabia or Iran, where they are forced by government edict to cover themselves from head to toe (they can risk arrest or physical attack if they do not) while men may walk freely, is a simple "religious" or "culture specific" matter. (After all, women in medieval Europe lived with many of the same restrictions.)

Clearly women's place in society is central to the clash of ideologies taking place.

During the last twenty-five years, Western women have changed society and the family enormously; this development has led to a backlash movement in the West that uses such phrases as "the collapse of family values" and "society has gone too far." Extremist groups in Iran and elsewhere point at "the new liberated Western woman" as symbolic of all that is wrong with the "decadent West." "Secularism" seems to mean, not only a government that is not ruled by religion, but also a government that allows many forms of religious belief; even more, it seems to mean equality of women, including sexual equality and freedom of sexual expression—even if that "sexual expression" as we see it today, as argued above, is not yet an authentic expression of "who women are" or "what sexuality is," but more a semi-pornographic version of "thumbing the nose" at past moral-sexual values.

Feminism is connected to the current world conflict in another way: it provides an analysis unlike that coming from other quarters. Feminist analysis asks why so often male psychology can feel such an urgent need to exclude women from power, even to exclude women from the streets, to make women almost invisible in the chador, as in the case of the Taliban rulers of Afghanistan in the 1990s.

Of course the Taliban leaders were all male, and they considered gender extremely important; one of the platforms of their "order" was to keep women out of work and only in the house. The question: why did/do such men wish to bond to exclude women, while women do not try to exclude men systematically—that is, women are not joining together to defeat "men"? The answer lies in the way boys and girls are socialized in our now international culture featuring tough-as-nails aggressive male heroes.

Boys learn at puberty in both West and East that they must not be "a mamma's boy" ("Don't stay home with your mother"!), that they must "get out and toughen up with the other boys," that "real men fight for dominance," are "not feminine," and so on. They learn that they should be in groups of men not "hanging out with a woman." This "education" is carried out largely by groups of boys at school who bully and taunt younger boys. As a society we could change the values we offer boys in these "initiation rites" and so achieve a less warlike society for adults.

The current escalation of tension and violence in international affairs may reflect the increased emphasis placed on these boyhood "be a man" rituals in recent years: for almost twenty years the amount of aggression put into boys' minds and personalities via video games, TV "cartoons" and other "entertainment" (seen worldwide) has been growing. These increased levels of "acceptable violence" were protested by educators, psychologists, and others, but few changes were undertaken. A constant diet of aggression and "toughness," broadcast around the world via movies and videos, was absorbed by boys who now have come of age. Did we think they would never use this violent value system, remain forever "young boys"? Certainly many of the "suicide bombers" probably believe "masculinity means a man is tough and can go it alone," even though they also probably believe themselves to be acting out of religious belief—"saving the world," "making a more pure society," or defeating "the evil money-war-Western group."

Although part of the global confrontation going on now is caused by the frustration millions of people all over the world feel at the seeming "ownership" of the global economy by the West—attitudes based on the belief that "the West" is entitled to world hegemony more than "others." But an even deeper problem may be the psychosexual teaching of boys. By this I do not mean to imply that the psychology of the "suicide bomber" is typically male but to point out that such behavior is not the consequence of "men having aggressive hormones" but of an ideology (common to both West and East) that repeatedly trains boys to adopt warrior-type behaviors while simultaneously training girls to adopt harmony-seeking behaviors. This ideology, currently being spread even more widely and restyled as "modern" by Hollywood films and Internet pornography (to name just two), could be modified to create more peace on earth.

In order to address the problem of violence on a long-term basis, it is necessary to think not only in terms of economics. We must change what boys and girls learn from movies, television, the Internet, and other media about "who a real man is." We must construct a new idea of heroism.

## CHURCH, WOMEN, AND FAMILY: A NEW DIRECTION

RESPONDING TO THE VATICAN LETTER TO BISHOPS ON WOMEN AND FEMINISM,
AUGUST 2004

In August 2004 the Vatican published a new document relating to women—in fact a letter to all the world's bishops about the status of women and the Catholic Church's position about it. There must be strong pressure on and within the Vatican—coming both from the human rights conventions of the European Union and from women within the Church who want to be priests, as well as from parishioners (both women and men) who question the teachings of the Church about birth control and women—to have made the Vatican publish such a document. Perhaps some of the pressure comes, too, from the recent scandals of child abuse bankrupting many United States and Catholic churches, calling into question the "family values" ethics of church fathers.

I believe that "family values" is a phrase that belongs to everybody, not only to the Vatican and certain political parties and that it needs more clarity.

The Vatican document seems to me, as a long-time feminist, to misunderstand the genesis of recent debates about the role of women in society. While the Vatican and I would agree on the value of women's childbearing work for society, we would disagree when the Vatican's opening paragraph (after the introduction) states:

> Recent years have seen new approaches to women's issues. A first tendency is to emphasize strongly conditions of subordination in order to give rise to antagonism: women, in order to be themselves, must make themselves the adversaries of men. Faced with the abuse of power, the answer for women is to seek power. This process leads to opposition between men and women, in which the identity and role of one are emphasized to the disadvantage of the other, leading to harmful confusion regarding the human person, which has its most immediate and lethal effects in the structure of the family.

This opening paragraph, which sets the tone for the rest of the document, starts the document with a false premise. Contrary to sowing discord, in fact the movement for women's rights is improving the relationship between men and women, not making it more antagonistic. The Vatican document is implicitly giving men the right to insist that women toe the traditional line, thus causing division between the two sexes, making their relationship more "antagonistic" by its seeming desire to ask women to stop looking at their wounds. If indeed women's rights groups have at times emphasized the legal and financial (as well as psychological) conditions of subordination, the purpose was not to "make themselves the adversaries of men"! The purpose was and is to help women (and men). The purpose of exposing injustices around the world is the same, whether it is in regard to the black civil rights movement or the South African antiapartheid movement, or indeed continuing to talk of the murders of Jews and others during Hitler's Nazi regime in Germany. The purpose of exposing the injustices black people suffered in the United States was not to make them adversaries of white people; rather, according to Martin Luther King and Nelson Mandela, who should know, it was to bring to light what black people have been through, to give them and others a sense of their courage in the face of adversity. Increase their pride and show their beauty. Or think of the Jews under the Nazi regime in Germany; current television programs and films highlighting Holocaust survivors and showing the suffering of the Jewish people during that period of Germany's history are not intended to make people adversaries of Germans, but rather to show that the Jewish people survived and that the world *has* changed; with such documentation, consciousness is changed so that it can never happen again.

It is totally legitimate for women's rights groups to expose the sufferings of women under past and present systems of nonequality—the very recent days when women did not have their own passports, the right to vote, and so forth—not forgetting that for centuries women in the Catholic Church were not considered to have souls nor to be able to ascend fully to heaven. (Mary became an important Catholic symbol only in the nineteenth century!) It is totally legitimate for women's groups today to expose current and continuing injustices to women, such as the outrageous prevalence of domestic violence, even the murder of women for "men's honor." For another example, today women still cannot hold equal positions with men in the church hierarchy. Women now are just beginning to take their place among world leaders, to be prime ministers, hold cabinet posts, be presidents of global corporations, and so forth, so that this situation as well as lack of equal pay needs to be addressed. Doing so does not mean that the result will be more division between women and men, but less. In fact, the division is artificial to begin with and was created/exaggerated by religious social systems that declared men to be superior to women in the family (he was the husband "shepherding her," she was the "helpmate"). We as a society are just now recovering from that unhelpful way of thinking.

I cannot think of many cases in which those who have campaigned against such abuses as female genital mutilation (excision and infibulation) or domestic violence (98 percent by men against women) have done so with the intention of creating "class warfare" between men and women, as the Vatican document would imply. If there is a chasm or distance ("opposition") between women and men, this is created by the situation and reality, not by those trying to achieve justice for women and society.

Men, not only women, gain from the campaign for equality between women and men; men gain better relationships and a broader spectrum of life. The Vatican document, in implying that its system (the traditional hierarchical family) represents harmony between men and women, while women's and men's equality and change/new style relationships represent division and fighting between men and women, is self-serving and false. In fact the opposite is true: couples are happier and closer when injustices are exposed so that they may become more equal and when men do not have to see women as "so different that they cannot be understood." Initiatives for change are most often undertaken by humanitarian and women's rights groups. The traditional ways of life prescribed by the church for married couples have more often than not led to cold bickering and silences, frequently followed by separation, and have cost society much of the energy and enthusiasm women can contribute, whether at home in families or outside the home at work— energy they give when they have full rights in the society to contribute in every way.

The good side of "family values" is best preserved by democratizing family structure (relationships between women and men), not retaining its traditional hierarchy.

### INCREASING DOMESTIC VIOLENCE AGAINST WOMEN—WHY NOW?

A 2004 European Union bulletin proclaimed that "there exists an increasing spiral of this type of violence to women, parallel to the process of women's independence. In certain sectors, there exists a macho culture calling for relationships of domination and possession of women, and now at times women are paying for their liberty with their very lives." Is it true that the increase in violent attacks on women in the twenty-first century are being "caused by" women's increased independence?

Women are facing an increasing climate of violence in many parts of the world. Although it is often said that "women's new freedom and independence is causing the problem of domestic violence," this situation is not the heart of the matter; it is not women's "independence" that causes a problem, it is an outdated mentality (glorified in films, novels, and media) defining maleness that is causing a problem (for both men and women) and needs to be updated. After all, to blame "independence" would imply that women should end the violence by becoming docile wives and mothers "again," not seeking "independence"—yet certainly the West today stands for equal dignity and human rights for women and men.

While it is commonly implied that women's increasing independence is provoking men to this violence, this attitude is unjust; society prefers to point the finger of blame at women rather than at the criminals or at an outdated ideology creating a certain formula of "masculinity," praising male dominance, that boys and men learn. Not every man is a "victim of male ideology," of course; many are independent thinkers who have innovated new, positive patterns of relating to women. Unfortunately others learned to take to heart militaristic slogans of "what being a real man means"—that is, "a real man tells his woman what to do, just like his father."

What about punishment for domestic violence as a solution? It did have a strong salutory effect in New York and elsewhere when batterers were arrested after police answered routine calls about domestic violence, and these men were shown on television handcuffed and being taken away by police; violence rates went down.

A long-term solution is to change the value system being absorbed by boys—that is, to cease the current glamorization of military behavior, which is causing a rebirth of the idea that "men should be tough," that same ideology that accepts bullies in schoolyards who prove that "might is right" by picking on smaller boys or ridiculing boys who do not "fight back" as "men should"—otherwise labeling them as "wimps who can't take it." We can change the social messages to boys about what it means to "be a man," offer better definitions.

An even deeper analysis may be this: the increase in violence to women also parallels the growth of the "family values" movement. As it is being asserted that the increase in violence parallels the increase in women's independence, the question is: why is that connection more logical than connecting the growth of violence with other trends in society? (Immediately I would like to say that the "other choice" from a family-values society is not a pornographic society! I am not against "family values" per se, but "family values" as usually interpreted means the traditional father-as-owner, woman-as-server situation, whereas by "family values" I mean a loving group in which both the male and the female contribute as much as they can to each other, giving love and support.)

Family-values pressures (defined in the old sense) may be causing some of the pressure and violence. For example, it may be the very pressure on women and men to "get into the right kind of marriage and be satisfied"—form a "perfect traditional family"—that is contributing to this violence. Many men are faced with a new situation "at home" and feel that they will gain approval for handling this "rebellion" with force or even violence—or they do not know any other way to deal with their emotions in the face of the situation. Indeed the violence is not so much a result of the increasing independence of women as it is a result of the current climate of social pressure insisting that women be "good wives and mothers" who "accept everything" and pressure insisting that men "take care of them all" and "be dominant"—so that if "the family" is dysfunctional, if neither role fits, violence is the result. This, of course, does not mean to condone or understand the violent behavior!

"Family values" proponents often turn a blind eye to the fact that the family has always contained domestic violence and that divorce was common in previous centuries, that our own century (or the last hundred years) has become increasingly moralistic about "the family," pressuring women and men to fit into it more than they were pressured in the nineteenth century, when fewer marriages took place. (There were no statistics on domestic violence kept during the 1950s, the heyday of the family; the family began to fall apart in the 1960s, not because of women's independence—men declared their independence of the family in the 1960s, the women's movement only started after that, in 1968–1969—but because the institution itself did not function properly).

In short, one could say that the self-righteous moralism of those who push

446 ~ THE SHERE HITE READER

"family values" is causing this violence to increase and that women are paying the price of submission once again. It is just as logical to say this as it is to assert a knee-jerk response implying that women are being "bad" and "rebellious" (that is, "too independent"!) and thus themselves causing the violence.

Blaming women themselves for the violence done to them ("they are too independent") is similar to the old mentality that used to judge women in rape trials: it was said that a woman was guilty herself or had caused the rape if she had been wearing a short skirt or bright lipstick (any sign that she wished to be sexually attractive), or if it could be shown that she had had sex outside of marriage with other men—rather than focusing "the problem" on the rapist himself. The unwritten law intoned that men were not responsible, since "they are male animals who cannot help it, they need to do it"; thus the ideology gave them carte blanche. Today we see things differently.

Women's increasing autonomy and belief in themselves ("independence")—not basically about the right to wear short skirts, no matter what some media imply!—is energizing and benefiting society, including each and every one of us, women, men and children—and must be encouraged! Not to do so is to betray the human-rights heritage and future that we stand for and to remove a great energy from our society.

The argument that women who are "rebellious" cause needless problems, that they should happily accept the role offered to them as mothers, is also heard in Middle Eastern politics, but such points of view are not realistic and do not include the view that women have as much right to self-determination as men do.

Another argument often heard is that violence against women is increasing because of the current climate of "sexual openness" and "women's freedom," which has come about during the last twenty-five years. It is said that if women today want to "go out and be free, sexually curious [like Eve?]," they deserve to be punished, these "devil women" need to be saved from themselves. It is also asserted that sex and violence are innately connected, that "what else can you expect when you don't impose a moral order on men's inevitable desires"?

In order to hide views "justifying" violence to women, some critics lump together "female freedom," "women's rights," pornography, miniskirts, consumerism, rock music, and drugs, often blaming "the new free woman" for them or using them as symbols of "the problem." Fundamentalist Islamists sometimes use images of Western "free women" in miniskirts to illustrate this attitude.

The litany against consumerism and drugs (illogically connecting them with the movement for women's rights, implying that somehow women are responsible or equally "decadent" and "negative" as are the drugtakers if they wish to change and create equality) appeals to people who feel a deep inquietude and alienation as they face a changing family dynamic; people may also be susceptible to these irrational arguments because they feel unhappy in today's cold market-values society, which seems to demand that the individual be productive or else irrelevant.

Although many people believe that the West has become corrupt, that women are "too free," too money-oriented, that sex is "too easy," that now women should "go back into the home where they belong," should stop having these independent ideas that things were better before ("when things were simpler"—or were they?), that one should turn the clock back. What simplistic notions these are! Of course society has always looked for easy explanations, especially when it has not understood the process of cultural change.

We are in the midst of a very profound period of change. The demand for women's equality and equal human rights with men has profound implications—in the areas of work, equal pay and advancement, access to top positions (such as prime minister), personal life (who cleans the house and takes care of the children), and sexuality (rethinking what we quaintly call "the sex act").

The legitimate desires of women and girls, men and boys, to create a new society in which women are equally valued with men are sometimes falsely linked to "the new world of pornography and cheap sex." You hear it said, "Women today don't know anymore how to take care of the family, or what real love is. They have lost their beauty, they just want quick sex, sex, sex! How superficial they are..."

To link women's new rights and autonomy with current market values or a superficial view of female sexuality is incorrect and insulting to women. Pornography, for example, does not represent "women's freedom"; most pornography is owned and directed by men and in fact depicts old values in which women are either "sexy devil-temptresses" or "good mothers at home." It reasserts the "devilish" view of female sexuality, which has hurt both women and men so much in the past. Pornography, under the guise of being about "the new sexual freedom," seeks to subjugate women even more than before while justifying men's violence to women ("He's lustful and gets carried away like all male animals, he can't help himself").

Women did not create "the sexual revolution" nor the current pornographization of so many parts of society, from art to advertising. To blame their "independence" is illogical. Rather, women have been agitating for their rights in general, not demanding pornography or "sexual freedom"; in fact they demanded sexual equality, which is a different matter, one that is still being worked out (of course). To be clear: the women's movement holds that women have the right to choose to be married or "single," to have children or not have children, and so on. Yet the old moral system holds that every woman who is not married by the time she is thirty must be "one of those women," that a woman who is not married after her early twenties and has a sex life is probably a "slut" or worse. . . . The women's movement has shown that this is part of an old system of values, not reality, part of the system oppressing women, and that it calls for change. This began at the same time during the 1970s when a differently oriented movement for "sexual freedom" (think of the hippies' 1960s "flower power" and singers like The Beatles) was making newspaper headlines; thus the two movements (related but different) were merged by the media, creating this confusion that remains with us today. Thus to blame "the women's movement" for "women's independence" and what is causing the violence to women seems to verge on the worst kind of scapegoating of women and to be irrational. The lurid pornographic styles so dominant in media and art now are signs of the end of the previous moral order, not a new "amoral order."

The movement to change society to include women as having equal rights with men in every area sees the future as enormously positive, based on an either male or female-headed household and on a new, evolving way of relating within a democratized family and at work.

The solution is not for women to become more docile and obedient—the Jews tried this in Germany before they were exterminated, thinking that surely if they would show that they were "fitting in," they would be accepted (but they were not, they were killed)—rather, the solution is for the "family values" and "traditional family" propaganda to be lifted. In these days of "fundamentalist revival," both West and East, there is increasing pressure on women to "return to the family," to "give up careers" and "independence and all that," to accept that "motherhood is better" (even though, according to recent Spanish statistics, quite a few parents are murdered by their children); there is increasing pressure on men to "be a man" in the miliary style—that is, to show dominance.

If some men's anger about change is coming to the fore, shouldn't there be a public debate about the traditional male value system/identity? If it is based on a desire for domination, shouldn't new types of values and identities be shown, other types of male heroes?

While it is understandable that in some moments we all feel uncertain and insecure about the changes taking place—will society become more pornographic—that is, will it value others only for their sexual prowess? Will we all act like "animals" and stop having long-term relationships? Where are we going with these changes, what is the future?—these fears are misguided because we have a great opportunity.

We are in the middle of a change that is unprecedented in the last centuries of our history: remaking the social order in a way that gives women equal status with men, reinventing sexual culture, work culture, and family culture—enormous tasks. Today's subtle changes in millions of individuals are aiming toward a new social order, one filled with more love, warmth, and caring than we know at present, yet no longer based on the antiquated family system, with its hegemony requiring that women submit to male authority or that men feel that they are "in charge" and "responsible" for everyone, not able to interact equally with the others but required to act "better than the others, and prove it." A democratization of private life. For the better.

What we can all learn here is that each individual is worth a lot, the value of being who they are: men do not need to dominate women to have value, nor do women need to be in a traditional family or have children to have worth.

## A NEW SEXUAL CULTURE TO GO WITH A NEW SEXUAL POLITICS

### SEX, GLOBALIZATION, AND PEACE

What are our values going to be in the new international, multicultural world? Unquestionably the values of the West are playing a big part in shaping global ideals. Although much lip service is paid to "respecting that the cultures of other societies are different" and that they "have as much right to their views as we do," in fact, the status of Western ideas has an undeniable glamour for many.

The omnipresence of modern, predominantly Western, media in the world, including the West's presence on the Internet and in advertising to a world market, seeming to be the partner of "the new global democracy" means that many younger people all over the world somehow wish to adapt to these fashions and products— even as they may protest Western policies of war and "economic imperialism." The "symbols of the West" carried in advertising and in internet pornography are highly visible and seductive for many.

In this context pornography currently seems to fill a void; whether seen in films, subliminally in advertising, or directly on the Internet, pornographic sexual values (both antimale and antifemale) are representing themselves as "new" and "part of the modern West." Pornography is the major vehicle spreading the values and definitions of private life and sex that have been created in the West.

Ironically, just when sexual values are changing in the West, the outdated sexual values of the past are becoming the "new thing" in other cultures, robbing them of their own right to create physical bodily expressions. Most cultures show much more diversity of expression than our own. It is indicative of our narrow, rigid, and straightjacketed view that the term "sex" has no equivalent in other languages, so that around the world the English word "sex" is being adopted (especially by those "young and hip"), as well as the word "fucking."

Yet the values of "human rights" and "justice" are also becoming strong around the world, often in the very same groups. How to account for this ironic combination? Just as in the West, there is a vast gap separating most people's idea of "sex" and the ideals of "human rights" and "global peace." One is not thought to be connected to the other. Human rights activists, for example, do not generally speak about "the details of sex," although sex trafficking is an issue that is very much alive. ("Yes, of course, there is the issue of women's rights, but this is an extremist idea that need not be addressed just at the moment when momentous matters of war and peace are at hand, and besides, this issue has already been addressed," it is often said; however, the inner definition of sex has not been brought up as a human rights matter, the idea that in the nexus of sex/coitus, the two faces of gender are formed, women learning that they are the helpers, that their orgasm is not so important—this is far from being on the agenda.) It is even said (in intelligent circles!) that pornography showing women as "dominatrixes" is the proof that our world's idea of sex is "modern" and "gives women equal rights"!

In fact, the values of human rights and world peace are much nearer to those of sex (as we need to redefine it; this does not mean showing women as either "submissive" or "dominatrix") than is usually imagined.

I believe that there can be a totally new way of seeing physical sexual interactions ("sex"), that includes eroticism and dignity for all, equality in "the sex act" itself. Changing what have been extremely damaging versions of "sex" will form an important fundamental basis for a new psychology, one that is more peaceful.

Both women's and men's rights are being violated by current ideas considered "trendy"; in fact the male psyche is being continuously constructed and reconstructed via propaganda about "male sexuality," through jokes about "male virility," and clichés about "who men are by nature," and the like.

My proposal, growing out of research with thousands and thousands of women and men, is for a new value system and a new way of defining the nitty gritty of sex and intimate exchanges. It can serve as a solid basis in daily life for a new system of global ethical values that is emerging.

Sex and human rights are connected. The globalization of values such as "human rights" means that whatever values of sex are disseminated (via pornography or pop media and culture) are the values of the new international global system—like it or not, say it's good or bad.

Therefore we should reevaluate sex, not only for ourselves, but in order to build a positive and lasting partnership with other cultures who receive their view of the West as much from pornography and pop media versions of sex (and all the values attached) as from the Western corporate presences and market mechanisms so much discussed (which at times do feature women in prominent positions—for example, Madeleine Albright and Condoleezza Rice).

Western society is not decadent, though it is going through the pangs of change. My best wishes to everyone on this journey.

# Afterword:
# Landscapes of the Mind

## A NEW EMOTIONAL LANDSCAPE[8]

It is said that "human nature' is a fixed phenomenon, that a new psychological-emotional landscape is not possible. Some point to the Athenian playwright Sophocles or to Shakespeare, claiming that their plays prove that "human nature has always been the same; all cultures are the same, humans love, hate, are jealous, greedy, and fear each other."

Yet isn't this merely a lazy justification of the status quo? Think of the Greek myths (pre-sixth century BC) and how hard it is for us to understand some of the myths in their original form. Our understanding of what was "natural," the meaning of human emotions, is different. Archaeologist Marija Gimbutas has proposed a worldview for "prehistory" that is quite different from the standard version; by showing many artifacts from these "primitive" times, she deduces that a psychological and political reality quite different in its basic structure from our own was possible; her evidence challenges the "real history starts with the Greeks, Sumerians, and Egyptians" view of history, instead outlining a "civilized history" that extends 20,000 years further into the past than is generally imagined, one with a sophisticated, complex and lively artistic tradition—and, in all probability, I would add, a different emotional and sexual landscape.

## UNDERWATER FRESCOES OF THE MIND: CAN WE MAKE A NEW PSYCHOSEXUAL AND EMOTIONAL LANDSCAPE?

A new emotional landscape is possible, even if it is unlike any that ever existed before. Today, it is very important for us to encourage a "humane nature" less focused on warlike behavior, one in which dominance and competition are not central. If a new psychosexual landscape is emerging, such a change can be very positive.

It is my contention that our individual psychologies are built not only on experiences we have growing up in our individual families, but also on a deeper substra-

451

tum of cultural beliefs and myths learned even earlier—generally referred to vaguely as "human nature."

People often prefer to claim that they have no myths; that myths are for more "stupid" or "primitive" people. Yet underlying the social system studied by sociologists, and the emotions studied by psychologists, lie myths of creation, myths of family, and myths of heroic behavior. These archetypes, currently unacknowledged or called "instinct," form the backdrop of our individual psyches and beliefs.

At present, the myths are undergoing change; a new psychological landscape is struggling to come into existence.

Based on my research, it would appear that a completely different emotional-psychological landscape is trying to emerge. The deepest layer of our psyches, often mistakenly called "human nature" or "instinct," is composed of all the myths and stories that create the human emotional landscape as we know it.

## MYTH PSYCHOLOGY (BASIC BRAIN SOFTWARE)

When you are born, you are offered a variety of mythologies with which to write the scenario of your life. Which you pick depends on various psychological factors built into your individual situation and family (your psychology, as discussed by Freud and other psychologists). Our sex lives, even more than our work lives, symbolize to us something profound about "who we are."

Today many people are torn between choosing what they consider "good behavior" and what they "really feel." (For example, 50 percent of people living in Western society today are "single," though most believe that people should be married and create happy families.) They worry that these choices are not legitimate, that they are not doing "the right thing," that perhaps they are immoral and degenerate. In fact, they may (unconsciously) be trying to create a "new morality," generally redesigning the entire package of available choices of mythologies on offer—thus, as in any transition period, they feel uncertain, "illegitimate"—living in "an alternative lifestyle," as we say today.

The four Hite Reports and this book examine—by measuring the counterpoint between what people say they experience and what society says they should be experiencing sexually—the repertoire of lifetime scenarios on offer: what are the new ways to interpret our experiences and emotions? Is a completely different psychosexual scenario possible?

Within most of us an intense battle is raging between "traditional values" and new beliefs. These new beliefs are the tentative beginning of an emerging new social system. Just as the early Greeks and Romans saw themselves differently from the later Christians, we now see ourselves differently yet again.

These essays, culled from in-depth research with thousands of people, have provided glimpses of the new psyche, the new emotional landscape emerging.

## NOTES

1 See the essay "Women, Church and Society" below.
2 Part of this essay appeared in an earlier form in L'Orgueil d'etre Une Femme (Lausanne: Favre, 2001).
3 See Part 2.
4 See Part 2.
5 See also *Robert Boyle: A Free Enquiry into the Vulgarly Received Notion of Nature* (Cambridge Texts in the History of Philosophy), ed. by Edward B. Davis, Michael Hunter (New York: Cambridge University Press, 1996).
6 See Part 2.
7 American Anthropological Association annual meeting: Controversies Over the Nature of the Family, 1981.
8 Parts of this essay originally appeared in Shere Hite, *Sex & Business: Ethics at Work*

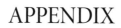

APPENDIX

# An Introduction to The Hite Reports: Theory and Importance

Naomi Weisstein, Professor of Psychology, State University of New York, 1987

These essays represent the theoretical structure of a series of three books (*The Hite Report on Female Sexuality*, 1976, *The Hite Report on Men and Male Sexuality*, 1981, and *Women and Love*, 1987) dealing with private life and gender definition in the United States. Through the essays (contained in these volumes), one sees a combination of discussion and impressive empirical research. Published internationally with widespread influence, these books comprise complex and fascinating portraits of a crucial fifteen-year period in American culture—a period in which society came into an extraordinary confrontation with the traditional ideas of home and family.

This confrontation is examined in the Hite Reports by looking at what really is there—i.e., documentation consisting of the responses of thousands of people to anonymous open-ended questionnaires—rather than at what reigning theory tells us should be there, and by a debate carried on sometimes among the participants, sometimes between Hite and the participants, a debate based on a coherent theoretical perspective. Perhaps we will look back and say that what is documented here is the ideological revolution in personal life of the end of the twentieth century.

## A. THE HITE REPORT ON FEMALE SEXUALITY: THE REDEFINITION OF SEXUALITY: SEX IS CULTURAL

Hite began this project in 1971 when, on leave of absence from graduate school, she became involved with the feminist movement, and taking seriously the idea that the personal is the political, undertook a major effort to find out what really happens in women's sexual lives.

From 1972 to 1976 she distributed a lengthy essay questionnaire to women all over the country; in 1976, on publication of the findings from the responses of 3,500 women, she explained her goals: "The purpose of this project is to let women define their own sexuality—instead of doctors or other (usually male) authorities. Women are the real experts on their own sexuality; they know how they feel and what they

457

experience, without needing anyone to tell them. This is not to say that Masters and Johnson's and Kinsey's work is not invaluable—it is. However, their work continued to view sex through certain cultural blinders which kept them from understanding the whole truth about female sexuality. In this study, for the first time, women themselves speak out about how they feel about sex, how they define their own sexuality, and what sexuality means to them." Hite's background in social and cultural history helped her to provide a cultural framework for this discussion, to see female sexuality for what it is, rather than how it fit into the prevalent patriarchal ideology.

Hite's basic finding was that seventy percent of women do not have orgasms from intercourse, but do have them from more direct clitoral stimulation. This testimony from thousands of women blew the lid off the question of female orgasm. Masters and Johnson had brought up the importance of the clitoris, but had emphasized that women should get enough clitoral stimulation from simple thrusting during intercourse to lead to orgasm; if they did not, they had a "sexual dysfunction." Kinsey had hinted at this issue by noting briefly that women like cuddling and that they have their highest rate of orgasm during masturbation, but he did not define masturbation beyond a few sentences, nor did he come to the logical conclusion implied, or reach the new understanding of women's sexuality that Hite formulated.

Anne Koedt had first questioned whether women have orgasms during intercourse and suggested that the issue involved a patriarchal definition of female sexuality in her ground breaking 1968 essay "The Myth of the Vaginal Orgasm."

Following publication of Hite's work, one commentator placed the discussion in historical perspective: "Anne Koedt's . . . 'The Myth of the Vaginal Orgasm' and Shere Hite's *The Hite Report on Female Sexuality* . . . are unique discussions of female sexuality because they treat sexuality as the unity of both human biology and psychology imbedded in a political formation." Advancing from the personal "sharing of experiences," Koedt and Hite both revealed how men have constructed sexuality to their advantage. In particular, Hite illustrated that within the dominant pattern of heterosexual interaction male pleasure is primary. The importance of her work lies in the fact that Hite clearly views sexual patterns as social constructions. Her book not only sheds light on contemporary sexual practice, but works to direct the creation of noninstitutionalized sexuality.[1]

Hite's documentation with such a large sample of exactly how women do have orgasms easily—during self-stimulation—and that they do not usually have orgasms during simple intercourse without additional stimulation, as well as her declaration that there was nothing "wrong" with this, that if the majority of women said this, it must be "normal" for women—no matter what "professional sexologists" said—was, after an initial period of shock among some in the sex research community, accepted widely, and eventually Hite received the distinguished service award from the American Association of Sex Educators, Counselors and Therapists.

Hite's findings that women could easily reach orgasm with clitoral stimulation (although society had said women had a "problem" having orgasms) also raised a further question—i.e., is sex as we know it (the basic set of physical activities with its focus on coitus) a social or a biological phenomenon? Hite had raised this question in the sense that she showed that for the majority of women, intercourse itself doesn't necessarily lead to orgasm, although clitoral stimulation does. Therefore we are forced to ask ourselves whether sex was "created" for pleasure and intimacy, or simply for reproduction. If the former, then the fact that the kind of stimulation the majority of women need for orgasm should be included in the definition of sex forces us to consider redesigning sex.

If women had been compelled to hide how they could easily reach orgasm during masturbation, then the definition of sex, it follows, is sexist and culturally linked. Hite, again, writing in 1976: "Our whole society's definition of sex is sexist—sex for the overwhelming majority of people consists of foreplay, eventually followed by vaginal penetration and then by intercourse, ending eventually in male orgasm. This is a sexist definition of sex, oriented around male orgasm and the needs of reproduction. This definition is cultural, not biological."

In other words, Hite's study showed that sex is part of the whole cultural picture; a woman's place in sex mirrors her place in the rest of society. Although, until that time, female sexuality had been seen essentially as a response to male sexuality, this was not a scientific or objective summation of the facts. It was a view of female sexuality through a certain ideological perspective.

Thus, *The Hite Report on Female Sexuality* linked the definition of sex as we know it to a particular society and historical cultural tradition, saying sex as we know it is created by our social system; it is a social institution.

While it is currently fashionable in academic circles to credit French philosopher Michel Foucault with the discovery that sex is cultural, that the way sexuality is defined is tied to a certain historical time and place, certain social structures, in fact, the idea grew out of early feminist discussions which were widely circulated both in the U.S. and France. *The Hite Report* contains the earliest full-scale statement of the clear connection between sexuality, its formation, shaping, and definition, and the society that channels it in certain directions.

Carrying these thoughts further, into an "un-definition" of sexuality, the first Hite Report continued, "Touching friends and sitting together intimately should be possible. . . . Intense physical contact should be possible in many varied ways. In short, our whole idea of sex must be reevaluated."

Not the least of the contributions of the first Hite Report was the presenting of women's own voices on this topic for the first time—as Hite said, "The statements women sent were full of beautifully written, moving descriptions of their feelings—an anonymous and powerful, deep communication, almost a soul to soul communication, from the women who answered to all the women of the world. Receiving these replies was one of the most emotionally fulfilling experiences of my life—and it is this I want to share with other women who read the book."

## B. THE HITE REPORT ON MEN AND MALE SEXUALITY: TOWARD A NEW DEFINITION OF MASCULINITY

The second Hite Report, *The Hite Report on Men and Male Sexuality*, was the first study of how men feel about themselves, their relationships and their sexuality: no such book had ever been done, certainly none using a data base approaching Hite's in size and representativeness. Although comparisons are often made with Kinsey, in fact Kinsey measured the frequency of sexual behaviors, not attitudes or feelings about sex, and he was dealing only with sexuality, not love or relationships.

Here also, Hite followed the format of anonymous essay questionnaires, asking men questions not only about sexuality, but also about love—about how it feels to fall in love for the first time, about their feelings concerning growing up with their fathers, their current relationships with women, their marriages, and what they would like to change about their sexuality and their lives if they could.

All told, *The Hite Report on Men and Male Sexuality* presents a staggering picture of men, told in men's own words. The heart of this book is about ideology, that is, about why people behave as they do—and specifically, about the patriarchal ideology and how it permeates men's behaviors in every area, including sexuality, which is supposedly biologically determined. In other words, what we call "sex"— as stated in the first Hite Report—comes down to a reflection of attitudes and values (i.e., an ideology) that extend through large segments of the overall society. These sexual behaviors are socially created, not just biological; further, this socially directed institution of sex does not equally value the needs and possibilities of women and men.

In effect, with this volume, Hite was beginning a reevaluation of "male psychology" and "male sexuality," which are so intimately linked —something rarely done,[*] since the assumption has been that the psychology of men is human psychology itself, that the way men are is "natural": not a socially constructed set of behaviors and perceptions, but "biological human nature in action."

To understand "male sexuality" it is necessary to understand the culture and what it informs men "male sexuality" and "masculinity" are —the whole context in which men are taught to see/express their "sexuality," and especially, to see their emotional world. Men are offered a very limited repertoire of admissible (or at least publicly admissible) emotions; if a man feels other emotions, he must hide them. Therefore, most men, if asked on the street for their opinion, are quick to say, "Well, I don't think I'm a typical male." And they are probably right; there are almost no "typical males," since few humans could live with the limited set of feelings they are "permitted." Furthermore, not being allowed to express their emotions, not even (in a way) being allowed to feel all the things humans feel, makes men confused and

---

[*] Psychologists earlier in the century such as Karen Horney and Beatrice Hinkle commented and wrote on these issues.

uncomfortable when asked to talk about their "feelings," and this, in turn, causes deep problems for them in their relationships with women.

While in this book Hite has sympathetically pointed out the difficulties for many men—the awkwardness of some male rituals, how many men are stuck in these ritual patterns, this system, and suffering from it—possibly all this was a shock to men, since they are not used to seeing themselves as the object of studies, not to mention a study done by a woman. Perhaps because it is so shocking for men to be treated as a specific group, rather than as a universal standard, the second Hite Report received dismayed and sometimes even lunatic reaction from some male critics.

Hite, in effect, was receiving criticism for her bold dissection of the current sociosexual system: by daring to claim that socialization pressures the male to adapt and perform in a particular sexual manner, she challenged the usual and highly touted idea that male physiology and evolutionary processes create and control male sexuality. As a result, she was subject to a deeply entrenched prejudice based upon her sex and the topic of her study. In effect, male critics attacked her expertise and her commentary on a matter which men consider to be extremely personal and important to their sense of being male. In other words, she was viewed as treading on sacred ground, daring to investigate an area which so greatly forms the male ego.

In this volume, Hite stressed again the cultural relativism of sexuality. In a section on the politics of intercourse, she argued that a man's "sexual drive" is not a biological imperative, but that our society's definition of sex is culturally created: if you can show that there are cultural pressures on people to behave in a certain way, then you cannot make the assumption that the behavior is a biological given.

What we know as "male sexuality," Hite explains, is not only a socially constructed but also a very limited version of what male sexuality might be. Just as men are offered a very narrow range of emotions by the culture, also their sexuality is narrowly defined and subtly inhibited. As she states in the preface to that work, society tells men to "define love as sex, and sex as penetration and ejaculation within a woman . . . [therefore] it is not simply by looking at the small details of men's sexual lives and understanding how they may hurt or give pleasure that will change our idea of what male sexuality is—discussing them rationally as if more 'pleasure' were the aim—because male sexuality is not based on simple pleasure. Male sexuality, and masculinity, is based on a larger ideology; [in fact, 'sex' in general] is not so much about pleasure as it is about a certain emotional symbolism that is a part of that ideology, a ritual drama reenacted over and over."[2]

Hite, in essence, is appealing for a redefinition of masculinity, for men to stop and look at what it is they are doing with their lives. This is a book full of possibilities for the future.

## C. WOMEN AND LOVE: A CULTURAL REVOLUTION IN PROGRESS
## (REDEFINING THE NATURE OF EMOTIONAL LIFE)

I have always felt that "love," perhaps because it is considered to be the center, if not the totality of a woman's life, is a risky business, and one to which feminists should address much energy and ingenuity. When I was in graduate school in the early 1960s, I was appalled by the abuse that my female colleagues sustained in the pursuit and achievement of love. Indeed, I organized a "syndicate" (modeled after Mio Minderbinder's in Joseph Heller's *Catch-22*) to resist such abuse, collectively taking the initiative in dating and blacklisting men who mistreated members of the syndicate. I continued this work later, when, as a member of the Chicago West Side Group, I led a drive to organize women in singles bars to rationalize and dignify the pursuit of love. But although the members of the group had previously demonstrated extraordinary courage, facing police, tear gas, going to jail in draft resistance demonstrations, when it came to the singles bars, their courage faltered. The project was abandoned because only two of us would regularly show up for planned actions at the bars, no matter how many had promised to come. At an early meeting of feminists from across the country in 1968, I spoke of the need for a task force of feminists to fight the oppression and dehumanization of women that went along with our pursuit and achievement of love.

But the politics of heterosexual love and romance have never been fully explored nor documented on a large scale. In the first Hite Report, in 1976, Hite had announced her intention of studying women's feelings about love, asking women to define the nature of love,[3] because "it is in the emotional dynamics of love relationships, and in the psychological assumptions, that stereotypes about women remain most deeply embedded."[*] And also, women have been defined by the society for a very long time in terms of "love"—i.e., told that they must raise a family, be loved by a man, married, or face being an "outcast."

This explains the explosion of popular psychology books in which the subject of relationships between women and men is now being talked about as women become more and more unafraid of the social system and of men, more independent financially and ideologically, yet find themselves in love with or living with men who still express (perhaps unconsciously) old stereotypes about women's "natures"—expecting women will be loving, take second place emotionally in relationships, not get angry when the man does not reciprocate with this emotional

---

[*] This explains the explosion of popular psychology books in which the subject of relationships between women and men is now being talked about: as women become more and more unafraid of the social system and of men, more independent financially and ideologically, yet find themselves in love with or living with men who still express (perhaps unconsciously) old stereotypes about women's "nature"—expecting women will be loving, take second place emotionally in relationships, not being angry when the man does not reciprocate with this emotional support—women wonder what to do about the situation, whether to leave or stay, what to think.

support—women wonder what to do about the situation, whether to leave or stay, what to think.

Much of this feeling, that women's basic function in life is to be loving and nurturing, still remains; it has not been fully accepted that women are complete above and beyond their biological capabilities, or ability to take care of, "service," others. This does not mean, of course, that it is "wrong" to be nurturing; the question here is whether all of the nurturing of society is supposed to be done by women.

In particular, there is a bias against women that often comes out in personal relationships—i.e., that men express by their behavior, actions and statements to women in private. Love between women and men is an area that needs to be analyzed more deeply than it has been. As Carol Gilligan has pointed out, "Among the most pressing items on the agenda for research on adult development is the need to delineate in women's own terms the experience of their adult life.[4]

Several earlier works broached these issues. Simone de Beauvoir's *The Second Sex* opened up some of the deeper areas of women's concerns about love, bringing out poignantly the mixed sense that love is great and yet somehow involves pain and humiliation for women—so that, according to de Beauvoir at the time, we finally may come to learn to love humiliation in love. In the 1970s, Kate Millett's *Sexual Politics* shook the world with its statements about love between women and men, exposing the violence in much of men's writing about women they love, or supposedly love. Ti-Grace Atkinson, in *Amazon Odyssey*, coined the phrase, "Scratch his love, and you'll find your fear." Shulamith Firestone and Laura X also presented interesting theoretical statements, and additional work was done by Elaine Walster-Hatfield and Dorothy Tennov.

However, after the early 1970s, issues of love between women and men did not receive as much attention as issues of sexuality (notable exceptions were Jessie Bernard, Letty Cottin Pogrebin, Barbara Ehrenreich, and Andrea Dworkin). Indeed, in a strange sort of reverse Victorianism, theorizing and writing about sex became more acceptable than writing about love, and some interesting theoretical works were produced by Alison Jagger, Catherine Stimpson, and a group of women editing *Powers of Desire*. But feminists rarely confronted the politics of heterosexual love head-on. Rather, two trends, both of which skirted the issue, arose. One went off men entirely, embarking on a stunningly revolutionary exploration of how women can love women without reservation. However, a sectarian part of this trend claimed that women still attached to males were "consorting with the enemy," thereby dismissing millions of women who had associations with men either by choice or circumstance. The other trend was of the position that "Men are changing, so why talk about it? There is no problem—a smart woman should be able to find herself one of the 'new men' out there."

Thus heterosexual love relationships became almost a taboo subject in feminist circles, not politically "correct" or "relevant." And yet this is one of the most important political topics there is, if one takes seriously the original slogan of the women's movement, that is, "the personal is political."

Academic psychological studies in recent years have come to focus on gender issues, but have also shied away from the study of love and emotion, perhaps since they are not easily quantified, and therefore the work might not be considered "scientific" by colleagues. Studying love, in other words, is difficult, and could easily leave one open to attack—as Elaine Walster-Hatfield found in 1972 when, after obtaining a government grant to study love, she was berated publicly by Senator William Proxmire, who thought the taxpayers' money was being wasted on such a frivolous topic, and as a result lost her grant. Nevertheless, in recent years, Pepper Schwartz and Philip Blumstein of the University of Washington have published in this area, as have philosophers such as Joseph Fell, Irving Singer, and Emilie Rorty.

In *Women and Love*, Hite and the 4,500 women participating begin the process of renaming what is going on in personal life, reseeing the emotions involved and the patterns of behavior, debating with each other the definition of love and various emotions felt for another.

We know that the home has been women's ghetto and were surprised when we first began to hear of the incidence of physical violence in these private settings. Now we see here something harder to pinpoint, that is, the terrible emotional draining of women that has been and is going on in relationships, the subtle ways women are badgered emotionally in private (even just by "standard" and "acceptable" usage of language which inherently puts women down)—and still expected to provide loving and nurturing.

Love relationships take place in private, there is no one to witness what goes on there, to name what is happening; each individual has to name it for herself, by herself—amid the confusion of also loving and perhaps being loved—and doubt that she is ever right in her naming. (If a relationship is painful, a woman may feel she cannot or "should" not complain, lest she be seen as having "problems.") So, many of these things are not said in daily life—in fact some of the voices we hear here seem almost to be voices from hidden bedrooms, sobs never before heard by anyone—or voices surfacing finally after months and years of numbness, of having almost forgotten how to speak because of the futility of it, since one's own "voice" was never heard. And yet there is also in these voices a great strength and determination to be heard, to speak, to no longer remain silent or be told what "reality" is.

The documentation women give here of their inner emotional lives should finally provide much of the material necessary to replace the Freudian-descended systems of "women's psychology."

Was Freud wrong about women? Yes, indeed, as I first argued in 1968:[5] Personality theory in general, whether Freudian or not, has missed the central importance of social expectation and culture in determining what we do and how we feel, and thus is largely irrelevant to an understanding of our lives and our behavior. As I showed, Freudians and others can neither predict what we do, nor seriously explain what we have done. Nonetheless, the idea of women's inherent "passivity" or "masochism" has remained a bedrock of the cultural myth about women, a myth strengthened by the cultural recidivism of the current era. Here this myth is annihilated by a large body of proof and documentation.

What women say in *Women and Love* supersedes Freud and many other current schools of therapy, none of which are based on large databases, and especially not on what women say. This book shows the fallacy of many of the stereotypes placed on women ("defining" women) by, as Hite describes it, "'Freudian Mysticism'—i.e., that particular brand of mystifying women Freud had which was a retort to the feminism of the 1900s; women are not 'dissatisfied,' he said, because of their secondary social status, or because they are in fact overworked; women are 'dissatisfied' for neurotic personal reasons." Hite goes on: "This line of 'thinking' continues today in abstruse academic theory and in popular advice books which tell women they 'love too much' and should change their 'crippled,' 'neurotic' patterns of behavior. But women are confronted by very real, negative situations in their lives. The question for any group in this situation is what to do about it. Women are trying to get men to see personal relationships differently, to change their values, but when they don't, women now feel forced either to leave, or if they stay, to become less committed emotionally—they feel psychologically divided and frequently confused and depressed. Freud may have, with his sample of three women, documented this stage of the process, but it was not correct to build an entire 'theory of women' or 'psychology of women' around it. What we are documenting here, by listening to women, is the whole panorama."

Hite's theoretical framework for understanding what is happening today in personal relationships and in the culture is neither Freudian nor Marxist, but builds on feminist analyses of patriarchy. As she says, Freud eventually came to believe that aggression was inherent in biology, and could not be eradicated from society in order to make a better society; Marx, however, declared that aggression was caused by the economic system, a system which should be changed; Hite, like many feminists, believes that the society we have, with so much emphasis on aggression and competition, is not necessary—we simply don't have to live this way—and what is needed to change it is a complete understanding and revision of the ideological system at hand. It is to this that her books are dedicated.

# Observations on
# The Hite Reports

Wardell Pomeroy, co-author with Alfred Kinsey of *The Kinsey Report*,
Society for the Scientific Study of Sex, 1982

When I learned I was going to appear here I went back to a review I did of *The Hite Report on Female Sexuality* made in November 1976 and published in S.I.E.C.U.S. To my surprise I found that I could almost have changed the word "female" to "male" and present the same review. *The Hite Report on Men and Male Sexuality* is a 1,129-page book, a 1,054-page paperback, about 95 percent of which consists of direct quotes from her sample of over 7,000 males who replied to her questionnaire.

Because I am used to and involved with a taxonomic, statistical approach in understanding human sexuality, I was originally disturbed by Hite's approach, which is quite different. I changed my mind after reading the female Report as well as the male Report and now believe that focusing on understanding behavior, feelings, and attitudes adds an important dimension to the overall understanding of human sexuality which cannot be obtained in other ways.

I have some minor quibbles, the most serious of which is Shere Hite's use of adverbs such as many, some, a few, a tiny minority, and so on. Whether something happens less than 1 percent of the time or whether it happens 10 percent or 30 percent of the time, one can only speculate.

I also quibble with Shere Hite about the advantage of a questionnaire versus a face-to-face interview—obviously I would because my Kinsey technique has been one thing and hers has been another. I really believe that for what we set out to do we were both right. It seems to me that for some things a direct interview is helpful, and in other cases, and in this case, it could not have been done in this way and needed a questionnaire approach. She points out that many people had told her that they would have filled out a questionnaire and would not have been interviewed. Of course my experience has been exactly the opposite, I have had people say they would be happy to be interviewed but not fill out a questionnaire.

I hope that by this time you are not turned off to the Hite Reports, because I believe they are very valuable pieces of work. I have suggested before and I will suggest again that I think there are five groups of people who need to read these books.

First I think that women who have sexual problems need to read the book, and secondly I think that women who don't have sexual problems need to read the book; and thirdly, I think that males with sexual problems need to read these books; and fourthly, males without sexual problems need to read these books; and fifthly, I think that therapists with or without sexual problems need to read these books.

The many quotes from respondents answering her questionnaires are an extremely valuable part of her book. The extensive use of direct quotes from the questionnaires on a particular topic provides knowledge that has been largely overlooked and has been badly needed. For example, to say that x-percent of females masturbate by clitoral stimulation is only the beginning. The many specific descriptions of clitoral masturbation given in great detail allow one to know what female masturbation is really like for these women, and do it better than any source that I know. Similarly, the many descriptions about what orgasm feels like are again the best and most comprehensive source in the literature. Previous reports have stated that orgasm can range from nothing more than a sigh to an epileptoid seizure, but here one is exposed to unique descriptions of many types of orgasm along this continuum. Almost all women and men will be able to find themselves in this book and this can be very reassuring.

Another of the contributions of the Hite Reports lies in the questions she is asking. Many of them are original, and hence the answers give us a unique insight into human sexuality. Let me just read an example of that for you. This is in the male book. She is asking about pornography: "Do you look at pornography? What kind? Did your father read pornography when you were growing up? Where and when did you see your first men's magazine? What is your opinion of the pornography you have seen? Do you feel it represents certain elementary truths about how men and women really are, both psychologically and sexually?

"What do you think of the sexual revolution? What do you think of women's liberation? How has it affected your relationship? What do you get from women that you don't get from men?"—and so on and on. I think that the very fact that many of these questions haven't been asked before, and have been asked in great number here, is another added dimension to this book.

In closing, I would like to highly recommend this book as a thought-provoking and insight-giving treatise on male and female sexuality.

# Write What You Want as Long as It's About Sex (Modern Mechanics of Censorship)

Shere Hite, *Index On Censorship Journal*

(Reprinted in Tagespiegel, Berlin), 1995–1996

"Oh! Do you paint freckles on your face? How do you do that?"

After twenty-two years as a researcher, I've arrived at a key interview to present four-hundred pages of new research to the press and this was the first question.

What would you make of it? Or of an article in a prestigious newspaper about an anthology of my work which states: "At age fifty, Shere Hite tottered down the stairs on remarkably high heels." This was followed by a discussion of whether or not a woman of "my age" has the right to "still" wear anything other than "practical clothing."

Sexual harassment in print, I guess. The reader is left to drown in oceans of "information" about my persona, while my ideas disappear in overexamined body descriptions.

Is it harmless? Could the journalist who asked—and kept asking—about my freckles really detect anything significant in my work, if her mind was geared to concentrate on my looks? And of course these incessantly body-ized articles (why discuss a woman's ideas when you can discuss her body?) have an impact on the attitudes of publishers and reviewers. They sense the inherent trivialization and don't always look further. They "know" who I am.

I am not the only woman to experience this by any means. The twentieth-century feminists Susan Faludi, Germaine Greer, Erica Jong, even Diana (of British royalty fame), or any woman who speaks out—all of us are called "colorful," "dramatic." Details of our bodies and appearances are hashed and rehashed in the press, while we write and write, and speak and speak, hoping to be heard.

Yet surely this trivialization, lamentable as it is, is not censorship. Censorship is political discrimination or punishment of those who have certain views unfavorable to the "establishment," those in power. But wait. This is not intentional censorship— but it operates just as surely to stop ideas from reaching people. And this repression can be worse than official censorship because it is invisible. It is not glorified by the noble martyrdom attached to the word "censorship."

The censorship of trivialization is also evident in some of the editing of my work over the years, influencing which books I have been "allowed" to write, i.e., those for which I have obtained contracts. *The Hite Report on the Family* is the fourth in a series of Hite reports. Some of my reports contain much more comment than my other works. Some editors encouraged me to expand my ideas, while others cut back almost everything but the bare bones of the research. Sexist denial that women have anything important to say is inherent in some editors' viewpoints, sexism I am sure they do not recognize. By excising my conclusions and comments, they would effectively silence me.

But, one always thinks, perhaps the editors are right and my words are not profound.

## CENSORSHIP FEELS CONFUSING TO THE INDIVIDUAL

Here are some entries from my diary, written while my last book was being edited and I was asked to cut large sections of my writing:

"I am nauseous, I cannot speak, my throat is so blocked I begin to think I must have cancer. Someone, a friend, says to me, 'Maybe you feel like you are being strangled because they are cutting your words.' My throat clears up but my nausea remains, to remind me of my revulsion. I can't swallow what is happening. I stay up most nights and sleep little, writing endless faxes to keep my words intact. Wondering, always wondering, if my work is really 'so valuable' (a woman's question about her worth), wondering how much is 'right' to fight for. I feel alone."

"The atmosphere [at the publishing house] is more and more impregnated with silence. There is fear all around, from those who would lose their jobs, from those who aren't used to fear, from those who hope to keep their heads down, be safe at all costs . . . like ducks lined up in a row, ready to be shot."

"I feel on trial, having to explain over and over again the simplest points, then still being 'misunderstood,' called names, accused of being an 'imposter' (in everything from my name to my research methods). Like Galileo, I'll say I never meant it: 'The sun goes around the Earth, women's oppression is their own fault—clearly!'

## CENSORING WOMEN'S THOUGHT

Men are called "geniuses" and women are not, Christine Battersby noted in her brilliant book, *Gender and Genius*. This is not to say that I am anxious for the "genius" label. But consider that I have traversed the same route as Freud and mapped a completely different territory; that my research is based on thousands of people, whereas he spoke with only a handful. I wonder whether people will be able to hear my conclusions or will insist on locating me within the confines of "sex and women's topics," while Freud's work is considered a profound commentary about the nature of human reality.

The very attitudes about women and men which I confront in my work also operate to confound my ability to speak and write freely. The media and publishing houses (but, fortunately, usually not the readers) converge to form an invisible net of entrapment and ghettoization.

In 1990 I attended a meeting of the women's committee of PEN in New York. Many women described being unable to get or renew publishing contracts. They lamented they did not make big enough profits for the company, saying "Only the real moneymakers get published." I said that a financial explanation is not sufficient: after all, every day hundreds of books on obscure topics are published. Further, though my books have a track record of making money, publishers tend to be nervous and do not always accept my projects (unless they are about sex). Indeed, feminist projects are having trouble for political reasons in this reactionary climate. The agenda of many large publishing conglomerates is not only financial but also political. These politics range from "Don't upset anybody, publish only safe books" to pushing a particular political philosophy. Financial decisions are also political: At one large conglomerate, no matter how much profit the feminist book division earns, it is not allowed to plow this money back into its own division nor to give more than small advances to authors, even those who made money for the house.

Even if a book has a chance of selling well, if it expresses radical political opinions (such as those of Noam Chomsky, Gore Vidal, or Salman Rushdie, as well as feminist activists) its publication may be hampered. But not overtly.

Even in overt censorship, the ripples can be subtle. During the McCarthy era, when Hollywood screenwriters and actors were investigated as "Communist sympathizers," some were jailed and most lost their ability to make a living in the industry. Hollywood films lost the complicated and interesting Betty Davis-type female characters of the 1940s to happy-girl or "innocent" characterizations of Doris Day and Debbie Reynolds types of the 1950s.

## MODERN MECHANICS OF CENSORSHIP

Censorship today is not a man in a suit with a big red pen. There is no formal bulletin on the six o'clock news that says, "Your news is now being censored" so that those watching can conveniently decide if they are prepared to do something about it. It just creeps around you, a vaguely unpleasant feeling. You have to be alert to see what it is before its mists engulf you.

Censorship happens in small ways, gradually. Only eventually does it amount to a big problem, a stifling way of life.

How serious a problem is it now in the West? We have our own "disappeared" here—authors and other political dissidents disappearing from public sight, going down for the third time with only a gurgle or two. For those who take a stand, questions of "Is it worth it?" and "How long can I carry on?" surface daily.

In fact, it is hard to recognize censorship or suppression when you see it—hard to know if it is really happening or just some kind of bizarre mistake, funny, not really serious, Kafkaesque.

Within the publishing houses, decisions are often made by committees, with unanimous agreement required: If even one person on the editorial board strongly disagrees with taking on a book another editor wants, it cannot be published. One person can blackball it. I do not know the rationale for this corporate policy, but new opinions and radical ideas almost never make it past these editorial boards.

Censorship today is increased by the consolidation of publishing, magazines, film, and television into a few hands. The term "free" market is Orwellian doublespeak when media conglomerates buy up book publishing houses not because they are so profitable but because books and their reviews are part of the creation of public opinion. The story is told in Ben Bagdikian's *The Media Monopoly*.

Another cause of decreasing diversity in publishing is that in the United States, the majority of bookstores are owned by two chains which control demand by cutting prices to a level with which the independents cannot compete. New publishing does spring up, but small new presses do not have the connections and the financial ties with the chains that will enable them to reach large numbers of people.

Finally, the last step of contemporary publishing can be the most censorious of all, as every author knows. Whether the media indulges in harassment and misinformation or simply ignores a book, it can be devastating. Modern democracy is closely linked to media politics. The first action in military coups in foreign countries is usually to take over the radio and television stations by force. Was it a coup in the West when behind-the-scenes financial interests bought up the media during the 1980s? They didn't need guns.

An aura of spreading censorship is hanging in the air, but the word, its name, is not spoken. People change the subject, feeling unsafe, nervous.

Despite the seeming plethora of "information," what is available to the public to read is more and more dictated by media monopolies, not by our own interests and tastes. Diversification of media ownership and programming control is key to keeping democracy running, keeping mass democratic twenty-first-century society from developing an Orwellian madness—without wit or humor.

As in previous centuries, the official canon of history will again make women invisible, except in decorative ways. Margaret Mead did groundbreaking research on Samoa, yet the *New York Times* front-page obituary a few years ago felt it correct to prominently note that "although she was never a scientist, nevertheless . . ." This would never have been said about a man who achieved what she achieved. Simone de Beauvoir mused from time to time about whether "the canons" would have seen her or accepted her if she weren't aligned with Jean Paul Sartre.

When the BBC and other worldwide networks sum up our era in their end-of-the-century programming, will including women mean only showing the reels of the suffragettes over and over, valuable as these are? Perhaps women need to buy their own stations or to control programming for half the hours of the day and create our own "canon." Then perhaps our women thinkers and authors will be remembered for more than wearing high heels at an advanced age.

# Dangers I Have Faced
# to Produce this Work
### October 26, 2002

I have faced considerable difficulty and danger in order to produce this body of work.

While I was not formally tortured for speaking out, I was in fact systematically held up to public ridicule for several years by an all-powerful consolidated United States media, or by a few individuals/groups in it.

As the committees defending me in both 1987 and 1994 pointed out in their statements,* the attacks on me did not relate to my work but to a general attempt to stop feminism and the spread of pro-woman ideas.

My documentation showing that women's human rights were/are being denied not only in the ways we know, but also in the previously nondocumented areas of "sex" and "love"—in the emotional dynamics and the physical acts accepted as "normal" (but in fact reflections of a social structure based on the devaluation of women)—triggered this defensive reactionary attack, unfortunately.

Fortunately, articles in several women's media supported my work and defended it, both in writing about me and in asking me to write articles about the situation. For example, the noted journal *Index on Censorship* asked me to write an article describing my experiences; this article, which was then republished by *Tagespiegel* in Berlin, Germany, appears above. The noted academic weekly *Chronicles of Higher Education* attended and covered my speech at the American Studies Association in 1987 as well as the simultaneous press conference held by twelve famous female writers who announced a statement in my defense at the conference that day. Susan Faludi's bestselling book *Backlash* in 1988 defended me in the context of the reactionary swing in the United States that she was documenting; *For Women Only*, Barbara Seaman and Gary Null's riveting book on health, explained the media frenzy, as did an article in *Ms. Magazine* by Jennifer Gonnerman. Other articles are noted later in this appendix.

To some extent these attacks (and personal threats to me) did "ruin" my reputation and that of my work and credibility—or drastically smeared it, put an aura of

---

* See below.

fear around it. It is still common to read in the United States that "while her work is not scientific and her research questionable, some of the voices she quotes are intriguing . . ." and such; the fact is that my research results are verified today by hundreds of other studies (verifiability is one of the criteria of good research, very little social science or medical research achieves this verifiability or predictability, even to 70 percent of its findings, whereas in my work almost 100 percent of the findings have been verified to date); my studies have stood the test of time, yet many who should know better still approach my work with a fear they mistakenly attribute to my work—or even to me personally—approaching my work as if it were shrouded with an air of danger. The danger is not my work but the groups of bullies who want to blacken the name of "feminism"; consider the 2001 speech of Jerry Falwell in Washington a few days after the September 11 attack, in which he declared that "feminists" and others are were to blame, because they had caused or enabled the attack to occur! Or consider earlier, Pat Buchanan's 1990 Republican convention speech in which he named feminism as "the real enemy we have to defeat now."

I hope that today the American public's independence of mind is strong enough that news corporations will not be able to distort what I am saying, so that people can think through for themselves the issues raised, agree or disagree with the theory on its own terms, in a calm and considered manner as is regularly done in other parts of the world, without "media hysteria" influencing their conclusions—thus inhibiting the personal progress of all of us in life.

This work is deeply anti-militaristic—Part Two detailing a theory about male psychosexual development at puberty and how a simple change on the part of "society" as a whole could lead to less militarism and aggression in the future. Even in this time of patriotism defined as militarism, my hope is that this theory will be heard, understood and debated.

## 1987 STATEMENT BY COMMITTEE

THESE DISTINGUISHED WOMEN HELD A PRESS CONFERENCE AT THE ANNUAL MEETING OF THE AMERICAN STUDIES ASSOCIATION (REPORTED IN THE *CHRONICLES OF HIGHER EDUCATION* OF DECEMBER 9, 1987) TO RELEASE AND READ THE FOLLOWING STATEMENT:

Terribly important issues that concern women's lives and health, in particular the emotional, psychological and physical abuse of women, are being obscured and trivialized by the media's assault on Shere Hite's new book, *Women and Love*. This is tragic at a time when the cases of Hedda Nussbaum and Charlotte Fedder, among others, are before us. There is a clear need to explore the hidden emotional dynamics between women and men. The attack on Hite's work is part of the current conservative backlash. These attacks are not so much directed against a single woman as they are directed against the rights of women everywhere.

*Barbara Seaman*
*Gloria Steinem*
*Ntozake Shange*
*Florence Rush*
*Phyllis Chesler*
*Barbara Ehrenreich*
*Naomi Weisstein*
*Ti-Grace Atkinson*
*Kate Millet*
*Sybil Shainwald*
*Ruby Rohrlich*
*Karla Jay*

## 1994 STATEMENT BY COMMITTEE

*The Hite Report on the Family: Growing Up Under Patriarchy*—the latest book by ground-breaking researcher Shere Hite—could be a major contribution to the U.S.'s ongoing debate over high divorce rates and "family values." Unfortunately, you cannot get a copy of this book in the U.S., although it has already been published to favorable reviews in Australia, Canada, Great Britain, the Netherlands and Germany. The fact that this work, by an author who has sold millions of books over the last two decades, is being withheld by the U.S. publisher suggests that the backlash against feminism is far from over.

*Phyllis Chesler*
*Naomi Weisstein*
*Jesse Lemisch*
*Barbara Seaman*
*Barbara Ehrenreich*
*Kate Millett*
*Ruby Rohrlich*
*Andrea Dworkin*
*Gloria Steinem*
*Susan Faludi*
*Stephen J. Gould*
*Christine Delphy*

## METHODOLOGICAL ESSAYS

There were unique challenges to be faced in devising the methodology for The Hite Reports, which comprise a three-volume study of over 14,000 women and men in the U.S., 1972–1986. First, although quantification was necessary as part of the final result, a simple multiple-choice questionnaire could not be used, since the theoretical concept for the project stated that "most women have never been asked how they feel about sex" and "most research has been done by men": therefore it was important not to assume predetermined categories, but to design an essay-type questionnaire, which would be open-ended. Also, the data gathering was designed to protect the anonymity of the respondent. Secondly, compilation of data from essay questions is very difficult, if the data is to be carefully and rigorously treated; the methods used in compilation, refined over the three Hite Reports, will be discussed. Finally, and almost as labor intensive as compilation and categorization of data, presentation of findings was planned to serve more than an informative function; rather than simply giving readers statistics plus the author's theoretical analysis of data, the aim was to create an inner dialogue within the reader, as s/he mentally conversed with those quoted. Therefore, large parts of text comprise first-person statements from those participating. The format of presentation shows how these fit into intricate categories of social patterns.

# Controversies Over the Nature of Love

### Dr. Linda Singer, Society of Women in Philosophy, Eastern Meeting, 1988

*The panic felt at any threat to love is a good clue to its political significance.*
*Women and love are underpinnings. Examine them and you threaten the*
*very structures of culture.*
     —Shulamith Firestone, *The Dialectic of Sex*, p. 21

In a current and widely circulated cultural script, love, especially the kind that bound women to love, was just fine until feminism came along. Up until that point, love was uncontroversial, universally valorized, celebrated, and sanctified, not only as the highest form of private personal gratification, but also as that which provided the possibility of civilization as we know it. Without love, we would be doomed to live by the law of the jungle, condemned to a nasty, brutish short life in the state of nature. In this version of the story, love was especially unproblematic for women, who were willing to devote their lives, energies, and bodies to it as expressions of their deepest yearnings and highest desires. Women were especially good at love by aptitude, talent or design. Then feminism, a discourse of the unloved and therefore chronically resentful woman, came along and threw a monkey wrench into what had been a smoothly running machine, by turning love into a battlefield and a political stomping ground.

My concern is not to try to contest this story. Fairy tales, like all fictional forms, are not subject to logical or factual refutation. Fantasies and dream discourses articulate themselves in other than a propositional logic. With respect to this phantasmatic projection, the language, as Shulamith Firestone has alerted us, is also a political language of power and privilege.

Like any other ideological construction, love, and the discourses which celebrate and proliferate it, operates by effacing itself, and the strategic utilities it is designed to serve. As a product of patriarchy, love, especially the heterosexist erotic variety, has functioned, at least for the last several hundred years, as a way of mobilizing women's energies in the service of men, under the guise of desire and self-fulfillment. In love, as Simone de Beauvoir pointed out nearly forty years ago, women freely choose their enslavement, eliminating the effort and expense of developing a technology of coercion. By constructing women as the emblems and exemplars of love, men are free to go off and pursue other ends—autonomy, separation, competition, success, war—while women are placed in a sphere outside, holding the place of love for men when they are ready and have time for it.

Because of the utility of this discourse for the maintenance of masculinist hegemony, there is a heavy investment in representing these arrangements as uncontroversial, i.e., not subject to serious challenge or contest from either side. This position is maintained even in the face of long-standing behavior and discourse on the part of men (including misogyny, battering, rape, familial desertion, and other practices clearly expressive of male contempt for women) that would appear to contradict this. But as with any ideological construct, it is less important that those receiving advantages by the political arrangements it naturalizes and solidifies believe in these projections, than it is to enlist the beliefs of those positioned so as to be dominated by it. In other words, it is culturally far more important to both represent and induce women to regard the sexual division of time, energy, and labor prescribed by the discourse of love as unproblematic and as something which could not or ought not be challenged or contested. Given the levels of social resources devoted to the construction of the discourse of love and systems for its circulation, we should not be surprised that this discourse succeeds in creating the kinds of subjects it works to produce. But we also should expect that its effects are not seamless and that the discourse of love has also produced critiques and resistances—specially, but certainly not exclusively, from women.

Feminist theory, at least in its second wave, has consistently questioned, challenged and critiqued the celebratory sanctity in which heterosexual erotic love has historically been cloaked. This critique is addressed both to the underlying logic which assumes that ultimate intimacy can be forged out of the union of opposites, and to its consequences, namely the claim that women become willful or desiring contributors to their own subjugation and effacement, on the ground that that is what love, especially love of men, demands. Armed with an array of unhappy material consequences of women's love for men including unwanted pregnancy, death and maiming through abortion, death and crippling side effects from contraception, battering, abuse and abandonment, as well as psychological suffering and trauma, feminist theory has sought to make love controversial, since failure to do so would amount to uncritical complicity with its fallout. As Firestone argued in 1972, "[a] book on radical feminism that did not deal with love would be a political failure."

The corollary of this position is that any book or thinker which seriously takes on the question of love, i.e., which challenges the cultural privilege and politics embedded in this institutionalized form of social relations, becomes a target for what is often a full-fledged hegemonic deployment aimed at trivializing or de-legitimating the very question raised. If the primacy of heterosexual love becomes questionable or, even worse, suspect, then so do all the forms of biological, social, and political distribution which are based on it including heterosexist privilege, male dominance, the nuclear family, phallocentrism, and a rigid separation between the private and the public, the personal and the political.

Historically, these latter oppositions have been used to justify forms of behavior and exercises of power in love relationships, like rape, assault, manipulation and exploitation that would not otherwise be considered acceptable, on the grounds that any form of direct social intervention into this sphere would violate the parties' right to privacy and free expression, even in cases where it is clear that such activity is designed precisely to limit the freedom of the female participant. Because the private sphere created by the logic of liberalism as the site for heterosexual erotic love is constructed as a space organized by the concepts of individuation and choice, social obligations are further reduced on the grounds that women have freely chosen the situations in which they continue to participate, and therefore, at least in a certain sense, consent to the consequences to which they are subjected.

In defense of this very vital thesis, numerous theories have been offered to explain women's willingness and, in fact, eagerness to freely engage in such relationships, including Freud's infamous theory of female masochism, the theory of woman's ego development in a context of relatedness rather than autonomy, and various formulations which emphasize the passivity of female eroticism.

The political utility of such theories in part accounts for their widespread proliferation and circulation, so much so that their truth is often taken for granted, even by writers like Carol Gilligan, who claim to be speaking on behalf of women. The use to which these theories are put reveals a lot about the political function of love in late patriarchy, since their effect is either to naturalize women's subjugation through love, or to blame the victim for the consequences she suffers, while protecting the prerogatives of the perpetrators on the grounds either that their behavior is also natural, and therefore not subject to moral censure, or on the grounds that they cannot be held accountable for women's complicity with their aggressive tendencies.

Examine love and you threaten the very structures of culture, the structures that depend on normalizing male dominance and aggression, in part on the grounds that this is what women really want, and then using the persistence of heterosexual coupling under the rubric of love as evidence in support of this truism. This in part explains why most of those who seriously questioned or challenged the discourse of love in the last century have been subjected to wrath, hostility, and trivialization. This would include not only the treatment given to feminist texts like Beauvoir's *The Second Sex*, Kate Millett's *Sexual Politics*, and the writings of radical lesbians like Ti-Grace Atkinson and Jill Johnston, but also works as distant from feminism as those of Sigmund Freud, Wilhelm Reich, Herbert Marcuse, and Norman O. Brown, each of whom raised questions about the organization of eroticism proffered by the rubric of love.

More recently we have the case of Andrea Dworkin's text, *Intercourse*, which was subjected to a range of socially conspicuous challenge and critique that might fairly be described as overkill, i.e., out of proportion to what would have been the likely readership for such a text. Dworkin's claim that penile vaginal intercourse as a mechanism of domination was challenged from a variety of directions by feminists, anti-feminists, women and men. The most common strategy employed was to invalidate Dworkin's thesis on the grounds that it was couched in an indefensible anatomical essentialism, which attached erroneous political significance to male and female body parts. What the media barrage failed to foreground, however, was the essentialist assumptions and motives underlying the combative discourse to which this text and author were subjected, namely that challenges to the hegemony of intercourse must be violently resisted, as conspicuously and publicly as possible, because the perpetuation of this practice is essential to the existing social order.

In popular media, any evidence of the waning cultural influence of love is subjected to a critical eye and ironic discourse, even when the phenomena in question are not cast in the context of an explicit challenge to existing social arrangement. As an example, there was *Time* magazine's recent cover story. "Is Love Doomed?", which focused on the life styles of urban professionals, which often leave little room for and attach only subsidiary priority to love and erotic relationships. Even though the motives here are represented in the conventional language of personal ambition and economic aggrandizement, the consequences are presented with irony and alarm, as they are also represented, albeit comically, in the recent Yuppie romance, *Baby Boom*, and the figure of the grotesque in another recent and very popular film, *Fatal Attraction.*

At a time when fear of AIDS and other sexually transmitted diseases would seem to offer both grounds and motives for revivifying the prospect of organizing eroticism as a monogamous practice undertaken as an expression of love, contemporary sexual politics is further destabilized by the persistence of contradictory theory and practice, theory and practice which, intentionally or not, resist, oppose or contradict the resolutionary rhetoric of love. To a certain extent, at least, these forms of resistance can be read as useful to the proliferative logic of the dominant position, offering occasions for its explicit articulation and defense precisely because it is under attack.

Because the discourse of advocacy depends on points of resistance to justify and occasion its evocation, the logic of this position demands a continual stream of appropriate targets in order to mandate its redeployment targets which have thus far included homosexuality, promiscuity, and teenage sexuality. Just as the saturation point with respect to these phenomena is being reached, in strides Shere Hite, with her new book, billed as the third volume in the trilogy of Hite Reports, *Women and Love: A Cultural Revolution in Progress* (UK title: *The Hite Report on Love, Passion and Emotional Violence*), a work that has been subjected to at least as much hostile treatment as any of those I have previously mentioned, as has its author. I think the degree of negative critical response to this text, a phenomenon which has received widespread attention from both the news and entertainment communities, provides some clue to its significance, as well as to the importance of its subject matter. Therefore I think it is worth examining the criticisms of Hite's work against the grain, which is to say resisting their implications that such critiques ought to result in a dismissal of Hite's conclusions because her methodology, or sample, or interpretations are flawed. I think that the heat this book has taken gives us reason for taking its claims more seriously, on the grounds that if there were not some significant fear, or temptation to believe that much of what is represented in Hite's text was true, there would be little or no need to devote so much time, energy, and space to refuting or contesting its findings, or the manner in which they were produced.

The subtitle of this book, "A Cultural Revolution in Progress," helps account for both the quantity and intensity of the critiques, both because it situates the text within an oppositional or critical context, and because it enlarges rather than minimizes the implicatory consequences of the findings and the interpretations Hite draws from them.

The findings from which these larger implications are drawn, and the ones that have been subjected to the most extensive and hostile challenges, are those that indicate not only that women are dissatisfied with their heterosexual love relationships, but also that they are no longer simply enduring it, as good women were supposed to, silently. Rather, women are doing something about it, including openly articulating their dissatisfaction and the grounds for it, as well as abandoning or decentering these relationships through divorce, extramarital affairs, and changing their erotic affiliations. The narratives Hite reproduces also make clear that many women no longer live for love, or consider it the most crucial factor for determining their happiness.

As troubling as this evidence is for those who wish to argue that heterosexual love still goes on uncontested, some of the conclusions Hite draws from this evidence of female resistance must be even more disturbing. Most striking, at least to me, if not the media, is Hite's claim that women's demonstrated willingness to leave relationships that disempower them can be read as part of a sustained, albeit unorganized, movement away from a society organized around male dominance and other masculinist values, toward a society which enfranchises feminine values like care and relatedness. Although much of what is represented as the grounds and consequences of women's dissatisfaction with love has already been articulated in earlier feminist theoretical writings, some of which Hite cites as support for her conclusions, Hite's book seems to pose an even greater threat, in part, because her book does not speak with a single authorial voice, but rather represents the voices of the several thousand women whose responses to Hite's questionnaire are reproduced in the text. While the conclusions of feminist theorists might be more easily dismissed on the grounds that they represented an elite, singular, idiosyncratic and therefore atypical point of view, Hite's work avails itself of empirical research technique, and thus claims to speak not only for its author, but for the collection of women whose views are offered and presented. This, unfortunately, also casts Hite in the position of the messenger who brings bad news, and she is being treated accordingly.

Rather than acknowledging their anxiety in the face of Hite's conclusions, most critics have attempted to challenge and undermine them indirectly, by caricaturing the manner in which those conclusions were reached. In an effort to displace the significance of what the women in Hite's book say, criticism has focused on representing these women as atypical, and the survey results as tainted, because the sample of women whose views they summarize was not sufficiently random: either because the surveys were distributed by women's groups (and the typical woman is assumed not to be a joiner) or because the voluntary conditions of response to what is, admittedly, a very extensive and therefore time-consuming questionnaire, already reflects a bias, namely that only women with an axe to grind would bother to respond to Hite's queries in the first place. The happy and contented women who do not supposedly appear in Hite's text are being constructed, by the reader critic— a silent majority with neither willingness nor ability to share their contentment with the rest of us. On the basis of this tainted sample, tainted by comparison to the constructed one, it is argued that Hite's conclusions ought to be dismissed, because the procedures for arriving at them were "unscientific."

Part of what is interesting to me about this critical strategy is the way it foregrounds contradictions within the operative politics of knowledge. Traditionally, love has been cited as one of the few phenomena that stands outside of the mechanisms of scientific discourse and objectification, a point of resistance to the hegemony of technological and informational objectification. For a long time culture has not only tolerated but valorized the assumption that love was not the sort of thing that could be subjected to or analyzed in terms of scientific method. As evidence one may simply point to the texts which have been most influential in constructing our social expectations for love, from Plato's *Symposium* and Ovid's *Art of Love*, to the Old and New Testaments, and more recent romantic literature from the nineteenth and twentieth centuries, as well as the work of popular psychologists like Erich Fromm and Leo Bascaglia, none of which are or claim to be scientific and yet continue to function as socially authoritative prescriptive and descriptive discourses. Unscientific approaches are unproblematic as long as the discourse produced confirms and validates dominant sentiments, and does not disrupt underlying social utilities.

When a text like Hite's comes along, and hers is clearly neither the first nor the last, which challenges hegemonic sentiments by claiming empirical evidence of their waning influence, methodological considerations are brought to bear in a way intended to discredit what has been said on the basis of who says it or on what basis, without ever having to challenge the truth or significance of the conclusions as such. The strategic utility of the methodological critique is double-edged: it casts doubt on the credibility and integrity of the inquirer, implying, in this case, that her methods were intentionally biased and designed to be misleading or unrepresentative, while concealing the ideological biases and allegiances of the critic and the criticism, by cloaking them in the language of scientific neutrality. Such a strategy allows the intended audience to believe that it is only the inquirer, and not the critic, who has an axe to grind, or preconceptions to protect.

The numbers game being played with Hite's book has also resulted in some interesting tactical reverses through which individual critics, or members of talk-show audiences, can, with a single stroke, make a claim that supposedly invalidates what thousands of women have had to say. How many women do there have to be before what we say is worth paying attention to?

But the numbers game is only one element in a larger strategic campaign to dismiss this text and thereby discourage a potential readership from confronting the text for themselves on the grounds that what the women represented in Hite's book write, whether or not they are typical, is not worth reading. It is worth remembering, however, that male entitlement to cultural visibility and authority is often construed on just the opposite basis. That is, by reference to some special and distinguishing mark that differentiates, hence privileges him with respect to the average observer on the basis of knowledge, access, or the uniqueness of his point of view. The authority of the critic comes from the fact that he is not an average Joe, but an expert.

I also cannot help but feel that this strategy represents another reversal, masking the concern that these responses are all too typical, and that too many women will identify and recognize parts of themselves in at least some of what the many women cited say. The critical barrage mounted against Hite's work has sought to operate as a self-concealing censorship mechanism, discouraging potential readers, on the ground that the text they are being offered is biased and therefore misleading. But the success of this strategy is predicated on a thin hope, and one that I take to be rather questionable, namely that if women are not presented narratives of dissatisfaction, such ideas or sentiments would otherwise never occur to them.

In re-reading the strategies used to try to discredit Hite's work, I do not want to leave the impression that the text is not open to certain kinds of critical readings. I myself question some of the language and logic operative in Hite's interpretations of the phenomena she recounts and their social and political consequences. But in the context of more immediate political urgencies, those differences don't seem all that important, and are better saved for another occasion. More important to address at this point are the reasons why any discourse of women's dissatisfactions with loving men must, it appears, be silenced, marginalized, or discredited. In examining those reasons we also come to realize how much and for how long the discourse of love as uncontroversial has necessitated and depended on women's silence. This can be an empowering as well as a painful insight, empowering to the extent that we recognize that the effort to silence women is also an indication of the power carried by our voices when we do speak. Powers to disrupt, intervene, and change the rules of the games women and men play.

Love in our age has been offered to an increasingly beleaguered, discontented, and anxious citizenry as a pacificatory moment of pleasure and solace in a world that is organized in increasingly inhuman and alienating ways. Love is therefore a significant mechanism in the apparatus of modern power which, as a number of social theorists from Marcuse through to Foucault point out, operates not through threat of coercion or death, but rather by the social construction and manipulation of pleasure, a technology of control by incitement. When women, who have been positioned as the emblems and place holders for love, confess to its failure, i.e., that we are not pacified in love but are rather mobilized in other ways by it, some crucial part of our social fabric starts to come apart at the seams. That is why Shere Hite has to be wrong. But if she is wrong, so is most of the feminist and other theory produced in our century that has challenged or criticized existing sexual and social relationships. If Shere Hite is right, however, about what's happening with women, there is some very confirming evidence for all of us who have been struggling to undermine the patriarchal organization of sexual difference. Evidence that our efforts at cultural revolution have not been in vain, they are in progress and may, in fact, have more power than we or the dominant culture and ideology usually give us credit for. At a time in our cultural history in which traditional codes of femininity are being recirculated as cutting-edge fashion, and where feminists are once again being caricatured as male bashers, any text that offers women a potentially empowering position within a discourse of love, that has historically been used for our domination, is worth taking seriously, not only as a mirror of the present, but also as a potential blueprint for building our future. If we fail to keep love controversial, we are doomed to the limits of the current situations and to forms of suffering and frustration with which many of us, I suspect, are all too familiar, because these disappointments are all too typical.

# Methodological Observations on the Hite Report Trilogy[6]

## QUANTIFYING THE EMOTIONS

Gladys Engel Lang, Professor of Communications, Political Science and Sociology, University of Washington, Seattle, 1987

Quantifications and analysis of attitudes and emotions is one of the most difficult tasks faced by social scientists—and one rarely attempted, almost never on such a large scale as in Hite's work. It has been one of Hite's contributions to devise an excellent methodology for studying the attitudes and emotions of a large population, while at the same time retaining a rich qualitative base: extensive data in people's own words about their deepest feelings.

When analyzing emotions and attitudes in depth, it has been customary in the social/psychological sciences to use extremely small samples; indeed, Freud based whole books on a handful of subjects. Thus for Hite to have used the small samples typical of psychological studies would have been quite legitimate. However, she also took on the more difficult goal of a larger and more representative sample, while still retaining the in-depth qualities of smaller studies. She does the latter by allowing thousands of people to speak freely instead of forcing them to choose from preselected categories—in essence, predefining them, as with so many studies. It is a method that is hard on the researcher, requiring analysis of thousands of individual replies to hundreds of open-ended questions, an analysis that involves many steps.

Hite's work has been erroneously criticized by some members of the popular press as being "unscientific" because her respondents, though numerous, are not a "random sample." However, scientists and scholars in the field of methodology and opinion sampling know that for many kinds of studies, and Hite's is one of them, the very large non-random sample generating rich data is preferable to a randomly chosen sample. A "random sample" does not guarantee representativeness; frequently, in practice, there is a problem of "who didn't respond." In this kind of sampling, to be perfectly mathematically "representative," all of those chosen must respond. However, in most cases, no such perfection is achieved. Thus, to put it bluntly, there ARE almost no random samples. Therefore most survey research today tries to match its samples demographically to the general population in other ways, by, for example, weighting responses to conform to the population profile, as Hite does.

John L. Sullivan, the noted research theorist, puts it, "Most of the work in the social sciences is not based on random samples; in fact, many if not most of the articles in psychology journals are based on data from college students, and then generalized. . . . Interestingly, these small and non-representative samples have not been criticized in the same way Hite's larger and more representative sample has been." Hite's large and rich sample of over 15,000 is an excellent achievement in itself. Moreover, Hite has matched her sample carefully to the U.S. population at large;* the demographic breakdown of the sample population corresponds quite closely to that of the general U.S. population.

Another hallmark of Hite's methodology is the anonymity guaranteed participants. It is this which makes it possible for her respondents to speak so freely about their most private feelings and thoughts, and ensures that they do not feel they must hold back any of the truth about these very personal matters for fear of being ridiculed, judged, or simply "known." It is in fact because the respondents are guaranteed anonymity (even from Hite and her team) that one can be confident of the accuracy of Hite's findings. And indeed studies in three other countries testing the findings of the first *Hite Report* have replicated her basic results.

As Robert L. Emerson of UCLA explains, "Hite's methodology is perfectly suited to her aims . . . the distinctive quality of her data is exactly that it allows men and women to talk about the subjective meaning and experience of a variety of personal matters. The purpose of her research is then to describe and categorize the varieties of such experience . . . so that the whole range of such experiences can be described . . . [she] has more than fulfilled this goal." Hite is straightforward about her procedures and has done as much and more than other researchers to explain her methods. She makes absolutely clear what she is doing methodologically—in fact, her degree of clarity is not frequently achieved in social science research.

Nancy Tuana of the University of Texas at Dallas writes: "For centuries, through the guise of science, men have been constructing theories of women's nature. Although women have been the object of study, our experiences and feelings have not been taken seriously. Shere Hite's work provides a model of a methodology that is based on women's experience. Hite has rejected the silencing of women by recognizing that a theory about women's ways of loving must be rooted in our efforts to give voice to our own experiences. Her work will be valued not only for the insights she provides, but also for her revolutionary approach." And Barbara Ehrenreich, whose background is in the biological sciences, notes that "Tables, graphs, correlation coefficients, etc., do not, in and of themselves, make a study 'scientific.' In fact, I would say that any study of human behavior that does not

---

* The samples for later research, beginning with *The Hite Report on the Family*, include European and other foreign replies as well as U.S. replies, they are no longer based exclusively in the U.S.

include—and highlight—the element of subjective experience is, in a fundamental sense, unscientfic. This was what was wrong with the Kinsey Report and Masters and Johnson's work, and what makes the Hite Reports so groundbreaking; at last (with Hite's work) we know something about love as women and men experience it and that is the most important thing we can know about it."

In summary, as a scientist and as a human being who obviously cares very much about her subjects (and those who may read and be affected by them), Shere Hite presents in the Hite Reports a deeply penetrating portrait of our culture, based on empirical data, giving us insights into who we are and where we are going. This work is an enormous contribution.

# EXPLICATION OF SCIENTIFIC METHOD AS USED IN RESEARCH FOR THE HITE REPORT TRILOGY

The main concerns of this research were described in the abstract of a paper presented at the American Association for the Advancement of Science annual meeting in May, 1985,[7] entitled "Devising a New Methodological Framework for Analysis and Presentation of Data in Mixed Qualitative/Quantitative Research: The Hite Report Trilogy, 1972–1987."

There were unique challenges to be faced in devising the methodology for the Hite Reports, which comprise a 3-vol. study of over 15,000 women and men in the U.S., 1972–87. First, although quantification was necessary as part of the final result, a simple multiple-choice questionnaire could not be used, since the theoretical concept for the project stated that "most women have never been asked how they feel about sex" and "most research has been done by men": therefore, it was important not to assume predetermined categories, but to design an essay-type questionnaire which would be open-ended. Also, the data-gathering was designed to protect the anonymity of the respondent. Secondly, compilation of data from essay questions is very difficult, if the data are to be carefully and rigorously treated . . . Finally, and almost as labor-intensive as compilation and categorization of data, presentation of findings was planned to serve more than an informative function; rather than simply giving readers statistics plus the author's theoretical analysis of data, the aim was to create an inner dialogue within the reader, as s/he mentally conversed with those quoted. Therefore, large parts of text comprise first-person statements from those participating. The format of presentation shows how these fit into intricate categories of social patterns.

## THE FOUR STAGES OF RESEARCH

### I. QUESTIONNAIRE DESIGN

One of the most important elements in the design of *Women and Love* was that the participants be anonymous, because in this way a completely free and uninhibited discussion could be ensured. For this reason, a questionnaire format, rather than face-to-face interviews, was chosen, with respondents specifically asked not to sign their names, although other demographic data were taken. That this anonymity was in fact an aid to communication with participants was verified in statements by respondents in each study, such as the following: "I would find it very hard to say all these things to another person, and I'm sure many women would feel the same as I. I am sick of reading various 'advice' columns about what I should be feeling, but I have not found another forum for saying what I think myself, taking my own time, rethinking, not feeling any pressure to be perfect or 'in' or anything. I am saving my answers; they have been very important to me."

The second choice to be made regarding format related to how the questions would be asked. In the sensitive realm of personal attitudes, a multiple-choice questionnaire was out of the question, because it would have implied preconceived categories of response, and thus, in a sense, would also have "told" the respondent what the "allowable"—or "normal" answers would be. Although a multiple-choice questionnaire is much easier for the researcher to work with, it would have given a subtle signal to the participant that the research categories were equated with "reality," or "allowable reality," whereas the intention here was to permit women's own voices to emerge, for women to say whatever they might feel on the deepest level to be the truth of their situation, with nothing to intervene or make them censor themselves.

Also, the development of the questions in this study has always been an interactive process with the participants. (In a way this was true of the Kinsey questionnaires as well, since Kinsey developed several questionnaires over his period of research.) In this study, questionnaires were refined and modified at the suggestion of those responding, so that, for *Women and Love*, there were four basic versions of the questionnaire used over several years.

Coming from an academic background with a strong awareness of the ideological elements in the definition of culture, and with a background in the women's movement that gave further emphasis to this idea, it was a constant matter for concern that questions are not simple questions, but always have several layers of meaning. For this reason, the methodology used here was designed to pay special attention to this issue.[8]

Many people hold the mistaken belief that multiple-choice questionnaires represent the height of scientific objectivity, in that they can be quantified and need no "interpretation." Nothing could be further from the truth. All researchers, no matter how careful or aware/unaware of their own biases, do have a point of view, a way of seeing the world, reflecting the cultural milieu in which they were brought up, and so on—and these assumptions are subtly filtered into categories and questions chosen. (Philosophically speaking, we are all/all life is "biased" and subjective; it is only by combining a mass of subjectivities—all of our "seeing," if you will—that we find, through collective sharing of perception, a "fact"; in other words, for example, we only "know" the sun will come up tomorrow because we have seen it come up every day, and we all agree that the probability is that it will come up again tomorrow.)

Thus, to design the categories of response for a multiple-choice questionnaire is a political act, unavoidably filled with subjective bias, whether consciously or unconsciously so, and whether the researcher considers him/herself to be "neutral" or "apolitical" and so on. If a study wishes to find out what's "out there," it cannot impose prior categories on that "out there"; it needs to develop its research instrument through an exchange with "them," the participants, before proceeding. This was done in the current study by listening to respondents' suggestions and, indeed, eliciting comments from them as to their feelings about the questionnaire. In other words, there was an ongoing interactive process of sequential refinement in designing the questionnaires for this project. Less meticulous care for research design may mean that a researcher only rifles through his or her pre-existing expectations as to the content of the opinions/answers "discovered."

As both Ellie Wiesel and John F. Kennedy have pointed out, to be "neutral" or "apolitical" is, in fact, to be highly political, because one is endorsing the status quo.

In the case of *The Hite Report on Female Sexuality*, for example, the point of view was woman-oriented, in that it let women define sex as they saw it rather than assuming that the male definition of sex which had been predominant for so long was the only possible "correct" definition. For this, the work was described by some as having a "feminist bias." In fact, much of the previous research into female sexuality had been less than "scientific"; rather than taking the information that most women could orgasm more easily during masturbation or direct clitoral/vulval stimulation than during coitus, and concluding that therefore this is "normal," previous studies had started with the assumption that if women did not orgasm during coitus, there must be something wrong with them—that they were somehow defective, "dysfunctional," psychologically or physically abnormal. Research was often geared to finding out what the cause of this "defect" might be. This was a nonscientific approach, not an objective way of looking at female sexuality.

In short, no study is free of bias, or a point of view; the important thing is to recognize this fact, and to clarify, insofar as possible, just what that point of view is.

## THE DIFFICULTY OF STUDYING SEX AND THE EMOTIONS

As Judith Long Laws has said, "Most social scientists still avoid the study of feelings and attitudes, because of the difficulty in quantifying such studies, and the belief that this is the'best' kind of social science. This is not always true; quantification is not always the best way to arrive at understanding. . . . *The Hite Report* was the first large scale set of data where women talked about their own experiences in their own voices."

For this reason, essay questionnaires—which are not less "scientific" than multiple-choice, and in fact are recommended for use whenever possible by methodology textbooks—were the research tool of choice. The goal of this study was to hear women's deepest reflections on the nature of love, and to learn how they see love relationships now in relation to the whole spectrum of their lives. The method was important also in that it enabled participants to communicate directly with readers sharing myriad points of view—in essence, debating with each other throughout the text.

### II. DISTRIBUTION OF QUESTIONNAIRES AND COMPOSITION OF SAMPLE

The questionnaire following this essay and similar versions were distributed to women all over the country beginning in 1980. Their purpose was to discover how women/we view ourselves and our relationships with men and the world now, how we define "reality."

Distribution of the questionnaires was extremely widespread and painstakingly done, in order to reach as many kinds of women with as many varied points of view as possible. In order to ensure anonymity, it was thought best to send questionnaires to organizations rather than to individuals, so that any member who wanted might be able to answer with complete assurance that her name was not on any list or on file anywhere. Clubs and organizations through which questionnaires were distributed included church groups in thirty-four states, women's voting and political groups in nine states, women's rights organizations in thirty-nine states, professional women's groups in twenty-two states, counseling and walk-in centers for women or families in forty-three states, and a wide range of other organizations, such as senior citizens' homes and disabled people's organizations, in various states.

In addition, individual women did write for copies of the questionnaire, using both the address given in my previous works and an address given by interview programs on television and in the press. However, if an individual woman did write for a questionnaire, whether she returned it or not was her own decision, therefore assuring her complete anonymity, as her reply was unsigned and bore the postmark and demographic information requested, such as age, income and education, but not name or address. All in all, 100,000 questionnaires were distributed, and 4,500 were returned. This number is almost as high as the standard rate of return for this kind of questionnaire distribution, which is estimated at 2.5

to 3 percent. A probability method of sampling might have yielded a higher rate of return, but then an essay questionnaire would not have been possible; the purpose here was to elicit in-depth statements of feelings and attitudes, and multiple-choice questions would have closed down dialogue with the participants.

Finally, sufficient effort was put into the various forms of distribution that the final statistical breakdown of those participating according to age, occupation, religion, and other variables known for the U.S. population at large in most cases quite closely mirrors that of the U.S. female population. See charts in the Statistical Data.

### COULD THE STUDY HAVE BEEN DONE USING RANDOM SAMPLING METHODS?

*There are many forms of scientific methodology besides the random sample; those of us in the field know that there is no such thing as a random sample in sex research, but this does not make the work unscientific if, as in the Hite Reports, the study population is carefully matched to the demographics of the population at large.*

—Dr. Theodore M. Mcilvenna, Institute for Sex Research

Almost no major research using essay questions today is done with the use of random samples. As Dr. Gladys Engel Lang has explained at the beginning of this section, most survey research now tries to match its samples demographically to the general population in other ways; for example, by weighting responses to conform to the population profile, somewhat similarly to the methods used here. But an even more important reason for not using random sampling methods for this study is that a random sample cannot be anonymous; the individuals chosen clearly understand that their names and addresses are on file.

Does research that is not based on a probability or random sample give one the right to generalize from the results of the study to the population at large? If a study is large enough and the sample broad enough, and if one generalizes carefully, yes; in fact, the Nielsen television studies and national political polls generalize on the basis of small, select, nonrandom samples all the time. However, in a larger sense no one can generalize from such findings, even if one were to somehow miraculously obtain a completely random sample—the reason being that variables such as psychological state, degree of religious or political fervor, and so on are not measured; thus there is no guarantee that those picked in a random sample, although they might represent the population at large in terms of age and income, would also represent the population in terms of psychological make-up.

### III. ANALYSIS OF REPLIES: MEASURING AND UNDERSTANDING ATTITUDES, EMOTIONS AND SELF-REPORTED EXPERIENCES

To go from essay statements to mixed quantitative/qualitative data is a long and intricate process.* Of course some portions of the replies received are already in quantifiable form—that is, questions answered with a "yes" or a "no." But the majority of questions were not so phased, since the intention, as discussed, was to open dialogue rather than to close it.

There is an ongoing and abstruse discussion in the field of methodology as to how best to study emotions, belief systems, and attitudes—not to mention how to quantify them. For example, not only is the question, "How do you love the person in your current relationship? What kind of love is it?" a difficult one to answer, but the answer is also every bit as difficult to analyze and compare with other answers received and, in some cases, build into statistical findings. Nevertheless, it is possible to do this if such statistics are attached for the reader to numerous examples of definition by the participants, such as is done in this study.

Specifically, the information was analyzed in this way: First, a large chart was made for each question asked. Each person's answer to the question being analyzed was then transferred onto that chart (usually many pages long), next to its individual identification number. The many months required for this procedure were actually very valuable in that they provided extensive time for reflecting on the answers.

Once the charts had been prepared, the next step was to discover the patterns and "categories" existing in the answers. Usually patterns had begun to stand out during the making of the charts, so that the categories more or less formed themselves. Then statistical figures were prepared by totaling the number of women in each category, following which representative quotes were selected. This procedure was followed for each of the 180 questions.

In addition one main chart was kept onto which much of the information from other charts was coded for each individual woman, so that composite portraits could be drawn and compared. Any attempt at condensation or computerization at an early stage of the analysis would have defeated the purposes of the study: to find the more subtle meanings lying beneath the more easily quantifiable parts of the replies, and to keep intact each individual's voice so that participants would remain in direct communication with readers, thus reinforcing the integrity of the study. After all the replies had been charted, and the process of identifying categories completed, with representative quotes selected, statistical computation was possible.

Analyzing data from essay-type questionnaires, then, is a complex endeavor, but there is no way, if one cares about accuracy and detail or wants to search out and understand the deepest levels of the replies, that lengthy testimonies such as these

---

* Thus, in this study, there were over 40,000 woman-hours involved in analyzing the answers, plus at least 20,000 put in by the women who answered the questionnaire. This, of course, does not include the time and effort needed to turn the resulting compilation of data into a book.

can be understood quickly—and it is precisely the possibility of reaching these deeper levels that makes the essay questionnaire more valuable for this purpose than multiple-choice. Although multiple-choice questions make the researcher's job easier, only through listening to an individual's complete and free response, speaking in her own way and with her own design, without restriction, can more profound realities be reached.

### IV. PRESENTATION OF FINDINGS: A NEW INTERACTIVE FRAMEWORK

As theorists have pointed out, simple presentation of people's statements is not a rigorous approach to documenting "reality"; people's statements do not "speak for themselves"; there are assumptions and things left unsaid. True analysis requires a complex presentation of subjective data—not just, "People say this, and so that's how it is." For example, in the study of male sexuality, if most men responded that they have extramarital sex and that it keeps their relationship/marriage working, while it does not bother them, must the researcher conclude simply that since the majority make this statement, this is "how men are"? It would be simplistic to draw this conclusion. There are many elements in every decision, and it is the researcher's job to search out all the variables.

As it was explained by Janice Green, "In standard social science projects, one researcher's unstated and often unexamined or unconscious point of view is projected onto a research design, and then later also onto the presentation and interpretation of findings in a rather undigested way. In oral history, at the other extreme (such as that by Studs Terkel), [each bit of] data is allowed to 'speak for itself'—but there is still no clarification of assumptions, biases or other hidden factors."

### DIALOGUE BETWEEN PARTICIPANT AND RESEARCHER

Most basic to the methodology of the Hite Reports is the separation of "findings" from analysis and interpretation. This is done by choice of research design, questions, and method of analysis and, in particular, the style of presentation of the final analysis—that is, separating the interpretation of what people say from what they do say. At times, in the text, participants debate with each other, in their own words; at other times, analysis of what people are saying can bring out several possible sides of a point; researcher and participants can agree or debate at different places in the text. In this way, the metaphysical dilemma of how much of what participants express is ideology, can also be addressed. As Janet Wolfe, director of the Institute for Rational Therapy, has explained, "This complex approach has confused some general media reviewers, especially as Hite's work is accessible to a wide audience. But this many-layered structure is another part of Hite's overall methodology, in that she means to involve as many people as possible in the dialogue (not presenting closed 'norms')—since it is, after all, a dialogue about social change."

## THE ISSUE OF CLASS AS RELATED TO PRESENTATION OF DATA

Much of the important work of the last few years in women's history and sociology has focused on class and economics as the major point for analysis; however, the purpose here is somewhat different.

Although it is important to write about women in terms of class and race, and not to see "all women" as "the same," the focus of this study is not class but gender and gender ideology—that is, the experiences women have in common because of their gender. Also, this book is not built around comparisons of the attitudes of women in the various traditional socioeconomic groups for the simple reason that differences in behavior and attitude are not the major dividing line between women on these issues that some have theorized they might be. But even more importantly, the intention here was not to focus on class differences between women and what should be done about them, but on men's attitudes to women and what should be done to change them, strategies women have devised for developing their own lives while still dealing with the overall society's view of them—and to find the similarities and dissimilarities in women's current definitions and redefinitions of their relationship with men and society.

Nevertheless, women in this study include a vast cross-section of American women from different socioeconomic groups and "classes." Great care was taken to ensure that statements by women from all classes are well represented throughout every portion of this book. Women's backgrounds will probably emerge to some extent through their manner of speaking/writing. However, perhaps unfortunately, some grammar and spelling was "corrected" so that answers could be more easily read. While some replies were very appealing when their original spelling reflected a personal style or regional accent, it seemed that in print these misspellings looked demeaning to the writer or might be seen as trivializing that respondent. It is hoped, however, that enough of the original syntax in the replies is intact so that readers will get a feeling of the wide diversity among the respondents.

Finally, it does seem that, based on this research, there are large areas of commonality among all women. While clearly the experience of a poor woman is different from that of a wealthy woman, and so on, in fact, the emotional expectations placed on "women" as a group by the society seem to be much the same. From the statistical charts and from women's statements here, it is clear that, with regard to gender relationships, variables such as "class," income, education, and race are not nearly as influential as the overall experience of being female.

## NOTE ON THE USE OF TERMS "MOST" AND "MANY" IN THE TEXT

For ease of reading, not every statement in the vast text is given with its related statistic, only the most important facts are given with a complete breakdown in terms of numbers; therefore, as a guideline for the reader, it will be useful to know that "most" refers to more than 55 percent, "many" to any number between 40 and 65 percent; "some" indicates any number between 11 and 33 percent; while "a few" will mean a number between 2 and 11 percent. In addition, tables giving a complete breakdown for all the major findings (of which there are 120) can be found in the statistical appendices below. This is the largest amount of precise data given in any study since Kinsey; certainly Freud never attempted any such large sample. Another comparison: the Schwartz/Blumstein data, also covering relationships, contained less intricate and less numerically coded data relating to the emotions, although theirs was an excellent study.

Even though, for ease of reading, these general terms are at times used, it is felt that the context makes their meaning clear; in addition, the extensive statistical appendices include the precise data.[9] The number of individual testimonies related to any given topic also reflect how widespread similar replies received were.

### REACTIONS BY THE MEDIA AND SCHOLARS IN THE FIELD

In the general popular media there seems to be a widespread misunderstanding of the types and validity of methodologies available in the social sciences—not to mention the subtle debates discussed earlier in this section. For example, even an important medical writer for the *New York Times* in 1976 opened a story on the first Hite Report with, "In a new, non-scientific survey of female sexuality . . ." The press has often made the mistake of equating "scientific" with "representative," and although both criteria are met by these studies, the press has at times insisted on the "non-scientific" nature of the work.

Many commentators in the scholarly community have tried to inform popular writers of their mistake:

Mary Steichen Calderone, MD, MPH; Founder, Sex Education and Information Council of the U.S. (SEICUS):

> The subject of human sexuality is one that closes many minds to any objective approach to it, so much so that panic and anxiety often cause people who have only marginal scientific information to repudiate such an approach to its examination. Hite's has been such an approach. Her studies have given ordinary women and men opportunity to verbalize their long-suffered panics and sexual anxieties, thus making it possible for other researchers and educators in this new field of sexology to understand better what has been going on in human minds, through the centuries, about a part of life that is universal and central to every human being born. We have an enormous store of information about the human reproductive system and its functioning, most of it gained in the past fifty years...Hite's research, as with all research dealing with thoughts and feelings, cannot be expected to be analyzed with

the same techniques as those that tell us what doses of what drugs give what results in what kinds of patients. . . . We are a scientifically illiterate people, and honest scientists such as Hite are bound to suffer as a result.

Robert M. Emerson, Ph.D., Professor of Sociology, UCLA, Editor, *Urban Life: A Journal of Ethnographic Research*:

> Statistical representativeness is only one criterion for assessing the adequacy of empirical data . . . other criteria are particularly pertinent when looking at qualitative data. This is primarily the situation with Hite's research, [in which the] . . . goal can be pursued independently of issues of representativeness, or rather, even demands a logic that is at variance with that of statistical representativeness. The logic is that of maximizing kinds of or variations in sexual experiences, so that the whole range of such experiences can be described; the frequency of any such experiences is another matter, one that is linked to the logic of representativeness. . . . Much of Hite's work seeks to organize qualitative comments in ways that do not involve an exhaustive set of categories, but again directly convey the more significant themes or patterns, in ways that also identify and explore variations in and from these patterns. Here again, range, breadth, and variation are more important than strict statistical representativeness.

John L. Sullivan, Ph.D., Professor of Political Science, University of Minnesota, co-editor, *American Journal of Political Science*, and editor, *Quantitative Applications in the Social Sciences*, Sage University Papers series:

> The great value of Hite's work is to show how people are thinking, to let people talk without rigid a priori categories—and to make all this accessible to the reader. Hite has many different purposes than simply stating population generalizations based on a probability sample. Therefore questions of sampling are not necessarily the central questions to discuss about her work. Rather, it is a matter of discovering the diversity of behaviors and points of view. Hite has certainly adequately achieved this kind of analysis. If she had done a perfectly representative random sample, she would not have discovered any less diversity in points of view and behaviors than she has discovered.
>
> Her purpose was clear: to let her respondents speak for themselves, which is very valid. . . . What purpose would it have served to do a random sample, given the aim of Hite's work? None—except for generalizing from percentages. But Hite has not generalized in a non-scholarly way. Many of the natural sciences worry a lot less about random samples, because their work is to test hypotheses. And most of the work in the

social sciences is not based on random samples either; in fact, many if not most of the articles in psychology journals are based on data from college students, and then generalized. Interestingly, they are not criticized in the same way Hite has been.

In short, Hite has used a kind of intensive analysis method, but not of individuals—of attitudes and feelings. One might say she is trying to put a whole society on the couch. Hers are works with many different purposes, and scholars and readers can use them in many different ways.

Gerald M. Phillips, Ph.D., Pennsylvania State University, editor, *Communications Quarterly Journal:*

The Hite studies are important. They represent "good" science, a model for future studies of natural human experience.... There have always been serious problems for social scientists involved with studying human emotions . . . they cannot be catalogued and specified . . . the most advanced specialists have difficulty finding and specifying vocabulary suitable for objective discussion of human emotions and their impacts on individuals and societies . . . Hite has acquitted herself of this task remarkably well.

The major share of published studies in the social sciences are done numerically under the assumption that similar methodology produced truth or reliable generalizations for the hard sciences.

What social scientists obsessed with "objective scientificity" do not seem to understand is that the hardest of scientists, physicists, for example, must engage in argument at the onset of their experiments and at the presentation of their data.... The problem with numeric measurement in the social sciences is, in the first instance, it works well only when the things being measured behave like numbers. Human data rarely stands still for measurement.... A major issue with which social scientists must cope in the future is how to describe and compare ephemeral numbers...It is also the practice of contemporary social scientists to [unnecessarily] obscure their methodologies in complex mathematical formulae...[it would be better to give] a statement of what was discovered, presented as simply and succinctly as possible a clear discussion of the theoretical basis for the study . . . and a clear description of the people studied [as in] the Hite model. Hite is a serious, reliable scholar and a first-rate intelligence.

Robert L. Carneiro, Ph.D., Curator of Anthropology, The American Museum of Natural History, New York:

Hite's work can definitely be seen as anthropological in nature. The hallmark of anthropological field method lies in working intensively with individual informants. And though Hite used questionnaires, they were questionnaires that invited long and detailed replies rather than brief, easily codable ones. . . . And from these responses, presented in rich, raw detail, deep truths emerge—truths which, in many cases, were probably never revealed to anyone else before . . . for every question she presents a broad spectrum of responses. . . . One comes away from Hite's books with a feeling that an important subject has been plumbed to great depths . . . of inestimable value.

In addition, "hard science" is still considered by many to be truly the province of the "male," as Evelyn Fox Keller points out in her article "Gender and Science":

The historically pervasive association between masculine and objective, more specifically between masculine and scientific, is a topic which academic critics resist taking seriously. Why? . . . How is it that formal criticism in the philosophy and sociology of science has failed to see here a topic requiring analysis? The virtual silence of at least the non-feminist academic community on this subject suggests that the association of masculinity with scientific thought has the status of a myth which either cannot or should not be examined seriously.[10]

# Additional Scholarly Papers

1977: Shere Hite, National Women's Studies Association Annual Meeting, "Is the Hite Report Scientific? Toward a New Feminist Research Methodology"

1982: Joseph P. Fell, Presidential Professor of Philosophy, Bucknell University, "Philosophical Reflections on the Hite Reports"

1984: Shere Hite, American Historical Association Annual Meeting, "The Ideological Evolution of Sexuality as Related to Gender"

1985: Shere Hite, S.W.I.P., "New Trends in the Social Sciences 'On The Uses of Hermeneutics For Feminist Scholarship': Devising a New Methodological Framework for Analysis and Presentation of Data in Mixed Qualitative/Quantitative Research"

1986: Shere Hite, American Anthropological Association Annual Meeting, "Controversies over the Nature of the Family in Human Pre-History"

1987: Nancy Tuana, Columbia University, "Women and Love: Toward a New Methodology"

1988: Prof. Linda Singer, Society of Women in Philosophy Eastern Meeting, Methodological Essay, "Controversies Over the Nature of Love"

1989: Cheris Kramerae, University of Illinois, "Shere Hite as Sociological Theorist"

1990: Shere Hite et al, Oxford Amnesty International Collected Papers

1999: Alison Jeffries, ed., *Women's Voices, Women's Rights: Oxford Amnesty Lectures 1996* (Westview Press)

1999: Shere Hite, *The Hite Report on Shere Hite*, (London: Arcadia Books)

## SCIENTIFIC METHOD AS USED IN HITE REPORT RESEARCH

1987: Laura Cottingham, *New York Observer,* "The Furor over Hite's New Study"

1988: Louise Armstrong, "Shere Hite and the Media," Women's Review of Books

1994: Dale Spender, "Introduction to Women as Revolutionary Agents of Change"

2002: Philippe Baraud, "Introduction to Hite's Work," in L'Orgueil d'être une femme

# Research Questionnaires on Female Sexuality, Male Sexuality, Love as Women Describe It, and Growing Up in the Family

Reprinted here are four questionnaires from the original Hite Reports. Hite's research continues, and readers are invited and encouraged to send responses (unsigned) to s.hite@hite-research.com, or Dr. Shere Hite, c/o Seven Stories Press, 140 Watts Street, New York, NY, 10013.

## A. RESEARCH QUESTIONNAIRE ON FEMALE SEXUALITY, 1970–1977

### I. ORGASM

1. Do you have orgasms? If not, what do you think would contribute to your having them?

2. Is having orgasms important to you? Would you enjoy sex just as much without having them? Does having good sex have anything to do with having orgasms?

3. Do you have orgasms during the following (please indicate whether always, usually, sometimes, rarely, or never):

    masturbation:

    intercourse (vaginal penetration):

    manual clitoral stimulation by a partner:

    oral stimulation by a partner:

    intercourse plus manual clitoral stimulation:

    never have orgasms:

    Also indicate above how many orgasms you usually have during each activity, and how long you usually take. Space for comments, if desired:

4.    Please describe what an orgasm feels like to you. How does your body feel?

5.    Is there more than one kind of orgasm? If you orgasm during vaginal penetration/intercourse, does the orgasm feel different than orgasm without penetration? How?

6.    Are you more aroused before or after orgasms? Would you use the word "satisfied" to describe your feeling after orgasm? "Loving"? "Elated"? A "feeling of well-being"? What word would you use?

7.    Is one orgasm physically satisfying to you? Do successive orgasms become stronger or weaker? Does the place to be stimulated change or "move around" slightly, from one orgasm to the next?

8.    Please give a graphic description of how your body could best be stimulated to orgasm.

9.    If you are just about to have an orgasm and then don't because of withdrawal of stimulation or some similar reason, do you feel frustrated? When does this tend to happen?

10.    What bodily "symptoms" do you show at the moment of orgasm? For example, does your body become tense and rigid, or are you moving? What position are your legs in? What is your facial expression?

11.    Is an orgasm something that "happens to" your body, or is it something you create yourself in your own body?

## II. SEXUAL ACTIVITIES

12.    What do you think is the importance of masturbation? Did you ever see anyone else masturbating? How did they look? Can you imagine women you admire masturbating?

13.    Do you enjoy masturbating? Physically? Psychologically? How often? Does it lead to orgasm always, usually, sometimes, rarely, or never? How long does it/do you usually take? How many orgasms do you usually have?

14.    How do you masturbate? Please give a detailed description. For example, what do you use for stimulation—your fingers or hand or the bed, etc.? *Exactly* where do you touch yourself? Are your legs together or apart? What sequence of events do you do?

15.    Do(es) your partner(s) stimulate your clitoral area manually? How? Is it usually for purposes of orgasm or arousal? If for orgasm, does it lead to orgasm always, usually, sometimes, rarely, or never? Is this form of sex important to you?

16.    Do(es) your partner(s) stimulate you orally (cunnilingus)? Is this stimulation oral/clitoral or oral/ vaginal, or both? Is it for orgasm or arousal? If for orgasm, does it lead to orgasm always, usually, sometimes, rarely or never? Do you like it?

17.    Is breast stimulation important to you? What kind?

18.    Do you like vaginal penetration/intercourse? Physically? Psychologically?

Does it lead to orgasm always, usually, sometimes, rarely, or never?

19. If you orgasm during vaginal penetration/intercourse, are other accompanying stimuli usually present? What would you say is your method of obtaining clitoral stimulation during intercourse: a) long foreplay, b) simultaneous manual stimulation of the clitoris, c) indirect stimulation from thrusting, d) "grinding" or pressing together during penetration, or e) some other method?

20. If you orgasm during intercourse, which kinds of movements do you like to make during penetration to increase your stimulation—soft or hard, slow or fast, complete or partial penetration, thrusting in and out or holding still, etc. Which positions do you prefer for orgasm? Are your legs together or apart at orgasm? Do you use vaginal or other muscles to help you orgasm?

21. Do you ever have physical discomfort during intercourse? Do you usually have "adequate" lubrication? Do you sometimes feel less excited the longer intercourse continues?

22. Is the emotional or psychological relationship more important during penetration than during other forms of sex? What is your emotional reaction to penetration?

23. Is it easier for you to have an orgasm by clitoral stimulation when intercourse is not in progress? If you had to choose between intercourse and clitoral stimulation by your partner, which would you pick? Why?

24. Do you like rectal penetration? What kind?

25. What forms of non-genital sex are important to you (for example, hugging and kissing? talking intimately? looking at each other? smelling?) Do you enjoy these activities as much as regular genital sex? Is the best sex genital?

### III. RELATIONSHIPS

26. Answer whichever are or were relevant to you: (Answer in space at bottom of page.)

   If you are *married*, how many years have you been married? Do you like being married? What is the effect on sex? Have you had "extra-marital" experiences (how many and how long)? If so, what was the effect on you as an individual, and on your marriage? Were they of the "open marriage" type, or unknown to your partner? What is your opinion of the "open marriage" concept?

   If you are *single*, do you enjoy being "single"? Or is it difficult? Do you think of "single" as a temporary way of life or a basic one? Do you have sexual activities very often? What kind?

   If you have a *regular sex partner* (not married), how does this compare with other life styles you have tried? Would you rather be married? Do you consider this temporary or permanent? Are you comfortable?

If you are a *lesbian* (relate sexually to women), please answer any of the preceding questions which may have applied to you, and also: How many years have you been relating physically to women? How do you feel sexual relationships with other women "compare" with relationships with men (or would compare, if you have never had heterosexual sex)? Physically? Psychologically? Please also explain how to relate to another woman physically, as this information is not always widely available.

If you are still *living at home* with parents or family, how do rules against sex for younger women affect you? Do they protect you or hurt you or what? Would you like less or more restrictions on sex? Are parents or relatives willing to discuss sex realistically with you? Friends? Teachers? Is getting information a problem? And finally, if you have had sex with a partner, do your parents know? How did they react?

If you have *not yet had sex with a partner*, what do you think sex will be like? What physical sensations have you enjoyed most so far?

If you are currently *asexual or celibate* (that is, you have no sexual relations except perhaps masturbation), how do you like this way of life? Would you recommend it to other women? How long do you plan to remain asexual?

27.  Which "life style" do you feel *would* be best for you? Extended periods of monogamy? Two or three or four regular lovers? Casual sexual relationships? Relatively long periods of no sex at all? "Swinging"? Or some other style which has not yet been invented?

28.  Rate the following in order of their numerical importance to sex (1, 2, 3, etc.), adding comments, if desired:

passion
romance
friendship
non-romantic love (deep caring)
long-term commitment, marriage
being "in love"
economics
hostility and feelings of violence

29.  Describe the first time you fell in love. How did you feel? How did the relationship develop and grow, or die? If you have fallen in love more than once, do you think there is a pattern of emotional developments which takes place in romantic sexual relationships?

30.  What have your deepest relationships been like, with both men and women? How were they satisfying or unsatisfying? Emotionally? Physically?

31. What are your deepest longings for a relationship with another person(s)?

## IV. LIFE STAGES

32. How old were you when you first masturbated? To orgasm? Did you discover it on your own, or did you learn how from someone, or somewhere else?

33. How old were you when you had your first orgasm with another person? During what activity?

34. What were your feelings about "losing your virginity"? Was there any pain or bleeding involved? How old were you?

35. Can you remember your sexual feelings during childhood? Grade school? High school? What were they?

36. Do you think that child and/or teenage sexuality should be repressed? Why or why not? Why is it presently repressed?

37. Have you had sexual feelings for members of your family? Brothers or sisters? Parents? Have your children (if applicable) ever shown sexual responses to your touch, or have you ever had sexual feelings for them? How did you react?

38. Did pregnancy and childbearing/birth have sexual aspects for you?

39. Have you had sexual contact with people who were quite a bit younger or older than you? Was it different in any way, either physically or psychologically, from other sex you have had?

40. How does age affect sex? Does desire for sex increase or decrease, or neither, with age? Enjoyment of sex? Does this have anything to do with age of your partners?

41. Does menopause ("change of life") affect sexuality, either physically or psychologically? How? Did it affect your partner(s)'s reactions to you?

42. If you have had a hysterectomy, did this affect your sexual activities or feelings? Physically? Psychologically? How?

43. What is your age and background—occupation, education, upbringing, race, or anything you may consider important?

## V. THE ENDING

44. Have physical sexual relations with men followed any particular patterns? What were they? (How have most men had sex with you?)

45. Is (are) your partner(s) sensitive to the stimulation you want? If not, do you ask for it, or stimulate yourself? Is this embarrassing?

46. Do you ever find it necessary to masturbate to achieve orgasm after "making love"?

47. Do you often feel your partner(s) is (are) not emotionally involved during sex? Or, what emotional responses do you most often feel from your partner(s)?

48. Do you ever fake orgasms? During which sexual activities? Under which conditions? How often?

49. Have you ever been afraid to say "no" to someone for fear of "making a scene" or "turning them off"? If so, how did you feel during sex? Would you define this as rape?

50. How do you feel about fellatio (mouth stimulation of the penis)? To orgasm? How do you feel about "performing" cunnilingus (oral sex) on another woman?

51. Do you think your vagina and genital area are ugly or beautiful? Smell good or bad? What other parts of your body do you like or dislike? Are you comfortable naked with another person?

52. Do you fantasize? (During masturbation, or during sex with a partner?) Is it to help bring on an orgasm, or just for general pleasure? Do you think of stories with plots, or just visualize specific images? What are they?

53. What do you think of sado-masochism (domination-submission)? Have you ever experienced them?

54. What books on sex have you read? What did you think of them?

55. What do you think of the "sexual revolution"?

56. Do you think that sex is in any way political?

57. Is there anything on your mind you would like to speak about which was left untouched by this questionnaire? If so, please add it here.

58. Why did you answer this questionnaire (*thank you!*), where did you get it, and how did you like it?

# B. RESEARCH QUESTIONNAIRE ON
# MEN AND MALE SEXUALITY, 1974–1982*

The purpose of this questionnaire is to better understand how men feel about their lives. Since so many of our society's ideas about who men are and who men should be (perhaps made most explicit in "sex") are so stereotyped, it is hard to know what men as individual human beings really feel.

Please answer and help us develop a more positive and caring way of relating to one another.

The results will be published as an extended discussion of the replies, including many quotes, in the same format as *The Hite Report on Female Sexuality*. The replies are anonymous, so don't sign your answers.

It is NOT necessary to answer every single question. Answer only those which interest you, but please answer!

---

* Research for *The Hite Report on Men and Male Sexuality* was conducted from 1974 to 1982: this questionnaire was used from 1979 to 1981, when a subsequent similar version was put in place.

We are looking forward to hearing from you. Send answers to S. Hite, c/o the publisher or hite2000@hotmail.com.

### I. TIME

1. What is the earliest sexual experience you can remember? How old were you?
2. How old were you when you first masturbated? To orgasm? How did you learn—by yourself, from someone else, or from books or movies?
3. At what age did you first orgasm? First ejaculate? Did you orgasm before you were old enough to ejaculate? Did you get intense pleasurable feelings from touching yourself? Have wet dreams?
4. Were you told about sex by your parents? What did they tell you? What did your friends tell you? What did you first hear about menstruation?
5. What were your sexual feelings as you grew up? In childhood? In grade school? In high school?
6. Do you think childhood or teenage sexuality should be repressed? Why or why not? Why is it repressed?
7. How has your sex life changed over the years? Does age affect sex? Has your enjoyment of sex changed? Have your attitudes and activities changed?
8. How big a part do sports and exercise play in your overall feeling of physical well-being and pleasure? What sports and exercise do you like? Swimming? Football? Running? Other?
9. How big a part do activities like sunbathing, cuddling up in a bathrobe on the couch, sleeping next to someone's warm body, petting your animals, etc., play in your overall bodily joy? What do you like especially?
10. How big a part does what we generally call "sex" (genital sex) play? Masturbation?
11. How big a part does talking to friends play in your overall feeling of well-being? Do you ever tell your friends how much you care about them?
12. Does home and/or family life play a part in your overall feeling of physical well-being? (This includes everyone, of course, not just those who are married.)
13. Do you enjoy touching and holding children? Do you enjoy snuggling with them? Wrestling? Giving them baths? Holding them? Rocking them? Feeding them?
14. Have you ever wished you could be a mother? How did you feel when you found out you couldn't bear children? How did you find out? How do you feel about it now?
15. What do you think of the role of being a father (whether or not you are a father)?
16. Do you enjoy physically caring for another human being, whether child or adult? How do you do it? Do you baby them? Were you prepared by your parents to nurture others?

17. Have you found the warmth and closeness in your life that you want? Where?
18. Would you like more time to yourself?
19. How do you feel about privacy in the bathroom? Do you close the door? Do you sometimes like for your partner to be in the bathroom with you during urination or defecation? Do you like to see your partner urinating, etc.?

## II. MASCULINITY

20. What is your age and your background—occupation, education, upbringing, religion, and race, or anything else you consider important?
21. What do you look like? Do you consider yourself handsome, pretty plain, ugly—or no comment? (Please forgive these words!)
22. How would you define masculinity? Are you masculine? How masculine are you?
23. What is the difference between masculine and "macho"? How high or low would you rate yourself on the "macho" scale?
24. What qualities make a man a man? That is, what qualities do you admire in men? Are you proud of your masculinity?
25. What did your father tell you about how to be a man? What did he tell you about women?
26. How can a man distinguish himself today? What is heroic in our time?
27. What can men as a group be proud of today? Ashamed of?
28. What is your biggest worry or problem in general in your life?
29. Is success important? Are you successful? In what way?
30. Do you believe in being ruthless when you have to?
31. Do you often feel hurt or sad when you don't show it? Do you force yourself to behave like a robot? Do you ever feel like a robot?
32. How would you feel if you were described as having something—anything—about your behavior or views that was "like a woman's"?
33. Were you ever called a "sissy"? Told to "be a man!"? What was the occasion? How did you feel?
34. Do you envy women's freedom to be gentle or emotional, or to have a temper? Do you envy them the choice of having someone support them, or the seeming lack of pressure on them to make money?
35. Do you have any strong resentments against women, or against ways any women have hurt you?
36. Are there ways in which you feel guilty for how you have behaved toward women, or toward a woman in particular?
37. Do you look at pornography? What kind? Did your father read pornography when you were growing up? Where/when did you see your first "men's magazine"?
38. What is your opinion of pornography you have seen? Do you feel it represents

certain elemental truths about how men and women really are—both psychologically and sexually?

39. What do you think of the "sexual revolution"?
40. What do you think of women's liberation? How has it affected your relationships?
41. What do males need from females? What do you get from women that you don't get from men?
42. Do you have more male or female friends? Why?

### III. RELATIONSHIPS

43. Do you prefer sex with women, men, or either—or with yourself, or perhaps not at all?
44. Do you think sex is important, or is it overrated? Is it interesting or is too much made of it? What other things in life are more important?
45. Does sex have a spiritual significance for you?
46. Answer one of the following:

A. If you are married, how many years have you been married? Do you like being married? Why did you get married originally? What is the effect on sex?
Do you love your wife? In what sense? Does she orgasm with you? From what stimulation? If you masturbate, does she know?
Do you believe in monogamy? Why or why not? Have you had/do you have "extramarital" sexual experiences? If so, how many and how long? Are you having one now? What was/is the effect on you as an individual and on your marriage? Did/does your partner know about them?
If you have children, why did you decide to have them? Did you want to be a father? How did you feel when your wife first told you you were having a baby? Do you love your children?
Do you feel you had to give up some things in order to be married and/or have children? Did being married/having children circumscribe your job and career opportunities? How would your life have been different?

B. If you are divorced, what are the reasons? How do you feel about it? Also please answer any of the questions above which apply.

C. If you are homosexual, please answer any of the previous questions that may apply to you and also: How long have you had physical and emotional relationships with men? How do they compare with relationships with women, if you have had any? Emotionally and physically? Are you involved with more than one man? Do you want to, or do you, live permanently with one man?

D. If you are "single," do you enjoy being single? What are the advantages and disadvantages? Do you plan to marry eventually? What is your sex life like?

E. If you are still living at home with parent or family, what rules are set up concerning your sexual and dating activities? Would you like more or less restrictions? Have your parents or relatives discussed sex realistically with you? Where have you gotten most of your knowledge of sex? From friends? Teachers? Books? Sex magazines? Family? Have you had problems getting accurate information on sex? If you have had a sexual relationship, do your parents know? If so, how did they react?

F. If you have not yet had sex with a partner, what do you imagine it will be like? Does it interest you, or does too much seem to be made of it? What physical activities have you enjoyed so far?

G. If you are living with someone, please answer any of the questions above which apply, and also how long have you been living with them? Would you rather be married? What are your plans for the future?

H. If you are currently uninterested in sex (except perhaps for masturbation), how do you like this way of life? How long do you plan to remain "celibate"? How long have you felt this way? Do you think this could be beneficial to other men? Do you find you relate more to nature or your pets or music when you are living alone?

47.   Perhaps you do not feel that any of these categories describe your life. If so, please describe yourself in your own way.

## Love

48.   Describe the time you fell the most deeply in love. How did it feel? What happened?
49.   Did you ever cry yourself to sleep because of problems with someone you loved? Contemplate suicide? Why?
50.   What was the happiest you ever were with someone? The closest? When were you the loneliest?
51.   How do your friendships compare with your love relationships?
52.   Do you feel you can truly love someone?
53.   What are your deepest longings for a relationship with another person?

### IV. ORGASM

54.   How important are orgasms to you? Can you enjoy sex without an orgasm? Can you enjoy sex if your partner does not have an orgasm?
55.   Please describe what an orgasm feels like to you—during the buildup? Before

orgasm? During the climax? After? Which moment feels best? How does the very best moment feel?

56. How often do you have sex without orgasm? Do you ever feel pressured to have orgasms? If so, when?

57. How does your body react when you are having an orgasm? Tighten up? Move a lot? Stop moving? Go out of control? What happens to your arms and legs? Your face?

58. Do you always ejaculate when you orgasm? How often do you orgasm or experience a sensation close to orgasm without ejaculating? Do you sometimes ejaculate without experiencing orgasm? How often? Or does orgasm mean ejaculation? Did you orgasm as a boy before you started ejaculating?

59. Do you have more than one orgasm during sex? Do you ejaculate each time? How do successive orgasms feel? Have you ever continued on to a second orgasm without losing your erection?

60. Is erection necessary for sexual arousal? Have you ever felt sexual without an erection? Did it bother you not to have an erection? What was your partner's reaction?

61. Is it O.K. to have sex with a soft penis? Are you embarrassed to continue sex with a soft penis if you don't have an erection?

62. Are you always aroused when you have an erection, or are there other causes of erection?

63. Do you like feeling aroused for extended periods of time, or do you prefer to go on to orgasm relatively quickly? Could you describe what arousal feels like?

### V. MASTURBATION

64. How often do you masturbate? How do you feel about it? Are you pleased? ashamed? satisfied? Are you secretive or open about it?

65. Do you enjoy masturbation? Physically? Emotionally? What do you find satisfying and unsatisfying about masturbation?

66. How do you masturbate? Please give a detailed description. For example, do you hold your penis with your hand and move your hand on your penis, or do you move your whole body—rubbing against something? Is stimulation important at the top or bottom of your penis? Do you mind the wetness of ejaculation? Is there any specific position you like to be in? Are there specific thoughts or fantasies you use?

67. Can you delay your orgasm during masturbation? Does this make it more or less exciting? What specific ways do you use to delay your orgasm?

68. Do you always want an orgasm when you masturbate? Do you ever stop short of orgasm when you masturbate to heighten your sexual feelings? Do you masturbate (but not to orgasm) to arouse yourself before sex? How often?

69. What is the importance of masturbation in your life?

VI. YOUR BODY AND YOUR FEELINGS

70. Do you like the way your genitals look, taste, and smell? Do you like the size and shape of your genitals? Your balls?

71. Are you circumcised? Do you like it, or wish you weren't? Did you, or would you, have your son circumcised?

72. What were your feelings when you found out about circumcision? About your own circumcision? Were you shocked? Pleased? Do you have a physical reaction in your genitals when you think about it?

73. Do you remember anything about the procedure? How old were you?

74. Has circumcision affected your attitude about exposing your penis to others? How? Does having or not having a foreskin affect your sexual activities?

75. Why are men circumcised?

76. Does your partner like your genitals? Has a partner ever commented adversely about your genitals? How? How did you feel about this?

77. Do you like fellatio (oral stimulation of your penis)? Can you orgasm this way always, usually, sometimes, rarely, or never? How often do you orgasm this way? How do you like it to be done?

78. Do you like mouth-anal contact?

79. Do you like manual stimulation of your penis by your partner? Do you often orgasm this way? What other parts of your genital area do you like your partner to touch?

80. Do you enjoy masturbating with another person present? Do you like having your partner masturbate him/herself when with you?

81. Do you like (or would you like) to be rectally penetrated? By a finger? By a penis? How does it feel? Do you orgasm this way? Exactly what does anal intercourse feel like—both physically and emotionally?

82. Do you like "foreplay"? What kind of "foreplay" is important to you for yourself? How do you like to be touched, and where? Kissed? Petted? Are your breasts sensitive? Your buttocks? Your testicles? Your mouth? Your ears?

83. Do you get enough foreplay from your partner? Does your partner touch and fondle you enough?

84. Do you sometimes like making out without having "real sex"? Do you prefer it?

85. Who makes the initial sexual advance? How do you feel if the other person makes the advance? Have you ever wanted the other person to make the advance and not gotten it? Do you feel unloved if your partner never makes the advance? Unwanted?

86. Have you ever approached someone about sex and been refused? How did you feel? Have you ever refused someone else? Why?

87. Are there certain times when you're not interested in sex? Is it O.K. to be celibate? Do you experience periodic highs and lows in your sexual interest? How often?

VII. FEELINGS ABOUT MEN

88. Describe your best male friend. What do you like about spending time with him?
89. Do you belong to, or socialize with, a group of men? What do you enjoy/like about it? What do you do? What do you talk about?
90. Do you value your men friends? Is it important to have male friends—or relatives you are close to? What do you value about their friendship? What do they mean in your life?
91. Were you in the Army or another branch of the military? Did you like the camaraderie? Did you have any close physical or sexual experiences with men during this time?
92. Do you like sports? Which kinds? Do you enjoy participating in sports with other men? Do you like the closeness with men in these activities?
93. Did you have a best friend in high school or college? What were your feelings for him?
94. Are you or were you close to your father? In what way? What was/is he like? What do you think of him?
95. Describe the man you are or were closest to in your life. In what ways are/were you close? Do/did you spend time together? Why is he valuable to you? Why do you like him?
96. If you have not had a physical or sexual relationship with another man, would you enjoy one?

### Sex with Men

97. How old were you when you had your first gay experience?
98. What was the first time you ever had physical contact with a man? Your father? A relative?
99. How is sex with men different from sex with women (if you have had sex with women, or based on what you think it would be like)?
100. What are your favorite things about sex with men? Why would you recommend homosexuality to other men? What are the advantages? Disadvantages?
101. Do you like anal intercourse? Exactly what does it feel like—both physically and emotionally? Do you orgasm this way?
102. Do you like giving a man fellatio? Do you swallow the seminal fluid? Do you like it?
103. Can you orgasm from just lying down together and kissing and rubbing crotches together?
104. Are you in love? In a steady relationship? How many men in your life have you had a sexual relationship with? Do you like monogamy?
105. Is gay "promiscuity" a myth or a reality? Do you prefer emotional closeness or casual sex or both?

106. Would you ever fall in love with a woman (again)? Why or why not?
107. Do people at work know you are gay? Do your parents?
108. Would you take an open stand on gay issues? Are you working for gay liberation? Or do you prefer the adventure of being gay in a straight world, the pleasure of belonging to a secret, elite society?

### VIII. FEELINGS ABOUT WOMEN

109. Do you have any close women friends? A sister you are close to?
110. Are you or were you close to your mother? In what way? What was she like? What did you think of her?
111. What things about women in general do you admire? Dislike? What do women contribute to society?
112. What do you think about women's liberation?
113. Are you currently in a relationship with a woman? What is she like? Why do you like her?

### Sex with Women

114. Has any woman discussed her sexual feelings seriously and openly with you? Did you ask?
115. When did you first learn about the clitoris? What did you hear from other men? From women? From books?
116. Do you like giving clitoral stimulation? Why or why not? When did you first do it? To orgasm? How did it feel? Do you feel comfortable now giving clitoral stimulation?
117. What kind of clitoral stimulation do you give? Please describe how you do it. Describe how you stimulate the clitoris with your hand or finger. Do you do this to orgasm?
118. Does your partner masturbate you to orgasm? How does she do it? If you don't know, would you like her to share that information with you?
119. When did you first hear/realize that most women don't orgasm from intercourse (coitus) alone? What was your original reaction?
120. Do you enjoy cunnilingus with a woman? What do you most dislike about it? Does it depend on your feelings for your partner?
121. Do you get sexually excited by stimulating your partner? Do you enjoy her orgasm? Physically? Emotionally? What aspects of touching, feeling, and kissing your partner(s) do you enjoy most? Least?
122. How do you give the woman an orgasm? Do you prefer the woman to orgasm from coitus?

## IX. INTERCOURSE

123. Do you like intercourse (penis/vagina)? Physically? Emotionally? How often do you have intercourse?

124. What position is most satisfying to you? Is this position all right with your partner? What position does she like? Do you like this position?

125. Why do you like intercourse?

126. Do you ever experience physical discomfort during intercourse? Afterwards? Do you ever experience boredom during intercourse?

127. After sex has begun, do you assume intercourse is expected next? Do you assume that every time you have sex, it will include intercourse?

128. Would you be willing to replace intercourse with other activities during some sexual encounters? How often? Or do you always want to define sex as intercourse?

129. Does your partner orgasm during sex with you always, usually, sometimes, rarely, or never? During intercourse? During other activities? Which ones?

130. Can you always tell if your partner has an orgasm? How can you tell? Are you ever in doubt? If in doubt, do you ask? If you ask and she says "yes," do you believe her? Do you talk about it?

131. Would you prefer to have sex with a woman who has orgasm from intercourse (coitus) rather than from clitoral stimulation? When does/do the woman/women you have sex with usually orgasm?

132. How do you feel if a woman stimulates herself to orgasm with you? During intercourse? How do you feel if she uses a vibrator?

133. Do you feel there is something wrong with your "performance," technique, or sensitivity if the woman does not orgasm from intercourse itself? That you're "not man enough," or at least that you did not do it right?

134. Does it matter to you if a woman orgasms during sex with you? Do you try to find out what stimulation an individual woman needs to have an orgasm?

135. Who usually orgasms first? You or the woman? During which activity? Do you orgasm when you want to? If not, why?

136. Has a woman ever expressed anxiety or been apologetic to you about how long she takes to orgasm or become ready for intercourse?

137. How do you feel if your partner does not have an orgasm at all, in any way?

138. Can you control when you come to a climax? How long can you hold off without losing your erection? Does it disturb you to lose your erection?

139. Are you embarrassed to have sex with a soft penis (i.e., if you don't get an erection)? Do you stop physical closeness and other activities if you can't have intercourse?

140. Do you ever ejaculate or orgasm "too soon" during intercourse? How long are you talking about? Is this ejaculation/orgasm satisfying to you? When does this happen? Why? Does it bother you?

141. Do you use any particular method to have intercourse longer without orgasming? Does prolonged thrusting dull the sensitivity or feeling of your penis?
142. When should a man ejaculate? Should the woman be consulted? Who decides when sex is over?
143. Do you control which activities sex consists of? Do you control when you come and how you have an orgasm?
144. Do you sometimes have difficulty having an erection at a time you desire one? When? Why? How often does it happen? What do you do at such times?
145. Do you talk to other men about sex? What do you talk about? Do you or other men tend to brag or exaggerate your exploits with women? Do you share practical information (how-to)? Feelings of insecurity?
146. What are the reasons why many women traditionally have not wanted sex as much as men? What kind of sex do women want most?

## X. BIRTH CONTROL

147. What contraceptive methods (birth control) do you use? Who decides what contraception will be used? Which kind do you prefer?
148. Are you aware of the possible side effects of the birth control pill?
149. Have you ever experienced physical discomfort from any form of birth control? Condom? The diaphragm? IUD? Foam? Have you ever used a condom to delay orgasm?
150. Do you feel responsible for discussing birth control before intercourse? If you are having a sexual relationship with a woman, do you protect her from becoming pregnant? Who is responsible if she does become pregnant? Do you ask a woman if she has taken measures to prevent conception before intercourse?
151. Do you fear impregnating someone? Does the possibility of pregnancy cause you problems in a sexual relationship?
152. Have you ever been a party to an unwanted pregnancy? What did you do about it?
153. Are you in favor of abortion? Have you ever impregnated a woman who subsequently had an abortion? Have you ever been involved in helping a woman secure an abortion? Did you share the expenses? Go with her? What was the outcome?
154. Did you have a vasectomy? (Do you have children?) How has having a vasectomy affected your sexual activities? What do your partners think about it? Have you ever wished to have it reversed? Would you recommend it to other men?
155. Do you know what vasectomy involves? Would you be willing to get one, and under what circumstances?
156. Have you ever witnessed childbirth?

## XI. VIOLENCE

157. Are you interested in violent sex? Has violence been part of a sexual relationship you had? What kind? How did you feel about it?
158. Have you ever been excited by a physical struggle or combat, or a fight—with a man or woman? Please describe.
159. Have you ever deliberately struck or hurt your lover? Why? What effect did it have on the relationship? Did you feel good when you did it?
160. Are you interested in bondage? Spanking? Why or why not? How does it feel?
161. Is it fun to force someone to your will?
162. Do you find kissing feet sexual? Golden showers?
163. Would you or have you had a sexual relationship with a very young person? How did you feel about it?
164. How do you define rape? Is it disturbing to you? How? How not? Where do you draw the line between consent and rape?
165. Have you ever raped a woman? If not, have you ever wanted to rape a woman? Why?
166. Have you ever pressured a woman to have sex with you, when she didn't seem to want to? How did you do it? Did you have a line? Did it succeed? Did you enjoy sex?
167. Is being forceful with your partner fun for you in sex? Do you usually control your partner during sexual activities? How do you develop the sexual relationship in the direction you desire? Is it easy to remain in charge of the situation?
168. If there is a power relationship involved in sex, who has the most power—you or your partner?
169. Is sex political?

### THANK YOU FOR ANSWERING THIS QUESTIONNAIRE!

A. Why did you answer this questionnaire?
B. Did you read *The Hite Report on Female Sexuality*?
C. Do you think other men will be as honest as you were in answering this questionnaire? How honest were you?
D. Please add anything you would like to say that was not mentioned.
E. Are you happy with your life, or do you want to change it?

# C. RESEARCH QUESTIONNAIRE ON WOMEN AND LOVE, 1975–1988[*]

The purpose of this questionnaire is to hear women's points of view on questions that were unanswered in the original *Hite Report on Female Sexuality*, such as how women feel about love, relationships, marriage, and monogamy. We would like to hear your thoughts and opinions on these subjects, as well as anything else you would like to add. The results will be published as a large-scale discussion of what was said, with many quotes.

The questionnaire is anonymous, so do not sign it. *It is not necessary to answer every question!* There are seven headings; feel free to skip around and answer only those sections or questions you choose. Also, you may answer on a tape cassette, if you prefer. Use as much additional paper as you need.

### HELLO!

1. Who are you? What is your description of yourself?
2. What makes you feel the happiest, the most alive? Your work? Your love relationship? A hobby or second career? Music? Going places (travel, concerts, dinner with friends)? Your children? Family? How happy are you, on a scale of one to ten?
3. What do you want most from life?
4. What was your greatest achievement personally to date?
5. What was the biggest emotional upset or disturbance you ever had to face— the greatest crisis, the thing you needed the most courage to get through?
6. Are you in love? Who is the person closest to you?
7. What is your favorite way to "waste time"?

### GROWING UP FEMALE

8. As a child, were you close to your mother? Your father? Did they love you? What did you like most and least about them?
9. Was your mother affectionate with you? Did she speak sweetly to you? Sing to you? Bathe you and do your hair? Were there any clashes between you? When was she angriest? What do you think of her today? Do you like to spend time with her?
10. Was your father affectionate? How? Did you talk? Go places together? Did you like him? Fear him? Respect him? What did you argue about? What do you think of him today?
11. Were your parents affectionate together in front of you? Did they argue? What did you learn from your father was the proper attitude toward your

---

[*] This is one of four versions of the questionnaire distributed over a period of seven years.

mother? What did you learn from your mother was the proper attitude towards your father?

12. Did your mother show you how to be "feminine"—act like a girl or a "lady"? Did you and your mother do things your brothers or father did not do, and vice versa? How would you define femininity?

13. Were you (are you) a "tomboy"? Was it fun? Were you warned against acting too rough, playing "boys" games, not acting "ladylike"? Were you urged to be a "good girl"? Were you rebellious?

14. Did you masturbate as a child? How old were you when you started? Did your parents know? Your friends?

15. What did/do you like and dislike about high school? Was/is there a lot of pressure to conform, be like everyone else? Dress a certain way? Be popular? To be a virgin, or to have sex?

16. Did/do you have a best friend? Did you spend the night at each other's houses? Talk on the phone? What about? Go out together? Are you still in touch?

17. How did you feel when you started dating? When you first kissed? Made out? Had sex? Did you discuss any of this with your parents? Friends?

### FALLING IN LOVE

18. Are you in "love" now? How can you tell?

19. How would you define love? Is love the thing you work at in a relationship over a period of time, or is it the strong feeling you feel right from the beginning, for no reason?

20. To live with someone, is it more important to be "in love" or to love them? What is the difference between being "in love" and loving someone?

21. When, with whom, were you most deeply in love? Were you happy? What was it like? Did the relationship last? Was this when you felt the most passionate?

22. Did you ever cry yourself to sleep because of problems with someone you loved? Why? Contemplate suicide? When were you the loneliest?

23. When were you the happiest with someone?

24. Do you like being in love? Is it a condition of pleasure or pain? Learning? Enlightenment? Joy? Ambivalent feelings? Frustration? How important is it?

25. What are your favorite love stories, in books or films?

### YOUR CURRENT RELATIONSHIP

26. Are you in a relationship now? For how long? Do you live together? Are you married? Do you have children?

27. What is the most important part of this relationship, the reason you want it? Is it love, passion, sexual intimacy, economics, daily companionship, or the long-term value of a family relationship? Other?

28. Are you happy with the relationship? Inspired? What do you like most and least about it? Can you imagine spending the rest of your life in it? Is your partner happy?

29. Are you "in love"? Or do you love them, more than being "in love"? What kind of love do you feel?

30. Do you love your partner as much as s/he loves you? More? Does one of you need the other more? Do you feel loved?

31. What is the biggest problem in your relationship? How would you like to change things, if you could?

32. What do you enjoy doing together the most? Talking? Having sex? Being affectionate? Daily life? Sharing children? Hobbies? Going out? Other?

33. How does your partner act toward you in intimate moments? Does your partner tell you s/he loves you? That you are wonderful and beautiful? Very sexually desirable? Talk tenderly to you? Use baby talk? Sex talk? How do you feel?

34. What things does your partner most often criticize about you? What do you most often criticize about him/her?

35. What is the worst thing your partner has ever done to you? The worst thing you have ever done to him/her?

36. Is it easy to talk? Who talks more? Would you like more intimate talk—about feelings, reactions, and problems? Future plans and dreams?

37. Does the relationship fill your deepest needs for closeness with another person? Or are there some parts of yourself that you can't share? That aren't accepted or understood? Or do you prefer to share every part of yourself?

38. Is the kind of love you are giving and receiving now the kind you most want? Have you seen another type in a friend's relationship or a movie or novel that you would find more satisfying?

39. Is this relationship important to you? How important? The center of your life? An important addition to your relationship with yourself and/or your work? Or merely peripheral—pleasant, but lacking somehow? What would make you leave it?

40. What are the practical arrangements? Who does the dishes? Makes the beds? Does the cooking? Takes care of the children? What is daily life like? Do you sleep in the same bed? Take baths or showers together?

41. Do you share the money? Who controls the money? Do you both work outside the home? Who pays the rent or mortgage? Buys the groceries? How do you feel about the financial arrangements? Do they affect the relationship?

42. What is the best way you have found to make a relationship work?

43. If you are married, how long have you been married? Do you like it? What is the best part of being married? The worst? Before you got married, did you expect it to be like it is?

44. Why did you decide to get married? Because of love? Sex? Social pressures? Economic pressures? Pregnancy? Companionship? To have children? A home

life? Emotional security? Was it a hard decision? Whose idea was it? How long had you known each other?

45. How did you feel immediately after you got married? Elated? Worried? Did your feelings for him change? His actions towards you?

46. If you have children, do you like having them? What was having your children like? Was your husband there?

47. How did you feel when you first knew you were pregnant? How did you lover/husband react? After the child was born? Does he take as much part in child rearing as you?

48. Would your life have been different if you had not had children? How? Would you do it over again?

49. Which is more important: Your job? Your love relationship? Your children? Yourself, having time for yourself?

50. Do you believe in monogamy? Have you/are you having sex outside the relationship? Known to your partner? How do you feel about it? What is it/was it giving you?

51. What was your original reason? Were you in love? Was there a lack of understanding or closeness at home? A desire to experiment sexually? Anger? Long absence? Other? Is/was the affair serious?

52. Do you think your partner is having sex with anyone else now? In the past? How do you feel about this? Do you want your partner to be monogamous? Do you want to know if/he is not?

53. Would you have sex outside the relationship in the future? Tell your partner?

54. Have you ever dated someone married? Did you mind that s/he was married? Did you want them to get divorced, and marry you?

55. Describe the biggest (or most recent) fight you had with your husband or lover.

56. What do you most frequently fight about? Who usually wins (if anybody)? How do you feel during? After?

57. How do conflicts or arguments usually get resolved—or at least ended? Who usually says they're sorry first after a fight? Who initiates talking over the problem? Making up?

58. Describe the time recently you were most happy with your lover, most joyous.

### BEING SINGLE

59. Do you like being "single"—whether you are single now or were in the past? Why are you single?

60. What are the advantages of being single? Disadvantages? Do you like going out alone, to a party, a restaurant, or shopping, etc.? Or do you sometimes get the impression people think there is something wrong with you when you are not in a couple? Do some people envy you for being single?

61. What is your sex life like? Do you enjoy periods of no sex with another person?

62. Is it easy or difficult to meet someone you like and are attracted to, and whom you respect?

63. Do you think most men today want to be married? Do single men find it difficult to accept the idea of marriage at first? Do they tend to avoid commitment? Do you think men today are less committed?

## BREAKING UP / GETTING A DIVORCE

64. If you have ever gotten divorced, or broken up with someone important, what was it like? Who wanted to break up—you or the other person? Why?

65. Were you glad or did you have regrets? Did you feel like a failure, or did you feel freer—or both? Did you hate the other person? Cry a lot? Or feel relieved, that now you could start living again?

66. How did you get over it, if you didn't want to break up? How long did it take? Did you talk to friends? Hide from them? Work harder?

67. While breaking up, what did you feel was the most permanent, solid thing in your life? Your parents or relatives? Friends? Children? Your work? Yourself?

68. Was there a time at which you gave up on love relationships as not being very important? You preferred to put more energy into work or children? You revised your definitions of what kind of love was important? Or have you always put love relationships first in your life?

69. Have you ever lost a loved one through death? What do you miss most about the person? Was a part of you not sorry? Did you feel deserted? Free? Did you grieve?

## SPECIAL PROBLEMS IN RELATIONSHIPS

70. Did you ever enter therapy to try to solve personal problems related to your love relationships? What were they? Did therapy help? What were your conclusions?

71. Do you sometimes think you pick the "wrong" lovers? What kinds of lovers do you pick?

72. Are you jealous? Of friendships? Career? Other women? Men?

73. Did you ever grow to hate a lover? Act violently? Scream? Hit them? Did a lover ever strike you, or beat you? What were the circumstances?

74. Have you ever loved someone who hurt you deeply, in spite of what had happened, and in spite of your desire not to love them any longer?

75. Who usually breaks up the relationship first—you or the other person?

76. Do you sometimes find you have to employ a "streak of manipulative coldness"—keep your distance, keep things "cool"?

77. Have you ever pretended you cared less than you did? That s/he was less important than they were? Put up a front? Did it work?

78. Are you afraid of clinging? Making someone feel tied down, "unfree"? Did you ever feel you were too emotionally dependent? Are men afraid of women's dependency? If you tell a man you love him, will he feel tied down?

79. Did you ever have a nagging fear of losing someone's love, or being deserted? That the other person would grow tired of you?

80. Do you ever feel you have "unhealthy" needs and cravings for love and affection? As one woman put it, "my love has usually been too blind, too desperate."

81. How do you feel if someone is very emotionally dependent on *you* in a relationship? Needs you more? Complains that you don't love him enough?

82. Have you ever felt that you were "owned" or suffocated, held down, in a relationship, so that you wanted out?

83. Do you think men take love and falling love as seriously as women do—if they do? What part does it play in men's lives? Are men more emotionally dependent, or women?

84. Were you ever financially dependent on a man you live with? Was this a problem? How did/do you feel about it? Did/does it affect the relationship?

85. How do you think men feel about women working outside the home? If you work, and are married/ living with someone, how does he feel about it? Does he share the housework?

86. Does your husband/ lover see you as an equal? Or are there times when he seems to treat you as an inferior? Leave you out of the decisions? Act superior?

87. How do you most men you know feel about the women's movement? How does your husband/ lover feel about it?

## SEXUALITY

88. What is sex with your partner (or in general) usually like? Do you enjoy it? Do you usually orgasm? During which activity? What is the worst thing about sex? The best?

89. Has your sexuality, or your style of relating sexually, changed over the last few years? In what way?

90. Have you read *The Hite Report* on female sexuality? Which ideas do you most agree with? Disagree?

91. Which is the easiest way for you to orgasm? Through masturbation? Clitoral stimulation by hand from your partner? Oral sex? Intercourse (vaginal penetration)? With a vibrator?

92. If you orgasm during vaginal penetration, how do you usually do it? (a) By added clitoral stimulation from your partner? Please explain, (b) By your own clitoral stimulation/masturbation during penetration? (c) By being on top and rubbing against your partner? (d) Friction of the penis inside the vagina, without other stimulation? (e) Other? Please describe.

93. When did you first orgasm—during sex with a partner or masturbation? (a)

Did you discover masturbation on your own, or did you read about it? How old were you? How did you feel? Did your parents know about it? Friends? (b) When you had your first orgasm with another person, which activity was it during? Did you learn to make it happen, or did it happen without trying?

94. Have you ever masturbated with a partner? During intercourse? During general caresses? Was it hard to do the first time? How did you feel? What was his/her reaction? Do you have to have your legs together or apart for orgasm?

95. Have you told a woman friend you don't orgasm from intercourse (if you don't)? Explained your sex life in any detail to her? What did you say? How did she react?

96. Have you told a man you don't orgasm from intercourse (if you don't)? What did he say? Did you tell him most women don't? How did you feel?

97. Have you talked with your mother, sister, or daughter about some of these things? Do they know if you masturbate? Do you know if they do? What else have you talked about? What would you like to talk about?

98. If you prefer sex with women, how did you come to this point of view? If you prefer sex with men, how did you come to this point of view? Have you always felt this way? What do you like best about sex with women/men?

99. Does sex with the same partner change over the years? Does it become boring, or more pleasurable? Or does it depend on how the relationship goes?

100. Is there a contradiction between sexual passion and a more long-term stable relationship? Do you have to choose? Do the daily details of living conflict with, or make difficult, feelings of passion?

101. When do you feel most passionate? How does it feel? Craving? Do you become more aggressive? Or want to be taken?

102. Do you usually like to be more passive or active, dominant during sex?

103. Do you like exploring a man's body? His chest? Penis and testicles? Anus and buttocks? Have you ever penetrated a man's anus with your finger? How do you feel about this? How do you feel about giving him oral sex? Do most men/does he like you to do this—or is he shy and uncomfortable?

104. Do you like, or would you like to try, exploring a woman's body? Her breasts? Her clitoris? Her vulva? Vagina? Anus and buttocks? How do you feel about giving oral sex? Do you like the taste and smell? Do most women like you to do this, or feel shy and uncomfortable? Do you like penetrating a woman's vagina? Anus?

105. Do you like to be stimulated vaginally? Penetrated? By a finger? Penis? Dildo? What do you like and dislike about it?

106. Do you like to be stimulated/ penetrated anally? By a finger? Penis? Dildo? How does it feel, and why do you like or dislike it?

107. Do you like oral sex to be done to you? What do you think about how you look and smell? What does the other person usually seem to think? How about during menstruation? Do you orgasm this way?

108. Can your partner stimulate you with his/her hand or finger on your clitoris? To orgasm? How does it feel? Do you have to guide his/her hand?

109. Have you shown someone how to masturbate you—that is, how to stimulate you to orgasm with their hand? Do most men offer clitoral stimulation by hand or mouth for orgasm, without being asked?

110. Do you use fantasies to help you orgasm? During sex? During masturbation? Which fantasies?

111. Do you ever feel pressured into sex? Into liking sex? Why? To be loving? To be "hip"? Have you ever been raped? Was this an important experience? How did you feel? Whom did you tell?

112. Do you like rough sex? What do you think of bondage-discipline? Spanking? Sadomasochism? Have you ever experienced them? Fantasized about them? Had rape fantasies? What were they like?

113. What do you think of pornography? Do you look at it? How did you feel when you first saw it? What does pornography tell you about what it means to be a woman?

114. Does your partner look at pornography? What kind? Men's magazines? Videotapes? How do you feel about this?

115. Do you use birth control? Which kind? What are its advantages and disadvantages? Do you think men should be involved in birth control?

116. Have you ever had an abortion? Why did you decide to have it? How did you feel after you had it?

### FRIENDSHIPS BETWEEN WOMEN

117. What is or has been your most important relationship with a woman in your life? Describe the woman you have loved the most. Hated the most.

118. What do you like about your closest woman friend? What do you do together? When do you see each other? Has she helped you through difficult times, and vice versa? How do you feel when you are together—do you have a good time? How much time do you spend together, or talking on the telephone? What does she do that you like least?

119. Were you close to your mother? Did she work outside the home, or was she a full-time mother and homemaker? Did you like her? Admire her? How did you feel about her taste in clothing? Are you like her?

120. Do you have a daughter? How do you feel about her? Have you talked to her about menstruation and sexuality? What did you say? What did she say?

121. What things about women in general do you admire? Which well-known women have contributed most to our society?

122. What do you think about the women's movement? Do you consider yourself a feminist, or in favor of the women's movement?

123. Have your feelings about the women's movement and its ideas affected your life?

124. Do you enjoy being "feminine"? How would you define "femininity"? Do you enjoy beautiful clothing? Dresses and lingerie? Do you spend time on your hair and makeup? How do you feel about the way you look? How "feminine" are you?
125. How do you feel about getting older?
126. If you could say just one thing to other women today, what would you tell them?
127. What do you think is the biggest problem in the United States today?

THANK YOU

Please give the following statistical information. A. What is your age? B. What is your racial background? Ethnic? C. What is your total amount of schooling? D. What was the approximate total income of your household before taxes in the past year? E. What kind of work do you do (inside or outside the home)? F. Where did you obtain this questionnaire?

# D. RESEARCH QUESTIONNAIRE ON GROWING UP IN THE FAMILY, 1975–1995

The purpose of this questionnaire is to better understand how children feel growing up, how they perceive the family and the world around them.

Teenagers, for example, are constantly *told* how to feel, think and behave—on the grounds that adults have "better judgement." But often teenagers completely disagree. What were your thoughts and experiences growing up? Can you remember how you felt, what it was like? Or can you describe what its is like, watching your own child grow up? There are many areas of this subject which are never talked about, especially the physical aspect, and your help in contributing information will be greatly appreciated.

IT IS *NOT* NECESSARY TO ANSWER EVERY SINGLE QUESTION! Answer only those that interest you—but please do answer some of the questions.

The results will be published as an extended discussion of the answers, including many quotes, in the same format as the Hite Reports on female and male sexuality, and *Women and Love*. The replies are anonymous, so *don't sign your answers*.

Looking forward to hearing from you!

1. When you were very little, around three or four, can you remember what it was like being close to your mother? Can you describe her presence, her sounds, her skin, her smell? How she touched you? How she looked?
2. Can you remember your mother breast-feeding your brother or sister? How

old were you? What were your thoughts? Were you jealous? Interested? Did you think it was beautiful or repulsive? Did you feel left out? Wish you would be a mother?

3. What things did your parents do that included body contact with you? Held and cuddled you? Bathed you? Washed your hair? Dressed you? Combed your hair? Spanked you? Gave you enemas? Please describe the kind of physical intimacy you had with your parents and how it felt to you.

4. As a child, did you think your mother was beautiful? Wonderful? In what way? Did you like to touch her and be close to her? Did you like in bed with her? Did she read to you, or did you watch television close together? Describe the feeling you had at these times.

5. Do you remember your mother coming into the room to kiss you goodnight? Was this a pleasant moment? What can you remember feeling?

6. What did your mother and/or father's bedroom look like? Did it have a double bed or single beds? Was it always neat or were the covers usually unmade? Were there lots of pillows? What was the atmosphere there (cold, erotic, friendly, etc.)?

7. What is your earliest memory of this room?

8. Did you spend time in her/his bedroom? Go there often? Or was it slightly mysterious, somewhat off limits? Were you allowed to play there as often as you wanted?

9. At what age did you begin to wonder about your mother's sexuality? Your father's? Or did you assume they didn't have any? Why did you think the bedroom was slightly off limits (if it was)? Or, did you know they did "something" together, but absorb the idea that you shouldn't wonder?

10. Would you have liked to know what your mother's sex life was like? If she masturbated? Your father's? If he masturbated?

11. Did you ever have fantasies of having sex with one of your parents? As a child? Later? What were the fantasies?

12. Did you ever run away from home? Contemplate it? Why?

13. Were you happy at home as a child? Did you have mixed feelings about your parents? Did you sometimes love them (or one or the other), and sometimes hate them? When?

14. Did you ever want to leave home and go and live elsewhere, but you stayed because you had nowhere else to go?

15. When you were a child, did you think it was a problem that you had no money of your own? That you had to ask your parents for money?

16. When was the time in your childhood that you were the angriest with your parents?

17. Who was more controlling of you, your mother or your father? How? Who had more power over you?

18. Did you like other friends' parents more? Other relatives?

19. Did you usually decide, during most conflicts with your parents, that they were right after all?

20. If you did not think they were right, but had to accept their decision anyway, how did you feel about this? Did you sometimes feel that you were living with injustice, but there was nothing you could do about it?

21. If you don't have one parent, how do you feel about it?

22. Do you know how your parents felt about having you?

23. If you are raised by a single parent, does she or he date? If your mother is dating, how do you feel about it is she has a man home with her? A woman? Or if you live with your father, vice versa?

24. Has anyone in your family become HIV positive or contracted Aids? Has anyone you know died? Do you know how to protect yourself against Aids?

25. Do you think your parents read pornography or watch sexy videotapes?

26. Do your parents (or partners) kiss in front of you? Are they sexually affectionate? How? Do you like or dislike it?

27. Do you have a boyfriend or girlfriend? Do you have sex together? Do your parents know?

28. When you fight with your parents, do your parents hit you? Speak a certain way to you? How? Spank you? Punish you? How? Is it usually your father or mother who punishes you?

29. If you were spanked, at what age was this? Were you slapped? Sent to your room? Told you were bad, not lovable, "not fit for human society," etc.? By whom?

30. If you were hit, who did this, and where, on what part of your body? With their hand, or something else? What?

31. Did they pull your dress up/trousers down? What were you wearing? Were you standing up, bending over, or lying down? Did it really physically hurt? Did you cry? Was it the physical pain that hurt or the humiliation?

32. How often did these things happen? Until what age?

33. How did you feel if a sister or brother was being punished?

34. Were there other forms of violence you experienced as a child? Physical? Emotional? Did you have friends who received physical punishment?

35. Were the girls in your family spanked more than the boys? Were boys "whipped", not spanked? Punished another way? Less or more often than girls?

36. What kind of relationship did you have with your mother by the time you were ten? Fifteen or sixteen? Can you remember conversations or arguments you would have? What did you like least about her? Most?

37. What was your relationship with your father like at that time? What did you spend time together doing? What did he talk to you about?

38. Did you admire him? Why or why not?

39. Did your mother know about any of your sexual activities (masturbation or

with a partner)? Did you know anything about hers? Did your father know? Did you know about his? Did you have sex magazines or other "adult" things in your room?

40. What was your parents' relationship? Did you feel comfortable with both of them together, or did you prefer to spend time with one or the other separately? Why?

41. Were you closer to your mother or father?

42. Were you close to a brother or sister? Were you "pals" or "rivals"? Did you do things together? At what age were you closest? Least close?

43. Who was treated better—you or your sister/brother (if there was a difference)?

44. Did your mother or father (or someone else) tell you about menstruation? Where/when did you first see a tampon? What were the circumstances?

45. What did your parents tell you about sexuality?

46. Did your father or mother look at pornography? When did you first see it? Where was it? What was your reaction, how did you feel?

47. Did you tell your parents you had seen it? Discuss it with anyone? What did you say?

### FOR WOMEN AND GIRLS

48. Are you like your mother?

49. How do you react when people say you look or act "just like your mother"?

50. If you don't want to be like her, what especially don't you want to be like? Do you look different? How are your looks different?

51. Was there any kind of (buried) competition between you and your mother? Was she ever jealous of you, or were you jealous of her? What for?

52. Did you ever get the message that looking for attention from your father was competing with your mother, that you shouldn't do it? That she could feel angry or left out? Did you try to get his attention anyway? How? Was this only when your mother was not around?

53. Did you sometimes feel you were emotionally in between your mother and father, and had to please both, not take sides? Did different types of behaviour please your mother and father—so that you had to behave differently with each one? Was it easier to relate to them alone than together?

54. Did you have a good relationship with your father? What did you do together? When were you closest?

55. Were you ever called your father's "little girl", or his "special girl"? His "girl-friend" or "best girl"? Did you have "dates" to go shopping, play sports, do errands? Did you enjoy these? What did you enjoy about them?

56. Did your father's behaviour to you change after the age of about twelve, for example, were you told (maybe a year or two later) that you shouldn't wear make-up or lipstick, that it made you look cheap and tarty? Did your mother

also tell you things like this? Did either parent warn you about girls with good "reputations" and "the other kind"?

57. Did anyone in your family touch you in ways which made you uncomfortable? How? Were you ever sexually molested by anyone in your family? Who? Please explain. Were you afraid you might be if you didn't watch out?

58. Should daughters sue their fathers in court for incest?

59. Did you have fights with your mother when you were in secondary school? What about? Did she comment on your hair? Your clothes? What did she say?

60. Did your mother or your father supervise your coming and going form the house, with whom, how late you came home, what you wore, etc.? How long you talked on the telephone?

61. What was your first experience buying a bra? Were you with your mother? Father? Friends? Alone?

62. Did anyone congratulate you at the time of your first menstruation? Or did you get the impression it wasn't too important or interesting? That it was supposed to be kept a secret, hidden, even that menstruation was dirty? What did you think?

63. Did you like your underwear? Did you pick it out, or did someone else? Was it practical? Athletic? Hip? Feminine? How did it make you feel?

64. What was your mother's underwear like? What did it tell you about her "femaleness" and sexuality? Did you like hers better than yours or vice versa?

65. Did you have a room to yourself, or did you share? Did you ever feel lonely, even frightened, getting into bed by yourself? or did you like having your own bed and your own room? Did you wish you could get in bed with your parents or your brothers or sisters (if you didn't)?

66. Did your parents expect you to have sex before you left home? Did they know if you did? Did they ask? Did you tell them? If you had a brother, was he allowed more sexual freedom around the house?

67. What was your main source of physical affection between ages seven and fifteen?

FOR PARENTS

68. When your children were living with you, were you closer to your son(s) or daughter(s)? Why? (Please answer this section in the present, if applicable.)

69. If you have a son(s), at which age(s) during his childhood was he closest to you? Which was the most satisfying period—infancy? Before kindergarten? During junior school? Secondary school? Why?

70. During which of these ages was your son least close to you? Most hostile and challenging?

71. Your daughter(s)? When were you closest? Most distant?

72. During which ages did your son(s) talk to you most openly and freely abut his thoughts and feelings? What did he talk about?

73. Your daughter(s)?
74. Did you like your daughter(s)? What did you like best? Least? What was your biggest complaint?
75. What did/do you most regret about your daughter's childhood/your relationship with your daughter? About your relationship with your son, his childhood?
76. When you punished your children, how did you do it? Physically? Emotionally? Both?
77. If you spanked your children, were these formal occasions, or spur of the moment outbreaks? That is, did you suddenly find yourself reaching out to slap your (screaming?) child, etc., or, after a certain level of misbehavior, did you say, "If you don't stop, you're going to get a good spanking?" Did you do it or ask your spouse to do it?
78. Would spanking or physical punishment be in the living room? Bedroom? Outside? Bathroom? Kitchen?
79. Is it different punishing a girl than a boy? How? If you have both, do you tend to hit one quicker, more often, than the other? In a different place? Which one? Why?
80. What do you think is the most important bond between parents and children?

### THANK YOU FOR ANSWERING THIS QUESTIONNAIRE

Please add the following statistical information for research purposes:

age

sex

occupation

in a relationship? married, single, coupled (living together or separately)

sexual preference

religious background

present religious identification

political inclination, if any

nationality, race or ethnic background

Please add anything else you would like to say.

NOTES

1 Rhonda Gottlieb, "The Political Economy of Sexuality" in *Review of Radical Political Economics* 16 (I): pp. 143–65.

2 *The Hite Report on Men and Male Sexuality* (New York: Alfred A. Knopf. 1981), p. xvii.

3 See *The Hite Report on Female Sexuality* (New York: Macmillan, 1976), Chapter 6.

4 Sandra Harding and Merrill B. Hintikka, eds., *Discovering Reality*, pp. 187–205, Copyright 1978 by Psychoanalysis and Contemporary Science, Inc.

5 An early version of this argument appeared in "Psychology Constructs the Female," published as a pamphlet in 1968 (Boston: New England Free Press); it was then reprinted as "'Kinder, Kuche, Kirche' as Scientific Law: Psychology Constructs the Female" in Robin Morgan's *Sisterhood is Powerful: An Anthology of Writings From the Women's Liberation Movement* (New York: Random House, 1970, pp. 205–20); and was later revised and updated as "Psychology Constructs the Female; or the Fantasy Life of the Male Psychologist—With Some Attention to the Fantasies of His Friends, the Male Biologist and the Male Anthropologist" (*Social Education*, April 1971, pp. 363–73).

6 From *The Hite Report on the Family*, U.S. edition, (New York: Grove/Atlantic, 1995); also distributed by Ms. Magazine Foundation.

7 See published proceedings, statistical abstracts, annual meeting, American Association for the Advancement of Science, May 1985, Washington, D.C.

8 Points presented at a speech to the National Women's Studies convention, University of Kansas, 1978.

9 See the original Reports for this data.

10 Sandra Harding and Merrill B. Hintikka, eds., *Discovering Reality*, pp. 187–205, Copyright 1978 by Psychoanalysis and Contemporary Science, Inc.

# INDEX

AASECT (American Association of Sex
   Educators, Counselors and
   Therapists), 19, 458
Abraham, Biblical story of, 121
active sex, for women, 29, 44
Adam and Eve, gender-role propaganda of,
   266
Adams, Abigail, 284
Afghanistan, oppression of women in, 440
Africa
   clitoredectomy in, 429
   infibulation in, 429
   sex outside marriage in, 405
aggression. *See also* passive aggression
   in boys, 441
   emphasis on, 465
   language of, 239–41
   Marx on, 465
   with masculinity, 157
   normalization of, 479
   against women, 239, 243
AIDS/HIV
   gay community focus on, 390
   in lesbian relationships, 357
   monogamy impact of, 480
Albright, Madeleine, 450
*Amazon Odyssey*, 463
*Amazon Odyssey* (Atkinson), 463
American Association for the Advancement
   of Science, 487
American Association of Sex Educators,
   Counselors and Therapists. *See*
   AASECT
*American Journal of Political Science*, 496
*American Studies Association: Statement By
   Committee*, 474–75
analingus, in homosexual couples, 376
anal stimulation, of male orgasm, 140
anorexia, in girls, 307, 336

arousal
   clitoral stimulation for, 64
   clitoral system during, *180–81*
   female anatomy during, 179
   orgasm in, 47
   orgasm v., 72
   pleasure of, 93
   sources of, 352–53
   in women v. men, 353
Atkinson, Ti-Grace, 463, 479
authoritarian model
   in family, 329
   in private life, 329

*Backlash* (Faludi), 473
"back to basics" movement, in traditional
   family values, 412
Bagdikian, Ben, 471
Bascaglia, Leo, 482
Battersby, Christine, 469
"battle of the sexes," social endorsement of,
   424
beauty, ideal of, 423
Bernard, Jessie, 293, 463
biblical tradition
   coitus rules in, 99–100
   on men's feelings, 121
biological difference, between men and
   women, 265
birth control
   acceptance of, 151
   in Catholic Church, 150
Blumstein, Philip, 352–53, 464
boys
   aggression in, 441
   bullying of, 334
   early sex lives of, 114
   emotional turmoil for, 222

## ABOUT THE AUTHOR

Shere Hite, Ph.D., is internationally recognized for her work on psychosexual behavior and gender relations. Visiting professor of gender and culture at Nihon University in Japan and professor of the American Academy of Maimonides University in the U.S., Dr. Hite is a frequent lecturer at universities around the world. She was director of the National Organization for Women's feminist sexuality project from 1972 to 1978. Since that time she has been the director of Hite Research International. Dr. Hite is the author of *The Hite Report: A Nationwide Study of Female Sexuality, The Hite Report on Men and Male Sexuality, The Hite Report on the Family, The Hite Report on Women Loving Women,* and *Sex and Business,* among many others.

*You may contact the author at hite2000@hotmail.com or c/o the publisher.*

Also by Shere Hite:

*The Hite Report: A Nationwide Study of Female Sexuality* (1976)
*The Hite Report on Men and Male Sexuality* (1981)
*Women and Love: A Cultural Revolution in Progress* (1987)
*Good Guys, Bad Guys and Other Lovers* (with Kate Colleran, 1990)
*The Divine Comedy of Ariadne and Jupiter* (1993)
*Women as Revolutionary Agents of Change: The Hite Reports & Beyond* (1994)
*The Hite Report on the Family: Growing up under Patriarchy* (1994)
*The Hite Report on Shere Hite* (2000)
*Sex & Business: Ethics at Work* (2000)
*Oedipus Revisited: Men Today* (2004)
*The Hite Report on Women Loving Women* (2005)

"Looking back from this end of the century we can begin to see how partial our views of its literary happenings have been: how time-bound, tongue-bound, often celebrity-bound. In an accurately titled *Poems for the Millennium* we can at last sense the scope of the Revolution of the Word that's been in process since—oh, 1895. There's no other anthology like this one, no other overview so venturesome."

**HUGH KENNER**

"This is not like any other anthology, not a collection of excellences, no absurd imitation of a canon. It's more like a Handbook of Inventors and Inventions, or of Explorers and Discoveries, that opens up all sorts of pathways for poetry from its past and future to a living present. This may be the only collection of modernist poetry that reveals its simultaneous connections to an archaic and ecological past as well as to a technological future, as it also wipes out rigid distinctions between poets and painters and sculptors and performers. It is above all a book of possibilities and invitations."

**DAVID ANTIN**

"A much broader, much more intelligent sweep, this anthology, than most. From real soup to real nuts!"

**AMIRI BARAKA**

"*Poems for the Millennium* is a riveting literary achievement of phenomenal scope and generosity. Kudos to Rothenberg and Joris for their passionate, discerning editorship, spanning cultures, sensibilities, and languages. This illuminating compendium displays the best of humanity's bardic inheritance and vision. It should be obligatory reading for all scholars, students, writers, and lovers of poetry. May the wisdom in these poems benefit us all."

**ANNE WALDMAN**

"The intermingling circles of poetries and cultures move outward to all continents and also open up to all times. True cosmopolitanism loves the specifics of little places and small societies—just the right gesture, the precise quaver of the voice, the exact variety of maize. Rothenberg and Joris's anthology gives us, by virtue of its organic structure and inspired choices, the possibility of a kind of situated internationalism, what "modernism" half wanted to become. This is a presentation of a poetics that is already here, but imperfectly recognized. It is a sourcebook for the future."

**GARY SNYDER**